Pediatric Oncology

Series Editors:

Gregory H. Reaman
Silver Spring, MD, USA

Franklin O. Smith
Cincinnati, OH, USA

Joanne Wolfe • Barbara L. Jones
Ulrika Kreicbergs • Momcilo Jankovic
Editors

Palliative Care in Pediatric Oncology

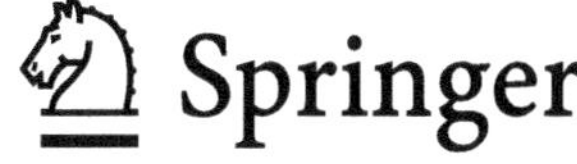

Springer

Editors
Joanne Wolfe
Department of Psychosocial Oncology
Dana-Farber Cancer Institute
Boston, Massachusetts, USA

Barbara L. Jones
School of Social Work
The University of Texas
Austin, Texas, USA

Ulrika Kreicbergs
Department of Caring Sciences
Palliative Research Centre
Stockholm, Sweden

Department of Women's and
Children's Health
Karolinska Institutet
Stockholm, Sweden

Momcilo Jankovic
Hospital san Gerardo
University of Milano
Monza, Italy

ISSN 1613-5318 ISSN 2191-0812 (electronic)
Pediatric Oncology
ISBN 978-3-319-87070-0 ISBN 978-3-319-61391-8 (eBook)
https://doi.org/10.1007/978-3-319-61391-8

Printed on acid-free paper

This Springer imprint is published by Springer Nature
The registered company is Springer International Publishing AG
The registered company address is: Gewerbestrasse 11, 6330 Cham, Switzerland

Contents

Introduction

Palliative Care in Pediatric Oncology is a novel textbook intended for all clinicians caring for children with advanced cancer. Several concepts are important to understanding this text, beginning with the definition of palliative care. According to the World Health Organization, palliative care is an approach that improves the quality of life of patients and their families facing the problem associated with life-threatening illness, through the prevention and relief of suffering by means of early identification and impeccable assessment and treatment of pain and other problems, physical, psychosocial, and spiritual. Optimal care of children with cancer involves the individualized blending of care directed at the underlying illness and the physical, emotional, social, and spiritual needs of the child and family with continuous reevaluation and adjustment.

Importantly, palliative care is *not* a phase of care and the term "palliative" should not be used to imply that a child's cancer is incurable. Misuse of the term "palliative" to imply a phase of care creates barriers to integrating a palliative approach into the care of all children with advanced cancer. Indeed, as editors, we would favor eliminating the use of the terms "curative intent" and "palliative intent" to describe cancer-directed therapies. Experience and research suggest that however cancer treatments are labeled; families continue to hope for cure, life extension, and even a miracle, up until their child's very last breath. Using these labels often serves to convey prognosis in a rather "short-hand" manner, rather than using optimal communication strategies as described in Chap. 4. Cancer-directed therapy labels should reflect family goals of care which typically fall into one of three approaches to helping the child to (1) live as long as possible, (2) live as long as possible and as well as possible, or (3) live as comfortably as possible. Needless to say, these goals evolve over time, depending on the child's illness outcome.

Notably, this textbook was written by oncology clinicians in collaboration with palliative care clinicians and this approach models how these subspecialists can effectively work together. Importantly, pediatric oncology clinicians all need to know basic, "primary" palliative care. Palliative care specialists should be invited into the care of children and families with more complex suffering to provide an added layer of support.

Palliative Care in Pediatric Oncology comprehensively covers the epidemiology of suffering in childhood cancer and the impact of distress on the child, families, the community, and the clinicians who serve them. The text emphasizes the critical role of the primary interdisciplinary oncology team and collaboration with a palliative care team, when indicated. Communication is a fundamental procedure in palliative care, an intervention that when optimally employed can facilitate easing suffering and enhancing well-being. The text also discusses the integration of cancer-directed therapy in pediatric advanced cancer as well as palliative care in stem cell transplantation. Individual chapters also focus on the various domains of distress including physical, psychological, spiritual, and social. Some children with advanced cancer do face end of life, and thus the text also focuses on this critical period of care as well as support for families in their bereavement. The text ends with a focus on caring for ourselves as clinicians as we care for children with advanced cancer and considerations about needed innovations to better support children with advanced cancer and their families.

It is our hope that this text provides an added layer of support to clinicians working with children with advanced cancer and their families. It has been a privilege working with such a talented group of authors in service to enhancing the well-being of children with advanced cancer and their families.

1 Epidemiology of Suffering in Childhood Cancer

Alisha Kassam, Kimberley Widger, and Franca Benini

1.1 Epidemiology of Advanced Cancer in Children

Survival rates for childhood cancer in developed countries have steadily improved over the last few decades from 58% in the mid-1970s to over 80% today (Fig. 1.1). These increased survival rates are due to high participation rates in large international collaborative clinical trials together with improvements in cancer-directed therapies and supportive care (Hudson et al. 2014).

Despite the tremendous progress in treating pediatric malignancies, 20% of children with cancer will still die from their disease. As such, death from cancer remains the leading cause of non-accidental death in children (ages 1–14 years) (Fig. 1.2). Figure 1.3 shows the distribution of childhood cancer deaths by cancer type. Leukemia accounts for a third of all cancer-related deaths, followed by central nervous tumors and neuroblastoma (Pizzo et al. 2011; Pizzo et al. 2016).

Pediatric cancer is a family illness (Patterson et al. 2004). Apart from the physical impact of the disease and its treatments on the ill child, there is also an emotional, social, and spiritual impact on the child, parents, and siblings (see Case 1). Particularly when a child dies, the experience may impact on the health of family members for many years to come. Much of the research to date are retrospective accounts primarily from parents as opposed to hearing from the ill child or siblings directly. As well, much of the research is more qualitative in nature or involves small sample sizes making it a challenge to determine the prevalence of distress and suffering in family members.

1.2 Prevalence and Patterns of Suffering in Children with Cancer

Children with cancer experience physical, emotional, social, and spiritual suffering as a result of the disease process, treatments for the disease, and treatment-related side effects. Not surprisingly, compared with children who have survived

A. Kassam, M.D., M.P.H. (✉)
Southlake Regional Health Centre, Newmarket, ON, Canada

The Hospital for Sick Children, Toronto, ON, Canada

University of Toronto, Toronto, ON, Canada
e-mail: akassam@southlakeregional.org, alisha.kassam@sickkids.ca

K. Widger, R.N., Ph.D., C.H.P.C.N.(C)
Lawrence S. Bloomberg Faculty of Nursing, University of Toronto, Toronto, ON, Canada

Paediatric Advanced Care Team, The Hospital for Sick Children, Toronto, ON, Canada
e-mail: kim.widger@utoronto.ca

F. Benini, MD
Department of Pediatrics, Pediatric Pain and Palliative Care Service, University of Padova, Padua, Italy

J. Wolfe et al. (eds.), *Palliative Care in Pediatric Oncology*, Pediatric Oncology,
https://doi.org/10.1007/978-3-319-61391-8_1

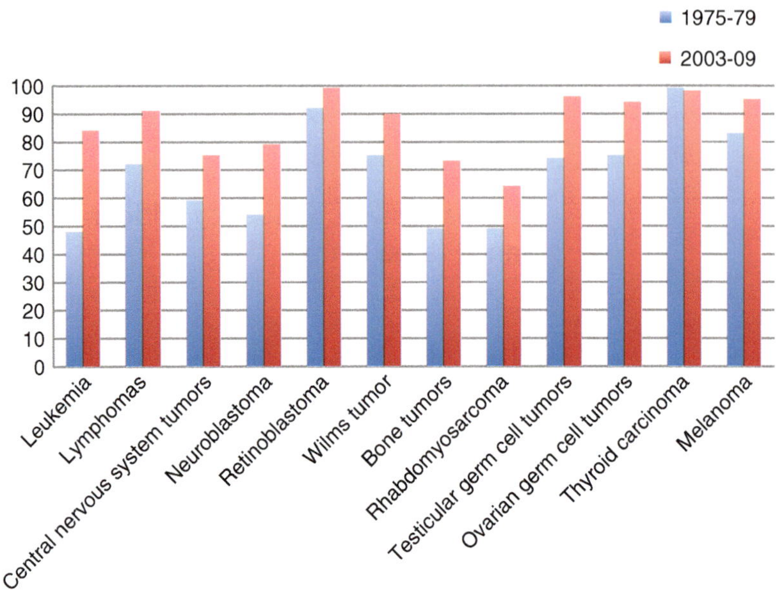

1975-79
2003-09
100
90
80
70
60
50
40
30
20
10
0
Leukemia
Lymphomas
Central nervous system tumors
Neuroblastoma
Retinoblastoma
Wilms tumor
Bone tumors
Rhabdomyosarcoma
Testicular germ cell tumors
Ovarian germ cell tumors
Thyroid carcinoma
Melanoma

Fig. 1.1 Pediatric cancer 5-year survival rates from birth to 19 years old for two time periods. Adapted from the American Cancer Society. Special Section: Cancer in Children and Adolescents (2014) https://www.cancer.org/content/dam/cancer-org/research/cancer-facts-and-statistics/annual-cancer-facts-and-figures/2014/special-section-cancer-in-children-and-adolescents-cancer-facts-and-figures-2014.pdf

Percent of Children
60%
50%
40%
30%
20%
10%
0%
Accidents
Other
Cancer
Congenital anomalies
Homicide
Heart disease
Infections
Suicide
Pnemonia/Influenza

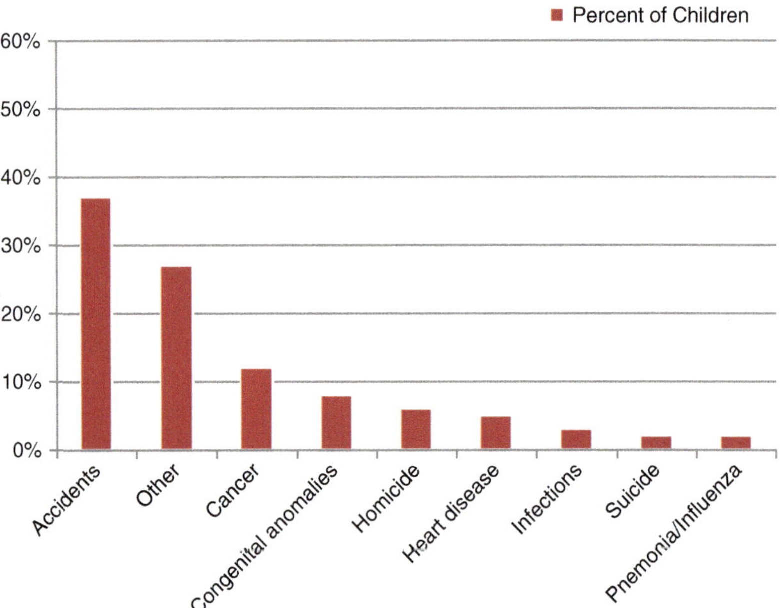

Fig. 1.2 Causes of childhood death in the USA, 2006. Causes of death among children 1–14 years of age

childhood cancer, children receiving cancer-related treatments have significantly higher mean scores for depression (49.0 vs. 45.9), anxiety (49.5 vs. 46.2), pain interference (50.2 vs. 44.7), and fatigue (52.9 vs. 43.8) and significantly lower scores for peer relationships (45.4 vs. 52.1) (Hinds et al. 2013). When there is disease progression, prospective parent-proxy reports of quality of life indicate in the last 6 months of life children had significantly worse physical health, more pain, and more fatigue compared to those who survived more than 6 months, while there were no significant differences in emotional or social functioning (Tomlinson et al. 2011).

Wolfe et al. (2000a) were the first to report a high symptom burden and substantial suffering

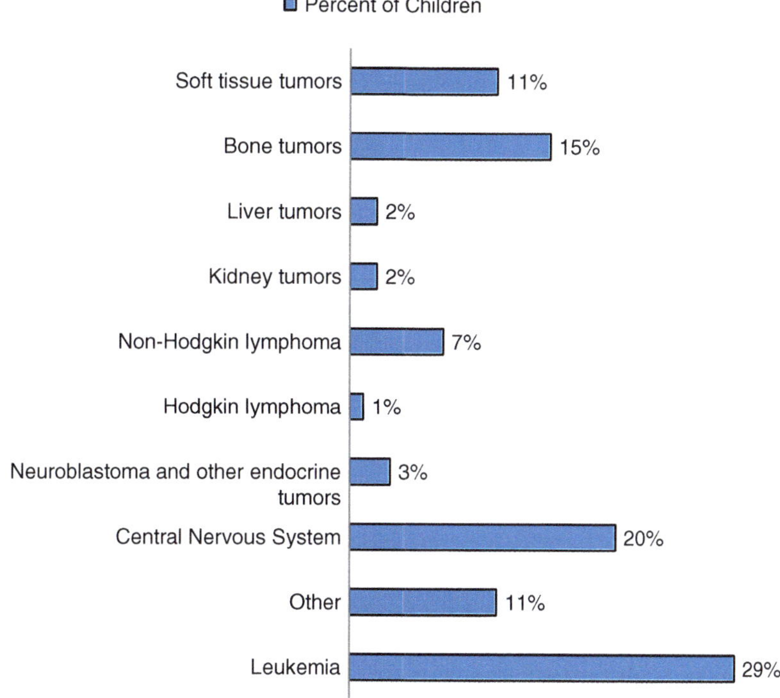

Fig. 1.3 Childhood cancer deaths by cancer type in children and adolescents 0–19 years of age, 2006

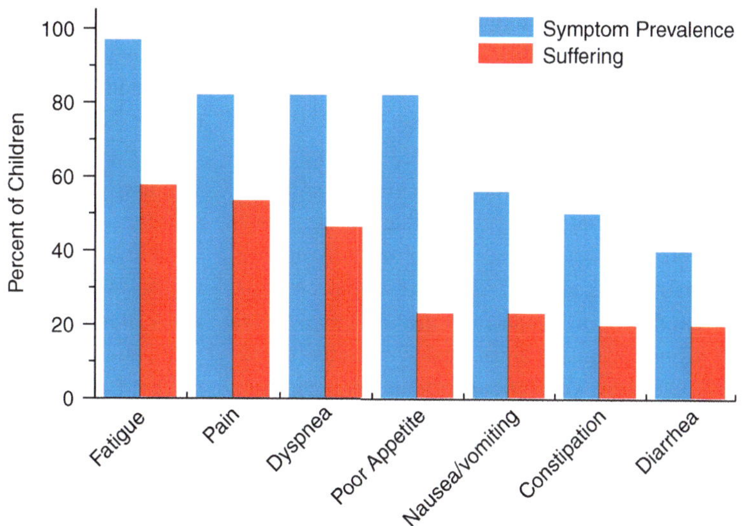

Fig. 1.4 The degree of suffering from common symptoms in the last month of life. The percentage of children who, according to parental report, had a specific symptom during the last month of life and who had "a lot" or "a great deal" of suffering as a result. Adapted from Wolfe J, Grier HE, Klar N, Levin SB, Ellenbogen JM, Salem-Schatz S, et al. Symptoms and suffering at the end of life in children with cancer. N Engl J Med. 2000; 342(5):326–33

in children who died of cancer. The proportion of children who, according to their parents, had a specific symptom during the last month of life and the proportion who suffered from the symptom are shown in Fig. 1.4. The most commonly reported symptoms were fatigue, pain, and dyspnea. Other prevalent symptoms included poor appetite, nausea and vomiting, constipation, and diarrhea. Worryingly, 89% of children experienced at least one symptom from which, based on parental report, they suffered "a lot" or a "great deal."

The finding of a high prevalence of symptoms in children with advanced cancer has been replicated over the last decade in studies across the world (Heath et al. 2010; Jalmsell et al. 2006). Health et al. (2010) examined the symptoms and level of suffering among Australian children with cancer at the end of life. They found that 84% of parents reported their child had suffered from at least one symptom in their last month of life. Pain, fatigue, and poor appetite were the most common. Similarly, Jalmsell et al. (2006) found a high prevalence of symptoms reported by parents of Swedish children with advanced cancer including fatigue (86%), reduced mobility (76%), pain (73%), and decreased appetite (71%). Symptoms like depression (48%) and anxiety (38%) were reported to a lesser degree (Jalmsell et al. 2006), while a study in the USA found higher prevalence of depression (65%) and anxiety (48.3%), along with fear (49.2%) and sleep disturbance (60%) during the last month of life from the perspective of bereaved parents (Friedrichsdorf et al. 2015). In Germany, bereaved parents indicated that 65% of children with cancer experienced severe suffering from pain and 63.6% from nausea during the last month of life; however, the majority (72.3%) of parents felt that their child was happy, in a good mood, and peaceful during the same time period (von Lützau et al. 2012).

The above studies evaluated symptoms in children with any cancer diagnosis; however, the underlying malignancy can influence the symptom profile. In addition to the common symptoms of pain, fatigue, and dyspnea, children with hematologic malignancies may also experience bleeding, coagulopathies, and symptoms of anemia. Children with central nervous system tumors are at risk of seizures and symptoms related to increased intracranial pressure. Children with solid tumors may experience symptoms related to compression of vital structures by the tumor such as bowel obstruction or spinal cord compression. The oncology team must be familiar with the symptoms of the underlying malignancy in order to provide anticipatory guidance to families. Preparing children and families for what symptoms to expect as the child's disease progresses, and educating them on how they will be promptly managed, can mitigate much of the suffering and distress.

In order to accurately understand the symptom experience of children with cancer, it is vital to also hear the perspective of the child when developmentally appropriate. Unfortunately, the majority of available literature about the symptom experience of children is based on clinician and parent observations (Hinds et al. 2007). A review article published in 2007 found that less than 17% of the published data about the end of life in pediatric oncology patients included actual patient reported outcomes (Hinds et al. 2007). The largest study to prospectively describe patient reported symptom distress in children with advanced cancer was published in 2015 (Wolfe et al. 2015). Symptom prevalence and distress observed in these children are shown in Fig. 1.5. Common physical symptoms reported by children with advanced cancer were pain (48%), fatigue (46%), and drowsiness (39%), while the most common psychological symptoms were irritability (37%), sleep disturbances (29%), nervousness (25%), sadness (24%), and worrying (24%). Pain was the most common highly distressing symptom. Similar to previous studies that have relied on parent report, symptom prevalence and distress were worse in the last 12 weeks of life. Children who experienced a recent disease progression or received moderate or high-intensity cancer therapy reported worse symptom scores.

While prevalence cannot be determined, some of the most poignant accounts of the suffering associated with having cancer come through qualitative research that include interviews with children and adolescents (Hurwitz et al. 2004; Weaver et al. 2016) or analysis of diaries or websites created by children living with or who have died from cancer (Suzuki and Beale 2006; Flavelle 2011). Table 1.1 includes a selection of quotes from these studies that highlight the experience in terms of symptoms, the desire to protect friends and family from the experience, and the thoughts about the future.

The research to date both from the child's perspective and through parent-proxy reports strengthens our understanding that children with advanced cancer experience distressing symptoms throughout their disease course and especially at

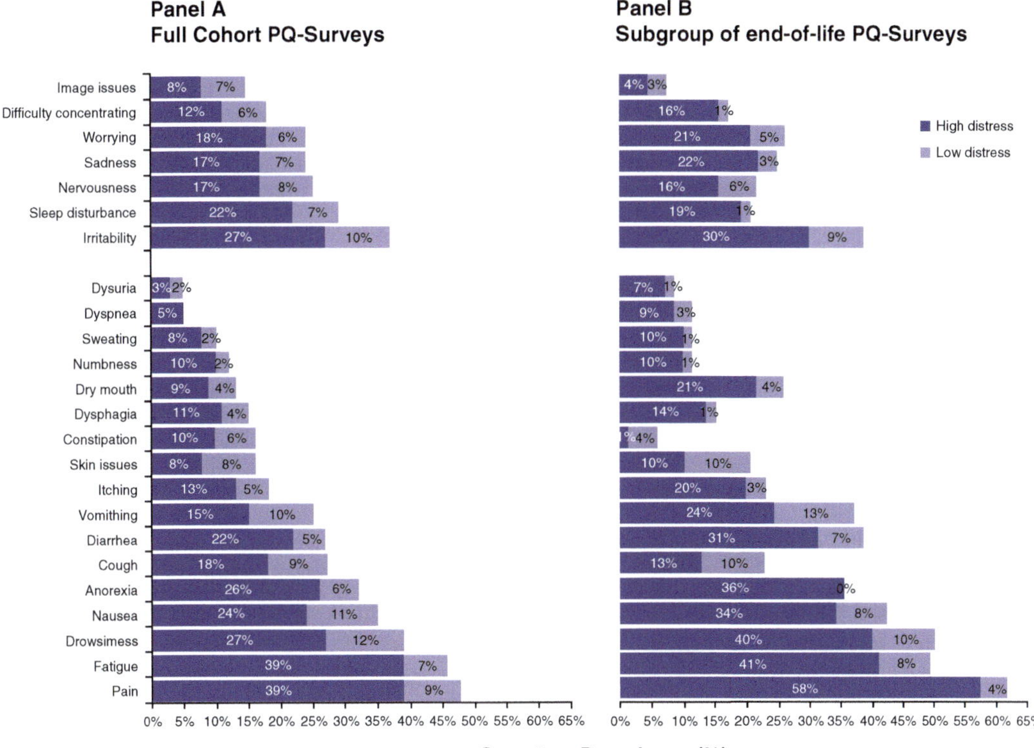

Fig. 1.5 Symptom prevalence and distress observed in 104 children with advanced cancer who completed 920 PQ surveys during 9 months of follow-up (**a**) and in the subgroup of 25 children who died and had completed 73 PQ surveys in the last 12 weeks of life (**b**). Adapted from Wolfe J, Orellana L, Ullrich C, Cook EF, Kang TI, Rosenberg A, Geyer JR, Feudtner C, Dussel V. Symptoms and Distress in Children with Advanced Cancer: Prospective Patient-Reported Outcomes from the PediQUEST Study. J Clin Oncol. 2015; 33(10):1928–35

Table 1.1 Quotes from children and adolescents about the cancer experience

Symptoms
"They ask you, 'you feeling any pain.' You know? Some people like to be macho…like, at the beginning I was kind of like that but I know it's…I have to tell them what's going on so they can help me more" (Weaver et al. 2016, p 4)
"Today was the worst out of all of them, my bone marrow biopsy. It feels like getting a tooth drilled without any pain meds except in your hip instead of your mouth. And afterward if feels like you fell down the stairs and landed on your ass really hard" (Suzuki and Beale 2006, p 157)
"Don't know if I want Emmie here. Sure, I love hanging out with her and just chillin' but I don't want her to see me like this either. I don't wanna get really mad at her cause I'm in pain or don't wanna sleep the whole time she visits" (Flavelle 2011, p 31)
"I think my spirits are getting low. I know they're getting low but I think I may be getting to a point where I'm getting depressed. It sucks" Flavelle 2011, p 29)
Protecting others
"I've had a lot of people compliment me on the way that I've been handling this … Well, I'm a good actor. This is the truth. I am scared, angry, and sad. All this positive (sic) stuff is mainly for my family and friends … What kind of messed up thing did I have to do to have God slap me in the face like this" (Suzuki and Beale 2006, p 157)
"That hard time is a seeing that my friends and family want to stress more. I am often trying to take things from them such as take the stress from them. So, that's personally what I try to do, to take away other people's stress and worries" (Weaver et al. 2016, p 4)
"I mean, I understand like being upset and not wanting to talk…but you just got to be like you were before, happy and respectful" (Weaver et al. 2016, p 5)

(continued)

Table 1.1 (continued)

Thoughts about the future
"Because your cancer, not all cancers, but it can take you away and you never know when you're going to get taken away" (Weaver et al. 2016, p 5)
"I understood very strongly that in order to die, you must first melt away physically. I had seen it happen to many other children. Kids who ate did not die. Therefore I ate; no matter how much my throat hurt or my gums bled. I would eat and throw it up, and then I would eat again" (Suzuki and Beale 2006, p 157)
"They had 3 different options, so I went with number 2. I do think they could have explained it better… the first time I heard it, it was pretty much, "You're going to die, and we can prolong your life, but you're going to die."… but then it was explained over and over again, and I know it is not the truth. I might die, there's a very big chance of that, and I'm scared of that, but there are people who make it, and I'm hoping I'm one of them" (Hurwitz et al. 2004, p 2144)
"I think the tumor is growing REALLY fast or the swelling has gotten worse … Maybe I just need more drugs. I don't really want to be on more drugs. Each time I go up a drug or get a new one makes me wonder who's winning. All I can do is get chemo and radiation and hope for the best. I pray every night for some strength and the strength to get through this" Flavelle 2011, p 31)

the end of life. This research highlights the need for comprehensive assessment of symptoms and a good understanding of typical worries and experiences in order to intervene appropriately to both prevent and address suffering in children and adolescents with cancer.

1.3 Prevalence and Patterns of Suffering in Parents of Children with Cancer

Regardless of disease outcome, the diagnosis and subsequent treatment of childhood cancer have a significant emotional impact on parents, which may result in poor psychosocial outcomes that may in turn impact on the well-being of the entire family (Patterson et al. 2004; Rosenberg et al. 2014). Posttraumatic stress disorder is evident across both bereaved and non-bereaved parents after childhood cancer; however, the prevalence is quite different with non-bereaved mothers' rates at 20% versus fathers' at 13%, while bereaved mothers' and fathers' rates were 53% and 33%, respectively (Norberg et al. 2011). For parents of children with advanced cancer, 50% experience high levels of psychological distress (Rosenberg et al. 2013). Distress levels were higher when parents felt that the ill child also had significant emotional suffering or the family was experiencing financial hardships. Levels of distress were lower when parents reported goals of care that aligned with their understanding of the child's prognosis (Rosenberg et al. 2013).

In a systematic review of quantitative research with parents of children who died from cancer, higher rates of anxiety and depression were evident compared with population norms or non-bereaved parent samples across three studies (Rosenberg et al. 2012). Other included research identified prolonged grief, poor physical and psychological health, and lower quality of life in bereaved parents. Factors associated with poor outcomes included the length of time the child received cancer treatment, with less than 6 months or more than 18 months being more difficult, the child having received a stem cell transplant, death in the hospital, little preparation for death, economic difficulties, and the child's quality of life (Rosenberg et al. 2012). The length of follow-up varied widely across the included studies from 1 month to 9 years after the child's death. One study with longer follow-up indicated that outcomes were worse 4–6 years after the death but then improved between 7 and 9 years after the death (Kreicbergs et al. 2004).

Despite the negative outcomes highlighted, some research also identifies positive outcomes for parents following the death of a child particularly in the areas of relationships, increased appreciation for life, greater empathy for others, and enhanced spirituality (Gilmer et al. 2012; Lichtenthal et al. 2013). The impact of a child's death on parents is clearly linked to relationships with health professionals and aspects of care that are provided both before and after the death (Kreicbergs et al. 2005; Snaman et al. 2016a, b), highlighting opportunities for health professionals to support parents and foster more positive outcomes. The responsibility of institutions that cared for children prior to death to continue to provide care to the family after the death has recently received greater attention in the research literature (Snaman et al. 2016b). The importance of this ongoing connection is highlighted in Case 2 through the comments of bereaved parents.

1.4 Prevalence and Patterns of Suffering in Siblings of Children with Cancer

Cancer and its treatment are generally unpredictable. Parents report living day by day and not making plans more than a day or two in advance. Sudden changes in the child's condition impact parents' ability to attend special events in their own lives or in the lives of the siblings. The ill child's needs must take priority leaving siblings feeling jealous, anxious, and insecure (Sidhu et al. 2005). In a systematic review of research about the psychosocial adjustment of siblings throughout child's cancer treatments, 65 papers were identified. Overall, findings indicated that siblings struggled particularly in the first 3 months after diagnosis with increased levels of fear, sadness, helplessness, worry, anger, and guilt as well as some evidence of posttraumatic stress symptoms (Alderfer et al. 2010). Findings from most studies indicated that siblings did not demonstrate psychiatric symptoms such as anxiety or depression. However, quality of life scores were lower than normal limits for at least the first year after diagnosis but returned to normal levels at 2 years (Alderfer et al. 2010). In some of the included studies, gender and age played a role in the degree and type of distress with females showing more difficulties overall, school-age children having more challenges with physical quality of life, and adolescents having more anxiety and overall lower scores for quality of life (Alderfer et al. 2010). More recent research also highlights the influence of the child's age and developmental stage on the prevalence and patterns of distress with younger bereaved siblings tending to express grief through temper tantrums and irritability, while adolescents tended to have more difficulty in school and engage in risk-taking behaviors (Barrera et al. 2013).

In a study of bereaved siblings an average of 12 years after a child's death from cancer, only about a quarter reported ongoing psychological distress (Rosenberg et al. 2015). For the majority of these siblings, anxiety, depression, and the use of alcohol or illicit substances increased in the first year after the death but over time returned to what it was prior to the child's diagnosis (Rosenberg et al. 2015). Similarly, Eilegard et al. (2013) found little differences in the prevalence of anxiety and depression when comparing bereaved siblings and age-matched non-bereaved siblings, 2–9 years after the death. The areas where there were differences between the two groups included sleep, maturity, and self-esteem with bereaved sibling reporting more difficulties with sleep and lower levels of maturity and self-esteem.

In a study, of 39 siblings, 44% felt they had experienced changes in their personality following a child's death from cancer, while 61% and 54% of their mothers and fathers reported personality changes in the sibling. The changes were both positive and negative with some becoming more compassionate and mature, while others reported being more withdrawn, fearful, sad, or angry. Interestingly, siblings tended to report more of the positive changes in themselves, while the parents tended to report more of the negative changes (Foster et al. 2012).

In one study, one third of 39 participating siblings indicated that their experience impacted on their relationships with friends. Some found it difficult to relate to their friends as they could not understand what the experience was like. Others found new groups of friends, sometimes becoming close to the deceased child's peers (Foster et al. 2012). In another study with 58 siblings, a majority (82%) reported that their relationships with others were not negatively impacted by the illness with median scores for social support similar to scores from the general population 12 years after a child's death from cancer. However, for the subset who did feel that relationships were negatively impacted during the illness, the effects were long lasting as, even 12 years later, reported levels of social support were significantly lower in this subset than in the larger group of participants (Rosenberg et al. 2015). Age at the time of the child's illness had a significant impact on long-term social support with those who were aged 13 years or more at the time of the illness experiencing greater difficulties over the long term (Rosenberg et al. 2015). Similarly, in a systematic review, Alderfer et al. (2010) found that across the included studies, measures of social functioning were no different than norms on mean scores, but a larger than expected subgroup fell into the clinical range for social difficulties.

For siblings in particular, it seems that the experience of living with a child with cancer and then experiencing that child's death has both positive and negative impacts in all aspects of their life. Distress is most prevalent in the first year after the death; however, the majority of siblings are able to work through their experience in a positive way. Unfortunately, some continue to struggle long after the child's death. An important consideration is how to identify siblings who are struggling or who are most likely to struggle so that additional supports can be put in place.

1.5 Addressing Suffering

For many parents, treating their child's symp toms is as important as treating their child's disease (Nass and Patlak 2015). Parental perception of poor symptom control at the end of life can lead to parental distress years after a child's death (Kreicbergs et al. 2005). Unfortunately, effectively managing symptoms at the end of life for children with cancer remains a challenge. A landmark study by Wolfe et al. (2000a) found that treatment of the most common symptoms at the end of life was rarely successful, even in the case of symptoms that are known to be treatable. In this study, only 27% of parents reported that the treatment of their child's pain was successful, 16% reported that their child's dyspnea treatment was effective, and only 10% reported that their child's nausea and vomiting or constipation was effectively managed. These concerning findings and other research about the prevalence of symptoms (Wolfe et al. 2000a, b, 2008; Drake et al. 2003) spurred international efforts toward improving the quality of care delivered to children with advanced cancer. One consistent theme arising from these efforts is the need to better integrate palliative care with oncology care. Palliative care is a philosophy of care aimed at preventing and relieving suffering for those living with a life-threatening or life-limiting illness. It includes the control of physical symptoms and addresses the psychological, social, and spiritual needs of children and their families (American Academy of Pediatrics 2000).

The American Society of Clinical Oncology has recommended the integration of palliative care into standard oncology care for any adult patient with metastatic cancer and/or high symptom burden (Smith et al. 2012). This recommendation was based on convincing evidence from clinical trials that demonstrated better patient and caregiver outcomes when patients received some element of specialized palliative care. Emerging evidence in the pediatric oncology literature also supports the notion that specialized palliative care is beneficial to children with advanced cancer. One study showed that children with advanced cancer who received specialized palliative care were more likely to have fun and experience events that added meaning to life (Friedrichsdorf ct al. 2015). Children receiving specialized palliative care also experienced less suffering from prevalent symptoms, such as pain and dyspnea, at the end of life (Friedrichsdorf et al. 2015; Wolfe et al. 2008).

Despite strong evidence supporting the integration of specialized pediatric palliative care, this model of care may not be feasible in many institutions that care for children with advanced cancer. A study published in 2008 reported that only 58% of Children's Oncology Group institutions have access to a pediatric palliative care team (Johnston et al. 2008). Furthermore, many of these programs had inadequate resources to provide after-hour palliative care coverage (Feudtner et al. 2013). Lack of after-hour coverage hinders effective symptom management, as uncontrolled symptoms require urgent assessment and intervention.

Access to palliative care remains a challenge even among institutions that have established pediatric palliative care programs. One study found that only 3 of 15 valued elements of palliative care were accessible to the families of children with cancer (Kassam et al. 2013). Elements included core tenets of palliative care, such as communication about end of life and preparation for death and dying. The same study found that only 56% of these children were referred to a specialized palliative care program. Low palliative care referral rates by pediatric oncology clinicians have also been previously reported (Widger et al. 2007). An additional barrier to children receiving high-quality palliative care is oncology clinician skill gaps. One study that surveyed a large group of pediatric oncologists found that nearly half of them felt anxiety about having to manage difficult symptoms in a dying child. Alarmingly, 92% of the pediatric oncologists also reported that they learned how to care for dying children through trial and error (Hilden et al. 2001).

The only way to eliminate all suffering associated with childhood cancer is to eradicate the disease itself from our world. While great strides have been made, children continue to get cancer and suffer from its effects. Even when the child is cured, the suffering endured by the child and family is significant throughout the treatment and beyond. When the child has advanced cancer and eventually dies, suffering increases both in the short and long terms for the child and family. Suffering can be addressed through provision of high-quality palliative care from the time of diagnosis of childhood cancer. While several models of palliative care delivery are possible in this setting, there is consensus that every oncology clinician should be equipped with the skills to comfortably provide basic pain and symptom management and family support (Kaye et al. 2016). Access to a specialized palliative care team should also be available to provide assistance in the management of more complex or difficult to control symptoms, complex family dynamics, and other challenging issues. Oncology and pediatric palliative care programs should work together to close the identified care gaps and ensure that physical, emotional, psychosocial, and spiritual distress in children with cancer and their families is anticipated and optimally addressed. Optimal care for children and families is likely to have not only immediate benefits in terms of a more peaceful or "good death" for the child but also on the long-term health outcomes for bereaved family members.

1.6 Keys Points

- Despite significant advances in the treatment of childhood malignancies, approximately 20% of children with cancer will die from their disease.
- Children with advanced cancer experience a high number of treatable symptoms that result in substantial suffering.
- Symptom prevalence and severity increases as cancer progresses and end of life approaches.
- The health and well-being of parents and siblings of children with cancer are affected in both the short and long terms. These effects can be both positive and negative.
- Subsets of bereaved parents and siblings may be at higher risk for negative health outcomes.
- Emerging evidence supports that integrating palliative care with oncology care leads to better symptom control and improved quality of life in children with advanced cancer and may impact on long-term health of family members.

Case 1

The mother of a 6-year-old girl diagnosed with very high-risk acute lymphoblastic leukemia (ALL) describes the impact of the diagnosis on the family:

We knew something was wrong with Elayna; she had been tired and pale and cold for several weeks. She had bloodwork done which showed low hemoglobin and white blood cells, but we were specifically told there were no cancer cells. We were awaiting an appointment with a pediatric hematologist and were expecting to confirm that a bad virus had wiped out her immune system. While awaiting that appointment, Elayna spiked a fever and was admitted to hospital. Two days later she was transferred to a larger hospital 2 h away to speed up the consultation with the hematologist.

It was October 16, 2012. We were sitting in a small room with a doctor and a social worker that we had just met. Elayna had been taken to a procedure room for the first of many lumbar punctures and bone marrow biopsies to find out exactly what was wrong.

We were still under the impression that these tests were to confirm the presence of a virus and to rule out anything serious. The doctor and social worker obviously knew that it was something more. The social worker started telling us about the Children's Wish Foundation, and the rest is a blur. I started to cry. Ugly, sobbing, can't catch your breath crying, sure that this was their way of telling me that my little girl was going to die. It was not until several hours later that they came back with the results of the biopsy to tell us that Elayna had ALL. We were told that she had a number of factors working in her favor and that with intense treatment her chances of survival were 85%. To most people, these would seem like pretty good odds, but when it is your child, anything less than 100% is utter devastation.

Elayna went along with surgery to install a port and the first few doses of chemotherapy without complaint. She kept herself busy in the hospital going for walks, playing computer games, coloring, and watching movies. It was 16 days before she returned home. In that time, my husband and I had taken turns staying in the hospital with her and staying home with our other two children. I remember my daughter Caitlyn, who was 10 at the time, crying on the phone, telling me that she wanted me to come home, that she needed me too, and that I loved Elayna more than I loved her. Could she really not see that I would be doing the same if it was her who had become sick? Cohen was only 3 at the time so he really didn't understand anything that was going on, but he was mad that we were gone all the time, he had temper tantrums and also started having horrible nightmares where he thought he could see Elayna as a ghost in his mirror. I couldn't bear the thought of what he may be foreseeing and eventually covered his mirror with a blanket. My marriage began to suffer. I wanted to be with Elayna all the time and wanted my husband to just stay home and look after the other two kids. We argued over everything to do with Elayna's care, about what she could and couldn't do, whether or not we should call a doctor, who would be taking her to her next appointment. We completely lost control of our other children, letting them do whatever they wanted, putting up with bad behaviour, losing any sort of rules or discipline we had once tried to maintain, and buying them gifts out of guilt for being absent parents. We tried desperately to "pause" the rest of our lives – we both stopped working, our lives revolved around bloodwork, counts, and chemo appointments. We sat in our house, hiding from the outside world as much as possible, anxiously watching Elayna for fevers or any sort of change or sign that the cancer was back. We tried to keep things somewhat normal for the other two kids, but worried so much about the risk of an infection, there were no more play dates or birthday parties at our house. It just wasn't worth the risk.

There was only once that I remember Elayna refusing to make the 2-h trip for an appointment. We always had to wake her up early and keep her fasting as we drove; usually the days were long and exhausting. Elayna was just tired of it all. I told her that she had to go to her appointment; there was no choice. She asked if she didn't go would she die? How can you possibly tell your 6-year-old that without the medications she most assuredly would die? How is it possible that life continues on, groceries need to be bought, meals made, bills paid? How can people smile, or laugh, or whine, or complain when my child has cancer?

Special thanks to Kelly Greenwood for sharing the story of the impact of her daughter's cancer diagnosis on the family.

Case 2

In a study of bereaved parents' perspectives on the quality of their child's end of life care, one parent highlighted the experience of leaving the hospital and not receiving any follow-up support:

> All of the help we've received with counseling, support groups, etc. we had to find on our own, which wasn't an easy process. After the insane rollercoaster ride, with crisis after crisis and agonizing decisions to make often on a daily basis, the trauma of watching our child get sicker and sicker, the hours spent at the hospital for 2.5 months and the decision to remove life support, we were a shell of our former selves, hardly able to cope with ourselves let alone our two [young] kids at home. Then suddenly it's all over and you go home and there is nothing. We felt as though we were dropped off an edge of a cliff.

Another parent highlighted the impact of even small efforts at continued contact made by health professionals:

> Staff who cared for her in two different hospitals sent notes to us about how they were affected by our daughter and her death. These notes were astounding to us, but even more, they made us feel less alone since we were a long distance from home and these health professionals were the only people who shared her death with us. We were very touched by their kindness. (Widger 2012, p 95)

References

Alderfer MA, Long KA, Lown EA, Marsland AL, Ostrowski NL, Hock JM et al (2010) Psychosocial adjustment of siblings of children with cancer: a systematic review. Psychooncology 19(8):789–805

American Academy of Pediatrics (2000) Committee on bioethics and committee on hospital care. Palliative care for children. Pediatrics 106(2 Pt 1):351–357

Barrera M, Alam R, D'Agostino NM, Nicholas DB, Schneiderman G (2013) Parental perceptions of siblings' grieving after a childhood cancer death: a longitudinal study. Death Stud 37(1):25–46

Drake R, Frost J, Collins JJ (2003) The symptoms of dying children. J Pain Symptom Manag 26(1):594–603

Eilegard A, Steineck G, Nyberg T, Kreicbergs U (2013) Psychological health in siblings who lost a brother or sister to cancer 2 to 9 years earlier. Psychooncology 22(3):683–691

Feudtner C, Womer J, Augustin R, Remke S, Wolfe J, Friebert S et al (2013) Pediatric palliative care programs in children's hospitals: a cross-sectional national survey. Pediatrics 132(6):1063–1070

Flavelle SC (2011) Experience of an adolescent living with and dying of cancer. Arch Pediatr Adolesc Med 165(1):28–32

Foster TL, Gilmer MJ, Vannatta K, Barrera M, Davies B, Dietrich MS et al (2012) Changes in siblings after the death of a child from cancer. Cancer Nurs 35(5):347–354

Friedrichsdorf SJ, Postier A, Dreyfus J, Osenga K, Sencer S, Wolfe J (2015) Improved quality of life at end of life related to home-based palliative care in children with cancer. J Palliat Med 18(2):143–150

Gilmer MJ, Foster TL, Vannatta K, Barrera M, Davies B, Dietrich MS et al (2012) Changes in parents after the death of a child from cancer. J Pain Symptom Manag 44(4):572–582

Heath JA, Clarke NE, Donath SM, McCarthy M, Anderson VA, Wolfe J (2010) Symptoms and suffering at the end of life in children with cancer: an Australian perspective. Med J Aust 192(2):71–75

Hilden JM, Emanuel EJ, Fairclough DL, Link MP, Foley KM, Clarridge BC et al (2001) Attitudes and practices among pediatric oncologists regarding end-of-life care: results of the 1998 American Society of Clinical Oncology survey. J Clin Oncol 19(1):205–212

Hinds PS, Brandon J, Allen C, Hijiya N, Newsome R, Kane JR (2007) Patient-reported outcomes in end-of-life research in pediatric oncology. J Pediatr Psychol 32(9):1079–1088

Hinds PS, Nuss SL, Ruccione KS, Withycombe JS, Jacobs S, DeLuca H et al (2013) PROMIS pediatric measures in pediatric oncology: valid and clinically feasible indicators of patient-reported outcomes. Pediatr Blood Cancer 60(3):402–408

Hudson MM, Link MP, Simone JV (2014) Milestones in the curability of pediatric cancers. J Clin Oncol 32(23):2391–2397

Hurwitz CA, Duncan J, Wolfe J (2004) Caring for the child with cancer at the close of life—"There are people who make it, and I'm hoping I'm one of them". JAMA 292(17):2141–2149

Jalmsell L, Kreicbergs U, Onelov E, Steineck G, Henter JI (2006) Symptoms affecting children with malignancies during the last month of life: a nationwide follow-up. Pediatrics 117(4):1314–1320

Johnston DL, Nagel K, Friedman DL, Meza JL, Hurwitz CA, Friebert S (2008) Availability and use of palliative care and end-of-life services for pediatric oncology patients. J Clin Oncol 26(28):4646–4650

Kassam A, Skiadaresis J, Habib S, Alexander S, Wolfe J (2013) Moving toward quality palliative cancer care: parent and clinician perspectives on gaps between what matters and what is accessible. J Clin Oncol 31(7):910–915

Kaye EC, Friebert S, Baker JN (2016) Early integration of palliative care for children with high-risk cancer and their families. Pediatr Blood Cancer 63(4):593–597

Kreicbergs U, Valdimarsdottir U, Onelov E, Henter JI, Steineck G (2004) Anxiety and depression in parents 4–9 years after the loss of a child owing to a malignancy: a population-based follow-up. Psychol Med 34(8):1431–1441

Kreicbergs U, Valdimarsdottir U, Onelov E, Bjork O, Steineck G, Henter JI (2005) Care-related distress: a nationwide study of parents who lost their child to cancer. J Clin Oncol 23(36):9162–9171

Lichtenthal WG, Neimeyer RA, Currier JM, Roberts K, Jordan N (2013) Cause of death and the quest for meaning after the loss of a child. Death Stud 37(4):311–342

von Lützau P, Otto M, Hechler T, Metzing S, Wolfe J, Zernikow B (2012) Children dying from cancer: parents' perspectives on symptoms, quality of life, characteristics of death, and end-of-life decisions. J Palliat Care 28(4):274–281

Nass SJ, Patlak M (2015) National Cancer Policy Forum (U.S.). Comprehensive cancer care for children and their families: summary of a joint workshop by the Institute of Medicine and the American Cancer Society. The National Academies Press, Washington, DC, 106 pages p 16

Norberg AL, Poder U, von Essen L (2011) Early avoidance of disease- and treatment-related distress predicts post-traumatic stress in parents of children with cancer. Eur J Oncol Nurs 15(1):80–84

Patterson JM, Holm KE, Gurney JG (2004) The impact of childhood cancer on the family: a qualitative analysis of strains, resources, and coping behaviors. Psychooncology 13(6):390–407

Pizzo PA, Poplack DG (2011) Principles and practice of pediatric oncology, 6th edn. Wolters Kluwer/ Lippincott Williams & Wilkins Health, Philadelphia, PA. xx, 1531 p 3

Pizzo PA, Poplack DG, Adamson PC, Blaney SM, Helman L (2016) Principles and practice of pediatric oncology , 7th edn. Wolters Kluwer, Philadelphia, xxiv, 1296 p 6

Rosenberg AR, Baker KS, Syrjala K, Wolfe J (2012) Systematic review of psychosocial morbidities among bereaved parents of children with cancer. Pediatr Blood Cancer 58(4):503–512

Rosenberg AR, Dussel V, Kang T, Geyer JR, Gerhardt CA, Feudtner C et al (2013) Psychological distress in parents of children with advanced cancer. JAMA Pediatr 167(6):537–543

Rosenberg AR, Wolfe J, Bradford MC, Shaffer ML, Yi-Frazier JP, Curtis JR et al (2014) Resilience and psychosocial outcomes in parents of children with cancer. Pediatr Blood Cancer 61(3):552–557

Rosenberg AR, Postier A, Osenga K, Kreicbergs U, Neville B, Dussel V et al (2015) Long-term psychosocial outcomes among bereaved siblings of children with cancer. J Pain Symptom Manag 49(1):55–65

Sidhu R, Passmore A, Baker D (2005) An investigation into parent perceptions of the needs of siblings of children with cancer. J Pediatr Oncol Nurs 22(5):276–287

Smith TJ, Temin S, Alesi ER, Abernethy AP, Balboni TA, Basch EM et al (2012) American Society of Clinical Oncology provisional clinical opinion: the integration of palliative care into standard oncology care. J Clin Oncol 30(8):880–887

Snaman JM, Kaye EC, Torres C, Gibson D, Baker JN (2016a) Parental grief following the death of a child from cancer: the ongoing odyssey. Pediatr Blood Cancer 63(9):1594–1602

Snaman JM, Kaye EC, Torres C, Gibson DV, Baker JN (2016b) Helping parents live with the hole in their heart: the role of health care providers and institutions in the bereaved parents' grief journeys. Cancer 122(17):2757–2765

Suzuki LK, Beale IL (2006) Personal web home pages of adolescents with cancer: self-presentation, information dissemination, and interpersonal connection. J Pediatr Oncol Nurs 23(3):152–161

Tomlinson D, Bartels U, Gammon J, Hinds PS, Volpe J, Bouffet E et al (2011) Chemotherapy versus supportive care alone in pediatric palliative care for cancer: comparing the preferences of parents and health care professionals. CMAJ 183(17):E1252–E1258

Weaver MS, Baker JN, Gattuso JS, Gibson DV, Hinds PS (2016) "Being a good patient" during times of illness as defined by adolescent patients with cancer. Cancer 122(14):2224–2233

Widger, K (2012) Initial development and psychometric testing of an instrument to measure the quality of children's end-of-life care. Dissertation, University of Toronto

Widger K, Davies D, Drouin DJ, Beaune L, Daoust L, Farran RP et al (2007) Pediatric patients receiving palliative care in Canada: results of a multicenter review. Arch Pediatr Adolesc Med 161(6):597–602

Wolfe J, Grier HE, Klar N, Levin SB, Ellenbogen JM, Salem-Schatz S et al (2000a) Symptoms and suffering at the end of life in children with cancer. N Engl J Med 342(5):326–333

Wolfe J, Klar N, Grier HE, Duncan J, Salem-Schatz S, Emanuel EJ et al (2000b) Understanding of prognosis among parents of children who died of cancer: impact on treatment goals and integration of palliative care. JAMA 284(19):2469–2475

Wolfe J, Hammel JF, Edwards KE, Duncan J, Comeau M, Breyer J et al (2008) Easing of suffering in children with cancer at the end of life: is care changing? J Clin Oncol 26(10):1717–1723

Wolfe J, Orellana L, Ullrich C, Cook EF, Kang TI, Rosenberg A et al (2015) Symptoms and distress in children with advanced cancer: prospective patient-reported outcomes from the PediQUEST study. J Clin Oncol 33(17):1928–1935

The Impact of Cancer on the Child, Parents, Siblings and Community

2

Myra Bluebond-Langner and Richard W. Langner

2.1 Introduction

The impact of cancer on families is ongoing and evolving. For some the impact extends into survivorship for others into bereavement. In this chapter, we focus on the impact of cancer from the time a child or young person falls ill up to the point at which he/she enters survivorship or the family enters bereavement.

Cancer presents children, parents and families with challenges to which they must respond to "problematic situations" which require a solution or an appropriate action in response (Wallander and Varni 1998). Our focus is on the active, constructive responses which parents and children make to the intrusion of cancer. We examine what families find problematic how they define the issues and sources of their perceptions. We also identify drivers of behaviour and the strategies families use to make their way through the journey. We provide a framework through which the experiences of children, parents and siblings with cancer can be understood. We see such an understanding as key to building and maintaining the relationships with various members of the family, essential for the delivery of palliative care at any level and at any point in the illness.

Our approach to understanding the impact of cancer is, like palliative care itself, multidisciplinary. While attending to results from psychology, our approach also relies upon sociology and anthropology. We stress the importance of understanding behaviour as relational and as social interaction.

Our aim is to provide an understanding of the impact of cancer which will enable clinicians to both assess the needs of children and families and to provide the necessary support. Our approach also can be used in developing further research in paediatric cancer as well as in assisting clinicians in picking their way through difficult discussions about disease progression, options for care and treatment.

2.2 The Approach Taken Here

2.2.1 Non-pathological Perspective

When a child becomes ill, it is not inevitable or even likely that the family will become ill as well. Many studies of the impact of cancer use the language of psychopathology, dysfunction and

M. Bluebond-Langner, Ph.D., Hon. F.R.C.P.C.H. (✉)
UCL Faculty of Population Health Sciences,
Louis Dundas Centre for Children's Palliative Care,
UCL Great Ormond Street Institute of Child Health,
30 Guilford Street, London WC1N 1EH, UK
e-mail: bluebond@ucl.ac.uk

R.W. Langner, Ph.D.
Louis Dundas Centre for Children's Palliative Care,
UCL Great Ormond Street Institute of Child Health,
30 Guilford Street, London WC1N 1EH, UK
e-mail: r.langner1@gmail.com

J. Wolfe et al. (eds.), *Palliative Care in Pediatric Oncology*, Pediatric Oncology,
https://doi.org/10.1007/978-3-319-61391-8_2

maladjustment. Our approach is to investigate how children (including siblings) and parents respond and carry on with life after the receipt of a cancer diagnosis. Studies show that they carry on with something like what life has been for them.

Some psychologists and psycho-oncologists take the view that in pushing back against the intrusion of cancer, most parents deploy healthy coping strategies and show resilience (Eiser 1990; Noll et al. 1999; Dixon-Woods et al. 2002; Noll and Kupst 2007; Van Schoors et al. 2015).

Most families in which a child is diagnosed with cancer are able to draw on their social, intellectual and emotional competencies to push back against the intrusion of cancer in order to maintain themselves and their lives. Despite the adversity to which they are subject, and despite what might even be traumas, in these children and families, "the prevalence of psychosocial dysfunction (i.e., psychopathology or social dysfunction) is similar to that found in the general population or appropriate comparison groups" (Noll and Kupst 2007). The term resilience is often used to describe these responses to the challenges of cancer which families display. Appropriate support for these families should always, of course, be a consideration.

The resilience model marks a shift away from deficit and pathology toward family's skills and resources, even capacity for growth. It focuses on families' competences (Last and Grootenhuis 1998).

2.2.2 The Family Unit as Central

In understanding the impact of cancer in a child or young person, the family must be kept central. This is a view shared by clinicians and by researchers from a number of different perspectives including those who study resilient families. Resilience is a "relational event" (Zaider and Kissane 2007). This has led to the view that family-centred care is the standard for all children "Central to family-centered care is the belief that a child is part of a family system and therefore both the child and his or her family are the unit of care" (Jones et al. 2011, p 135).

The family is a unit "led" by the parents. This is not to diminish or underestimate the competencies of even young children who must deal with cancer. Even less does it minimize the competencies of adolescents who are part adult and part child. We recognize and it has been shown in previous work that children do have their own social worlds and that they have social relations in their own right which can be studied in their own right (Bluebond-Langner 1978). Our view is that in the present context of serious and life-threatening illness, the family is the place where these various competencies are exercised and as such the family, as led by parents, is crucial for understanding the impact of cancer.

Parents' behaviour is often the focus of studies of the impact of cancer. This does not mean that focus has shifted from a family perspective to a focus on the experience and behaviour of individuals. The strategies or management behaviours which have been reported in the literature can affect the entire family. These are relational strategies and not purely personal ones. They are aimed at maintaining the integrity of the family, maintaining the order of everyday life in the family and seeing to the needs of all of the members of the family. They are about parents fulfilling their roles within the family and fulfilling their responsibilities to the ill child and to their other children and the responsibilities between spouses.

2.2.3 The Impact of the Disease Over Time: A Biopsychosocial Illness Trajectory

The impact of cancer on families and with it the experiences of the different members of the family change in important ways as disease-related events unfold. The illness trajectory of children with cancer and their families is driven by clinical events and the related experiences which children, parents and siblings have as a result of these. The psychological and social aspects of this trajectory include sentinel events, knowledge about and understanding of the disease, parents' narrative of or construction of the ill child and the ill child's disease-related self-concept.

Both quantitative and qualitative researches support a complex picture of the impact of cancer, a picture that is not simply a linear procession from diagnosis onward (Bluebond-Langner 1998). Psychological studies show that parents are challenged at diagnosis but that over a period of 6–18 months, they adapt to the challenges which the diagnosis presents. Being overwhelmed and confused may be followed by the reassertion of control and understanding-only to be overwhelmed again and to find uncertainty returning. From the perspective of psychopathology, parents, for example, may appear as in distress and dysfunctional only to return to normal after experience with the disease (Patenaude and Kupst 2005; Phipps 2007).

Grootenhuis and Last (1997) found that relapse presents renewed challenges. Stress which had returned to normal levels increases again. Long and Marsland (2011) report in their review that "variations in family functioning paralleling the cancer symptom course more closely than time since diagnosis or treatment protocol" (Woodgate and Degner 2004, p 78).

Qualitative research confirms these findings. Qualitative researchers have described a psychosocial natural history of the disease or what could also be called a psychosocial disease trajectory. Bluebond-Langner (1978) found that children's understanding of their illness (typically leukaemia at a time when chance of cure was low) and associated self-concept changed throughout the course of the disease. Their understanding of the disease progressed from viewing cancer as serious but treatable to a disease which cannot be cured and finally as a disease from which they would die. The catalysts of change were illness events such as relapse or the appearance of new symptoms together with experiences in the hospital and clinic, especially with other similarly ill children.

In a later study, Bluebond-Langner (1998) mapped well siblings of children with cystic fibrosis, understanding of the disease and prognosis. As their ill siblings progressed from being chronically to terminally ill, the well siblings' views changed. The views changed gradually and incrementally from seeing the illness as a condition to a series of potentially acute episodes to a progressive life-limiting illness and finally to a terminal illness. Transitions in understanding were related to significant disease-related experiences, and so the same transition might occur after a year for one sibling and within a week for a sibling of a different ill child.

This process of a changing and increasing understanding reflects the fact that ill children and well siblings may acquire information about the disease over a protracted period of time. It also indicates that information needs to be available as well as assimilated or internalized. This assimilation/internalization of information, Bluebond-Langner (1978, 1998) found, is mediated by disease- and treatment-related experiences.

This is not unlike the distinction Valdimarsdottir et al. (2007) make between parents' intellectual and emotional awareness of a child's inevitable or imminent death. In the case of parents and children, "internalization" can occur years or hours before the child's death. Valdimarsdottir et al. found that two of the mediators of the transition from being intellectually aware to emotionally aware were time spent with the ill child and interaction with healthcare professionals, a finding which aligns with the view that disease-related experience is a key factor in the internalization of information.

2.3 A Biopsychosocial Trajectory of Cancer

2.3.1 Seeking and Receiving a Diagnosis

Children's and parents' experience of cancer often begins with the occurrence of symptoms which could be normal and transient, symptoms which any child might occasionally experience and which general practitioners or primary care paediatricians frequently see in healthy children. If symptoms persist and their import is missed, concern and anxiety escalate. If there is a significant delay and parents' concerns have been dismissed, parents can arrive at a diagnosis of cancer with feelings of anger, mistrust and guilt (Eiser et al. 1994; Dixon-Woods et al. 2005).

Though parents of children with cancer have lived for some time with a sense that there is something significantly wrong with their child and so have pursued a diagnosis, the receipt of it is nonetheless difficult. A number of studies report that at diagnosis parents feel overwhelmed (Day et al. 2016; Eiser et al. 1994; Levi 2000; Bluebond-Langner 1998; Martinson and Cohen 1989). Young et al. (2002) state that hearing the news is catastrophic. At this point parents can be "unable to think and act effectively" (Salmon et al. 2012).

Parents find it difficult to absorb much of the information which they are being given (Eiser et al. 1994; Day et al. 2016; Young et al. 2002; Should be Gogan 1977b). They may later have difficulty recalling the time surrounding diagnosis (Eiser et al. 1994). "Although all parents reported that they were encouraged to ask questions, many felt quite unable to do so" (Eiser et al. 1994, p 201).

Following quickly upon diagnosis, sometimes within hours, some parents must make decisions about participation in clinical trials. Given their state, they may find this extremely difficult, if not impossible (Levi et al. 2000; Stewart et al. 2012).

In addition to the threat to the child's health and even life, the diagnosis carries another less apparent, less tangible impact. Cancer is a threat to how parents and children define themselves, to their identities and to their understanding of themselves as a family. The role of a parent, how parents see themselves in this role and how parents view or construct what it is to be a child and a child in a family is crucial to the understanding of the impact of cancer.

Over 40 years ago, Futterman and Hoffman (1973) stated that:

> The onset of leukemia in a child represents an assault on a parent's sense of adequacy as guardian of his child, and, more generally, as a person with a meaningful control over his own and his family's destinies. (p 132)

This remains true today. A parent's very existence as a parent is threatened and in turn so is the integrity of the family.

Significant in this statement by Futterman and Hoffman is the link between what a child is, what a parent is and what a family is. By their very nature fathers, mothers and children are connected. The intrusion of cancer affects both the individuals in a family and their life together. The distinction which is sometimes proposed between individual and family factors does not arise here because who the members of the family are as individuals essentially involves relations, connections to others.

The idea of the parental role—some have used the term "good parents" (Woodgate and Hinds)—has often been employed in understanding the behaviour of families of children with cancer over the last four decades (Bluebond-Langner 1978, 1996; Woodgate 2006; Hinds et al. 2005, 2009, 2010; Day et al. 2016). The parents' role is that of advocate and protector. Parents advocate in a number of ways. They become vigilant observers of their child's condition and report changes to their clinicians. They also search for information about the disease and its treatment in order to understand what is happening to and being done for their child. In addition, they also may raise questions about the appropriateness of therapies they have read about for their child.

While the pursuit of information has become easier for parents in the wake of media coverage and, of course, the Internet, it is not a recent phenomenon. Pursuit of information and treatment options has been reported as a fundamental part of parental response to a cancer diagnosis going back to the early 1970s. Then Futterman and Hoffman (1973) pointed out that as advocates parents are driven to make sure that nothing has been held back from their child and that nothing has been overlooked. They leave no stone unturned. At the same time, however, charged with responsibility of protecting their child from maltreatment and harm, they strive to protect their children from pain, both physical and mental.

The threat to the family lies not only in the ways that cancer challenges what it means to be a parent but also in the ways it challenges what it means to be a child. In Western society, the child is a being with a future. Cancer threatens this defining characteristic. Essential and defining activities for children such as being in school are interrupted. Sacrifices which children and families make and the discipline to which child is subject are all for a future benefit. Cancer calls this future into question.

The two aspects of parental role—advocate and protector—are in tension and can come into conflict with each other. The treatments and investigative procedures can be harsh and painful. Yet it is such procedures which give children with cancer a chance—sometimes an excellent chance and sometimes barely a chance—at cure or living substantially longer than without them. So what is often called the weighing of risks and benefits in decision making takes on a personal and even existential dimension for parents. The parent as advocate focuses on the benefits; the parent as protector sees the risks. But when seen as a conflict of aspects of a single role, this is not a matter of weighing or calculating, but of while deciding for one's ill child also defining one's parenting, something which is an essential part of the person.

2.3.2 Post Diagnosis Through Beginning of Treatment

Parents and the family begin to re-establish control and respond to the various challenges which they face in a number of ways. Children and parents alike learn to understand the "foreign" language of cancer care as well as the customs and rituals of the hospital, the new world of which they are becoming a part. The initial feelings of being confused and overwhelmed give way to a perception of order and routine (Stewart 2003; Bluebond-Langner 1978).

Normalizing, being normal is a term which parents and children themselves use in talking about their experience with cancer. It is also used by researchers. Sometimes being normal is having the opportunity to do simple things which are typically associated with children and childhood but which have been missed out on because of the illness (McGrath 2001).

Compartmentalization and selective awareness are strategies which parents use to manage information. The term compartmentalization (Bluebond-Langner 1998) recognizes a difference in the way in which bits of information figure in a person's awareness. There is information which is in focus rather than peripheral; as with vision, items on the periphery are part of the field but only come into play under special circumstances. There are thoughts which are present as opposed to those which would require a deliberate act to access and make present in awareness. Hinds et al. (1996), using the term "selective awareness", report a similar phenomenon. In selective awareness, parents focus on what they have to know, that is, what is necessary to care for their child and fulfil their roles. By calling it selective, Hinds et al. acknowledge that parents who adopt this practise are aware of other pieces of information but keep them out of focus.

It is apparent that central to the families' response is information. Information plays an important and multifaceted role in the response parents, children and others make to the cancer. Information is both sought after and a source of comfort in some contexts but can be disturbing and disruptive in others. Mack et al. (2005, 2006) found that parents want information about treatment and prognosis and that this is an important part of establishing a relation with their child's oncologist. Parents rated care highly when honest and ample information was provided which suggests that information is crucial for them in their role as parent. Parents desired information even though it might be upsetting to them, indicating that it is a sort of double-edged sword.

Parents and children must manage information carefully. There is a crucial balance to be struck. Though some information can bring control and a sense of fulfilling one's role and order, other information can be threatening. Certain information can undermine the order which parents have worked hard to establish. Parents carefully manage information and their vision of the future. They manage their interactions with clinicians and other families so as not to disturb the equilibrium they have created.

Relapse, recurrence and deterioration threaten that equilibrium. The carefully constructed post diagnosis balance must be recalibrated. The new adaptations are once again balancing acts between what parents have been told about the longer term while focusing on the present.

2.3.3 Relapse and Deterioration

Relapse is a complex and critical event. It is also one which has received little attention in the literature (Hinds et al. 2002; De Graves and Aranda 2008). At relapse parents are once again faced with a challenge to which they must respond. Some researchers have reported the stress at this point to be greater than at diagnosis (Hinds et al. 1996; Gogan et al. 1977a, b). Parents experience hopelessness and uncertainty (Grootenhuis and Last 1997; Hinds et al. 2002; De Graves and Aranda 2008). Parents' ability to process information is again compromised (De Graves and Aranda 2008).

Though this may sound as if it is a repeat of the experience at diagnosis, there are important ways in which relapse or recurrence differs from diagnosis. De Graves and Aranda (2008) describe the families at recurrence/relapse as going through *a process of understanding the implications of relapse* and realizing that the child may not survive. Hinds et al. describe this as a *cognitive shift* to entertaining the possibility of death. Hinds et al. (2002) point out that the various components of their central construct "Coming to Terms" all took place within *a context of* "Sensing difference" (Hinds et al. 2002). Her team observed "parents' strong sense that all important aspects of their lives changed…". This is parallel to what Bluebond-Langner reports for ill children (1978) and well siblings (1998) in the context of the biosocial disease trajectory which is facilitated by clinical changes in the ill child and significant experiences with the child and with others around that child in hospital or clinic. In this context, the ill child's own self-concept changes as does the construction of that child by other members of the family (discussed above and below).

De Graves and Aranda (2008) describe decision making after relapse as having become a "contested process" in that parents have to manage competing goals: saving the child, protecting the child and minimizing harm. Treatment decisions become "impossible choices". Hinds et al. (1996) recognize the same dilemma within the construct "eyeing treatment limitations". This captures the parental recognition that competing goals are in conflict and that the choice seems impossible. One parent commented that though she knew choices may have to be made, she didn't want to be the one to make them, a sentiment echoed by 7/33 (21%) of parents in their study.

De Graves and Aranda (2008) stress that parents live with both fear and hope at the same time. They take the position that this establishes the uncertainty that is essential for allowing parents to go on and at the same time not despair. Hinds et al. (1996) find something very similar using the term "alternating realization's" in describing one mother as "thinking at both ends". Hinds et al. (1996) also speak of parents doing their best to help their child survive—fighting while "simultaneously" contemplating and even preparing for the child's death. As the mother referred to previously said "I think about them *both* a lot" (italics added) (p 150). Notably, DeGraves stresses that hope is not incompatible with understanding the life-threatening nature of the child's illness and the very real possibility of death (Mack et al. 2007a, b; Bluebond-Langner et al. 2007).

We also see in the studies by De Graves and Aranda (2008) and Hinds et al. (2002) that understanding the likelihood of the child's eventual death does not deter parents from the pursuit of treatment. De Graves and Aranda (2008) report parents invariably "pursuing the hope for cure" and that the thought of losing the child outweighed the possibility for suffering and harm. All parents in Hinds et al.'s (1996) study of children at first recurrence pursued treatment. At recurrence, there is on the part of parents an "immediate need to consider and select a new treatment option". We see a similar phenomenon in parents of children with high-risk brain tumours at recurrence when cure is no longer possible (Bluebond-Langner et al. 2017).

Hinds et al. (1996) comment that parents report that they were helped by willingness of clinicians to present treatment options and by their willingness to keep parents aware of the child's response to treatment. Mack et al. (2008) point out that in their study even parents who would not recommend treating to other parents recommended that all options be presented to parents.

De Graves and Aranda (2008) note that "The uncertainty of treatment regimens, febrile neutropenic episodes, or other periods of ill health made future planning difficult". Yet, maintaining uncertainty they go on to point out is key to maintaining hope. Hence parents in this state may be reluctant to commit themselves to specific decisions. Dussel et al. (2009) concluded that the opportunity to plan for the location of a child's death is a better indicator of quality care, specifically palliative care, than the actual place of death. If we take a step back from this finding, one might say that it is the discussion of critical issues in the care and treatment of children with cancer that is more important than arriving at a decision in advance.

For some children, the disease will progress and the child's condition will continue to deteriorate. As successive lines of therapy fail, further changes take place in the lives of parents and children; the impact of the illness changes.

2.3.4 When Standard Therapies Fail: Last Recurrence to Death

We do not use the term "end of life" in our discussion of the progress of disease. This stems from our goal of trying to capture the impact of cancer from the ill child's and the family's point of view. "End of life" is a term which is more meaningful to clinicians than to ill children and families. And even for clinicians, it is a time which is often more accurately recognized in retrospect. In seeking to capture the impact of cancer and understanding children's and families' experience of that impact, we find examining the period of time from when disease-directed options have been exhausted and child and parents realize the child will die from the disease, often coinciding with last recurrence, through to death, a more useful interval.

At this point in the illness trajectory, some children may still be eligible for further experimental therapies or off-label use of particular medications. Typically these offer no significant chance of either a meaningful extension of the child's life or cure. They may also burden the child with significant side effects and require that the child be hospitalized. This is truly the time of choiceless choices for parents. It is a time when as Bluebond-Langner et al. (2007) found "Parents will accept something with infinitesimal odds, because the prize they seek is of infinite worth".

At some point during this period, though not necessarily simultaneously, the ill child, well sibling and parents do come to the realization not only that there is no cure and the child *could* die from her disease but also that disease-directed options have been exhausted and that the child *will* die imminently from the disease. This is the culmination of the process of the assimilation of information and the move from an intellectual to an emotional awareness of the child's prognosis described above in Sects. 2.2 and 2.3.

Sometimes without evidence of deterioration in the child's behaviour as opposed to just scan results, for example, parents are reluctant to see the child as terminally ill (Bluebond-Langner et al. 2017). This is one example of how and why parents' awareness of the child's condition may lag behind the clinician's (Mack et al. 2007a, b; Bluebond-Langner et al. 2017).

2.4 The Impact of Cancer on Children and Adolescents

2.4.1 Children

The impact of cancer on young children as well as their experience is not routinely studied (Hinds et al. 2012). Most accounts of the experience of young children are provided by proxies, most commonly by mothers (Dixon-Woods et al. 2005). Yet the experience of cancer is a defining characteristic of those very young and young children and adolescents who are affected by it. Some children literally grow up with it, as noted in this parent-clinician dialogue about a child who was 5 at the time and diagnosed at 18 months:

> Clinician: "Jane [child with cancer] has a remarkable capacity to deal with this," Mother: "…it's a sad but true part, which she's not unhappy about but is, is that she's grown up with this. Since she was 18 months of age she's lived with chemotherapy. And she's lived with her disease". (Bluebond-Langner, M. (2002). Medical Decision Making. Unpublished data)

The use of child-centred methods together with participant observation—observing and audio recording the children's interactions with parents, clinicians and peers—has been used as effective ways to study young children with cancer (Carnevale et al. 2008; Bluebond-Langner 1978). Engaging in participant observation and actively following the children in hospital, clinic and home, Bluebond-Langner found, in contrast to many studies of the time, that children as young as 5 could come to understand the disease and its prognosis. Further, as discussed earlier in this chapter, that knowledge was linked to particular experiences in the illness experience and changes in self-concept (Bluebond-Langner 1978; Sisk et al. 2016). Finally and not insignificantly, the children did not necessarily share their views with parents and professionals. Instead they engaged in mutual pretence (for further discussion, see Chap. 4 Communication in Paediatric Palliative Oncology). While the study was conducted at a time when the overwhelming majority of children with leukaemia did not survive, the model has stood the test of time suggesting, along with studies of young children who go to cancer camp, that children's experiences are a better predictor of what children know, how they see themselves and the ways in which the disease has affected them and their lives than their age.

There are good reasons to think that perhaps the best approach to understanding the impact of cancer in children is a mixed method approach. Using a mixed method case-controlled study of children with mean age of 11.5, Noll et al. (1999) were able to show not only the impact of cancer on several domains but also to definitively move the field on from pathology-deficit-based perspective which held sway for a not insignificant period to one which better reflected the overall impact of cancer overtime. Noll and colleagues found that:

> Children with cancer currently receiving chemotherapy were remarkably similar to case controls on measures of emotional well-being and better on several dimensions of social functioning. These findings are not supportive of disability/stress models of childhood chronic illness and suggest considerable psychologic hardiness. (Noll et al. 1999, p 77)

2.4.2 Adolescents

Adolescents with cancer have been recognized as a distinct subgroup for a number of reasons. First, the profile of incidence of different types of cancer changes from younger children to adolescents. Second, these cancers are often more difficult to treat and toxicity is often more of a problem. Third, in the psychosocial domain, cancer intrudes upon and alters a life which is engaged in a variety of pursuits and relations. It comes at a time when an increasing desire for and possibility of greater independence is very much at the forefront of their lives (Day et al. 2016).

Like their parents, at diagnosis and again at relapse, adolescents are shocked and keenly aware of a loss of power and control (Stegenga and Ward-Smith 2009). Wicks and Mitchell (2010) found that at diagnosis adolescents reported a greater loss of control in the medical rather than in personal or social spheres. Some adolescents stated that all control had to be surrendered to doctors. They are understandably angry and frustrated; they report feeling inadequate (Wicks and Mitchell 2010).

Adolescents react to the diagnosis as a loss of normality. They strive to regain a sense of normality, to define a new normal (Taylor et al. 2013; Gibson et al. 2005, 2016; Stegenga and Ward-Smith 2009; Rechner 1990). They employ strategies which enable them to establish a new normality such as scheduling treatments so that they did not conflict with important activities in the adolescent's life (Gibson et al. 2016). In this way they kept the cancer world separate from the normal world (Rechner 1990).

Finding normality meant resuming previous activities—attending school, driving a car and resuming sports as they were able. "To walk to school with their friends, which meant learning to walk less aided, or socializing when feeling unwell, which required more effort became even more important" (Gibson et al. 2016). Remarkably this study found that some adolescents sought normality even when facing death. Descriptions of what was important to young people in their diaries where death was inevitable were similar to those receiving curative therapy: hospital environment, peer support and being in control of treatment and care choices (Gibson et al. 2016).

In this quest for normality, this new normal did not mean, however, distancing themselves from their family. Both Wicks and Mitchell (2010) and Stegenga and Ward-Smith (2009) report that despite the adversity they face, adolescents experience and value increased closeness with their family.

2.4.3 Symptoms and Side Effects: The Burden of the Illness

Cancer and cancer treatment bring with them serious symptoms and side effects. Therapy is daunting. Nausea, vomiting, loss of appetite, mood swings and loss of motivation are not uncommon. "The simplest of activities became challenges" (Gibson et al. 2005, p 655). Having a bath and getting dressed required pauses for rest (Gibson et al. 2005).

The impact of symptoms, both effects of treatment and from the disease itself, can be understood not only in terms of how they shape the child or young person's view of the disease and themselves but also in terms of the child or young person's relation to the rest of the family (Woodgate et al. 2003). Indeed, symptoms and side effects become part of the experience of cancer for all members of the family. They belong to the child but they become part of the family's life as well. Not surprisingly, symptoms take on different meanings at different points in the illness trajectory (Woodgate et al. 2003; Bluebond-Langner 1978). For example, during treatment a certain level of symptoms becomes normal and unremarkable. Symptoms consistent with what oncologists have explained as the side effects of treatments are accepted as normal (Dussel et al. 2016). Children perceive themselves this way, as do others around them. As one mother remarked:

> I call Freddie a healthy sick kid... you know it's the inside of his marrow that's sick. He still fools life. (Bluebond-Langner, M. (2002). Medical Decision Making. Unpublished data)

At this time, symptoms such as nausea or hair loss are taken by some children, young people, parents and well siblings as evidence that the treatment is working (Woodgate et al. 2003; Bluebond-Langner 1978). At other times, however, these symptoms can represent the hold that cancer has on the child and that it may be progressing. Some children will come to see particular symptoms as indicators that medicines are "running out" and that they are dying (Bluebond-Langner 1978).

Symptoms of both the disease and side effects of treatment were one of several factors which brought about renewed reliance on others, family members. This process is highlighted by researchers in part because it is seen as reversing a core experience in adolescents' lives—negotiating independence from parents (Gibson et al. 2005). This can, according to Gibson et al. (2005), lead to frustration and guilt for not fulfilling normal family obligations, for interrupting family life and for getting angry with family members. Thus, during treatment, adolescents can experience guilt toward family members for the burdens they have placed upon them.

2.4.4 Peer Relations and School

Peers are perceived by children and adolescents as a source of support (Christiansen et al. 2015), and so continuation or resumption of these relationships is an important aspect of their experience as they are dealing with their disease. School attendance plays several important roles in the lives of children and families. Schooling is closely associated with what it is to be a child in many places in the world. Education is a future-oriented process leading to benefits years in the future. In this respect, it is also a mirror of the image of children in many societies, an image of becoming.

Next to the family, the school is the most important social institution in the lives of many children (Sullivan et al. 2001). For some children and adolescents, school attendance acts as a marker of their health (Stewart 2003). For most, it is the place where peer relations are formed and maintained. Rechner (1990) found that maintenance of relations with schoolmates was "part of what adolescence is all about" (Rechner 1990). Chekryn et al. (1986) describe school as a "normalizing environment".

Absence from these relations, the changes in the children as a result of therapy and well children's perceptions of and ignorance of cancer all work to complicate the process of resuming peer relations and school attendance. Studies of the success of young cancer patients in returning to school and resuming relations with peers are mixed in their findings (Vance and Eiser 2002; Katz et al. 2011; Christiansen et al. 2015). Noll et al. (1999) reported that school-aged children receiving chemotherapy did not show more social problems or lower well-being than case-controlled classmates. Katz et al. (2011) using different methods assessed interaction in the form of free play with best friends and found differences which suggest that cancer survivors experience some disengagement in these interactions as compared with healthy children, a finding which they note is consistent with previous reports of social isolation in cancer survivors (p 244). One widely reported and unsurprising finding is that cancer patients and survivors report lower athletic competence in the context of peer relations and school attendance (Noll et al. 1999). In children who have had CNS-directed therapy or HSCT, however, poorer social functioning is reported (Christiansen et al. 2015; Emond et al. 2016). Noll et al. (1999) excluded children with CNS malignancies, reflecting their belief that it is well established that children with CNS malignancies have "significant behavioural and emotional problems that are uniquely related to tumor location" (Noll et al. 1990, p 46).

Qualitative and mixed methods studies found that adolescents with cancer reported that their healthy peers didn't know how to talk to them (Choquette 2016). The mutual exchange of information, thoughts and feelings which had once been commonplace had been replaced by one-sided conversations. Friends might ask about treatments and the ill friend's current status, but when the answers had been given, the conversation ended, often leaving them feel as outsiders and rejected. Both younger and older children felt a degree of exclusion or avoidance (Bluebond-Langner et al. 1991; Vance and Eiser 2002) by healthy peers. Some well children worried about issues such as possible contagion (Suzuki 2003), especially when faced with signs of the illness such as hair loss (Bluebond-Langner et al. 1991). In spite of these difficulties, Suzuki (2003) concluded that "relationships with classmates mitigate the negative experiences" (p 163).

In a study of children and adolescents attending a cancer camp, Bluebond-Langner et al. (1990, 1991) found that with cancer peers, these children and adolescents could speak openly and freely about their experiences, often gaining knowledge in the process. Their cancer peers understood in an instant and required no explanation of what they were going through. Whereas healthy peers who lacked shared experiences were limited in their ability to understand or empathize with their friends with cancer.

At the same time, however, relations with ill peers presented their own set of challenges. Ill peers are valued friends who could relapse and die. They worried about how to deal with an ill peer who was doing poorly when they were relatively well. Relapse or a second cancer in a friend could feed or reawaken the uncertainty which affects all children with cancer and their families. Bluebond-Langner et al. concluded, based on camp attendee reports, that relations with cancer peers were an important, enduring source of support for children and adolescents with cancer, but that they did not displace for them the importance of their relations with healthy peers.

2.5 The Impact of Cancer on Parents

2.5.1 Consultations, Out-Patient Clinic Visits and Hospitalizations

A core component of the cancer experience for parents is the clinical consultations, the meetings with clinicians. It is here where parents both receive and give critical information about their child's condition, care and treatment. While communication in consultation is discussed further in Chap. 4, it needs to be pointed out here in considering the impact of the illness that learning how to participate in the consultation is just one of the ways in which parents manifest the impact of cancer on their lives (Bluebond-Langner et al. 2017); learning how to make decisions is another.

In addition to dealing with consultations and decision making, there are also tasks of care and treatments to be managed including chemotherapy or radiotherapy, while at the same time maintaining a household, looking after other children, cooking, cleaning and earning a living. Some of the treatments would require hospitalization and at the very least the frequent or constant presence of a parent/guardian. Often one parent would spend a considerable amount of time in hospital with the ill child. Young et al. (2002) report that many mothers in their sample ($N = 20$) lived practically full time on the ward with their children in the weeks or even months following diagnosis, returning home for brief visits, while fathers assumed responsibility for the well siblings (Young et al. 2002). A similar, though not necessarily desirable for the patients, pattern was reported by Hinds et al. (2005) for adolescents.

2.5.2 Marital Relations: Marital Satisfaction and Divorce

Although cancer can strain marital or couple relationships, parents of children with cancer do not appear more likely to divorce over the long term, even in the case of bereaved couples (Schwab 1998; Syse et al. 2010; Eilegard and Kreicbergs 2010; Gerhard and Salley 2016). In fact, marital satisfaction in couples with a child with cancer is comparable to those who do not. Pai et al. (2007) in a meta-analysis found small but statistically significantly higher marital distress in parents of children with cancer at diagnosis compared to parents of healthy children. These differences decreased after 1-year post diagnosis (Pai et al. 2007).

Long and Marsland (2011) in their study of marital relations in couples with a child with cancer reach only qualified conclusions about marital quality. They find that illness or treatment stage is likely a factor in perceptions of quality. In addition, as with assessments of individual satisfaction with one's life, precancer marital functioning must be taken into account. They allow that partners may put the demands of their prescribed roles in the marriage on hold, especially when treatment is intense or the child's condition is worse. There are also studies that report that spouses find increased closeness over time (Silva-Rodrigues et al. 2016) and that their spouse is their primary source of support (McGrath 2001).

2.5.3 Single Parents

Children with serious illness who live in single-parent homes are a growing concern for policy makers (Brown et al. 2008). The US Census Bureau Current Population Survey for 2015 shows 27% of children 0–17 in single-parent living arrangements (U.S. Census Bureau n.d.; *Current Population Survey*, Annual Social and Economic Supplement). These families are an overlooked, understudied group (Brown et al. 2008). However, defining what makes someone a single parent is not a straightforward matter. As Brown et al. point out, much of the demographic data fail to reflect the support system which is actually involved in the care of a child whose parents indicated on a questionnaire that they were single. They may have a cohabiting partner or an ex-spouse still involved in the care of the child.

These situations are not typically captured on forced-choice questionnaires used in research.

With this caveat, two studies have found inconsequential differences between single or lone and married or partnered parents. Iobst et al. (2009) reported that maternal distress after a diagnosis of cancer did not significantly differ between the two groups of mothers. Klassen et al. (2012) found that reported caregiving demands and physical and psychosocial HRQOL were similar for single- and two-parent families. Mullins et al. (2011) found higher perceived vulnerability and parenting stress, yet the differences disappeared when income was introduced as a mediating variable. These somewhat surprising findings may be explained in part by the methodological discussion above: parents classified as single parents may not be parenting alone.

2.5.4 Financial Issues

The impact of cancer on the family is not limited to the social and psychological. There is a financial impact to be considered as families face increased expenses for travel, food, accommodations and telephone, especially in the 6-month period following diagnosis as well as disruption in employment, which is common. Bona et al. (2014) found 92% of families experiencing disruption and in 42% of the study families at least one parent quit their job. Other studies reported similar significant cessation of employment or reduction in hours, especially amongst mothers (Eiser and Upton 2007; Fluchel et al. 2014; Limburg et al. 2008; Tsimicalis et al. 2013).

Eiser and Upton (2007) found that 68.3% of parents in their study reported financial worries. Heath et al. (2006) reported that 74% of parents experienced moderate to great economic hardship following diagnosis, leading in turn to parental distress and other symptoms. It is not surprising then that Rosenberg et al. (2013) would find higher parental distress scores in parents experiencing economic hardship and that Creswell et al. (2014) report an association between negative economic events and parental depression.

Single parents are even more likely to experience financial hardship. Lower-income families bear the brunt of economic hardship. Dussel et al. (2011) show families in the USA and Australia with incomes of less than 50% of national median losing 40% or more of their income due to cancer-related work disruption.

Even in countries with a number of government-provided healthcare and benefits, parents encountered hardship. Eiser and Upton (2007) described parents' experience in the UK. There, families must wait 3 months before applying for benefits—the very time when expenses are highest. Parents often relied on professional help to complete applications. Approval of applications and receipt of benefits could be delayed. Further studies found that government support was unable to offset cancer-related economic stress and hardships (Heath et al. 2006; Miedema et al. 2008). A longitudinal Swedish study, however, found that after a decrease during treatment at a year after end of treatment, family income in a majority (>75%) returned to at least pre-diagnosis levels (Hovén et al. 2013). The authors recognize that their findings need to be understood within the context of Swedish state welfare policies and social insurance which they describe as generous and "family friendly".

While studies of financial issues have been cross sectional and have not plotted changes in financial strains against the disease trajectory, there is reason to think that the financial strains of the first 6 months might recur at relapse, with or at deterioration, whenever hospitalizations become more frequent (e.g. with haematological malignancies) or as families move for treatment (e.g. UK families to the USA for proton beam therapy) or as home care intensifies (e.g. high-risk brain tumours after first recurrence).

2.6 The Impact of Cancer on Well Siblings

Cancer disrupts the lives of well siblings as well through the effect that it has upon the people to whom they are closest. Parents become distraught, preoccupied with the ill sibling and distracted from what was normal family life. Well siblings lose parental time and attention. One fears that they become almost forgotten. Yet, psychological studies, report that:

> Siblings of children with cancer do not experience elevated mean levels of psychiatric symptoms such as behavioral problems, anxiety disorders, or depression However, the percentage of siblings falling into at risk/clinical ranges on these indices is elevated in some samples typically soon after diagnosis. (Alderfer et al. 2010, p 796)

With the passage, of time most of these siblings return to normal levels (Alderfer et al. 2010, 2015).

As with parents, there is a group which shows an enduring cancer-related post-traumatic stress (Alderfer et al. 2010, p 800):

> Although we, along with others [9,10], have established that most siblings do not exhibit elevated levels of psychopathology, qualitative descriptions indicate a pattern of adjustment that differs from normative developmental processes. These qualitative descriptions, along with elevations in post-traumatic stress and negative mood states and lower scores on quality of life measures, indicate that the sibling experience is unique and worthy of further investigation.

Along with reports of enduring cancer-related post-traumatic symptoms, several studies report positive gains for siblings as well, such as increased maturity, responsibility, independence, resiliency and empathy (Alderfer et al. 2010). Positive and negative outcomes may be found in the same individual.

2.6.1 Relationships Between Well Siblings and Other Family Members

Central to the experience of well siblings are their parents' responses to the disease; they both observe these and experience their effect on life at home. Well siblings' adaptations to the disease thus follow from and mesh with, at least in part, the adaptations which their parents make. Both in studies of well siblings with cancer and studies of well siblings of children with other life-limiting conditions and life-threatening illnesses, researchers have found it useful to explore the impact of the illness on relationships in terms of allocation of resources, communication about the illness and ill child's condition (Bluebond-Langner 1998).

Disease-related events—diagnosis, relapse, deterioration and remission—and disease-related experiences drive the parents' behaviour toward the ill child and the well siblings. As discussed in other places in this chapter, time since diagnosis is crucial. As in the case of parents of children with cystic fibrosis, parents of children with cancer are more anxious and report being less patient with well siblings at the time of diagnosis (Bluebond-Langner 1998).

Well siblings report a number of negative experiences at time of diagnosis and at periods of relapse and deterioration including loss of attention or status within the family when material and emotional resources are focused on the ill child. At such times, well siblings report feelings of exclusion, marginalization or being an outsider and being peripheral to the parent-ill sibling dyad (Yang et al. 2016).

Contributing to these feelings of exclusion is the fact that well siblings are often given little information about the ill sibling's disease and treatment (Lövgren et al. 2016) and, especially, the prognosis. Well siblings are not necessarily part of discussion of child's condition and decision making, yet in the case of bone marrow or stem cell transplant, they may be a major participant, or in situations where parents' first language is not English, they might come along and act as translators for both clinicians and parents (Bluebond-Langner et al. 2017).

It is important to note that the parents' lack of discussion with well sibling is not unique to that relationship. Strategies parents use to contain the intrusion of the disease into family life make conversations beyond the subject of current treatment and tasks problematic for parents. They similarly limit topics in discussions amongst themselves. Studies also report a lack of discussion by parents with well siblings for reasons of age and maturity (e.g. too young, will tell them when they are older, not now when they have exams). Also parents may regard well siblings as uninterested or unwilling to talk about the ill sibling and so do not open conversation (Bluebond-Langner 1996). In addition there is a concern that well sibling might say something outside the home that will change the way others regard the ill child (Bluebond-Langner1996).

Not surprisingly, siblings with one parent absent, caring for child in hospital or staying with other family members also report a loss of order, routine and normalcy in the home (Yang et al. 2016).

Well siblings can feel loss of attention or neglected (Chesler et al. 1992; Wilkins and Woodgate 2005; Alderfer et al. 2010). These feelings are often accompanied by an understanding or acceptance of the reality of the ill sibling's needs and worry about their condition and what the future holds. Such worries can lead to difficulties concentrating in school and poor school performance. Alderfer et al. (2015) note that peer relationships of well siblings of children with cancer are "similar to classmates, though they experience a small decrement in activity and school performance".

Understanding of the well siblings' situation and needs does not take away the sting of neglect. Lindsay and McCarthy (1974) find that well siblings understand their ill siblings' needs but still feel resentful and angry and yet in response to that guilty for those same feelings. Bluebond-Langner (1998) found that in siblings of children with cystic fibrosis, a distance can develop in their relationship. Wallin et al. (2015) found that "siblings who were not satisfied with the amount of time they talked about their feelings with others in their brother's or sister's last month of life were more likely to report anxiety than those who were satisfied".

Parents are aware of and worry about neglecting their well children (Bluebond-Langner 1998). They find that while they are striving to fulfil the parental role with regard to the ill child, they neglect that role with respect to well siblings telling themselves they will make it up to them later. Parenting the well sibling is deferred.

All these findings need to be understood with the recognition that the literature on the impact of cancer on well siblings is the least settled in its findings and consistency. It is difficult to reach firm conclusions about the size and duration of impact in educational, social and emotional domains. Provisionally, at least, there is more indication that they may be more at risk than parents or ill children (Alderfer et al. 2010, 2015).

2.7 The Impact of Cancer on Grandparents

Several researchers have looked beyond the nuclear family in assessing the impact of cancer on the family. Wakefield et al. (2014, 2016) reporting on two cross-sectional studies that also looked at child's stage of the illness found that grandparents of children with cancer had high stress. Moules et al. (2012a, b) described grandparents as having doubled worry, for both their children, the parents, and for the ill grandchild. Grandparents "silenced" their various worries in order not to burden the ill child's parents with concern about them. Grandparents reported that they contributed to retaining a sense of normalcy in the ill child's home; they recognized it as an approximation to normalcy, a new normalcy.

Notably in some families, the grandparents and other members perceived that the grandparents were paying less attention to the other adult siblings of the ill child's parents and to other grandchildren, a mirror image, so to speak of what is seen in the parents of the ill child with respect to the ill child's well sibling.

2.8 Differences: Individual and Cultural

It is taken for granted today that culture informs behaviour. Precisely how this happens and what it means for the behaviour of a given individual, however, are less than clear. Culture informs but does not dictate behaviour. Hence while trying to respect the different perspectives which ill children and their families may have, we must also recognize their individuality and avoid stereotypes. Addressing this issue, the psychiatrist and anthropologist Arthur Kleinman wrote:

> We can say of illness experience that it is always culturally shaped. But conventional expectations about illness are altered through negotiations in different social situations and in particular webs of relationships. Expectations about how to behave when ill also differ owing to our unique individual biographies. So we can also say of illness experience that it is always distinctive. (Kleinman 1988)

As such, while we might thoughtfully and carefully use generalizations about culture to understand children and families dealing with illness, we cannot simply turn those individuals into generalizations, into stereotypes (Wiener et al. 2013). Not all individuals from a particular culture display predictable traits, especially when they have been educated or have lived in different societies with a different culture. "Beliefs and practices vary along the spectrum of education and Western acculturation" (Wiener et al. 2013, p 64). Information about cultural practices should be used heuristically rather than to prescribe approaches which clinicians can employ in dealing with children and families of a particular culture or ethnicity.

We must also remember that everyone involved in a clinical consultation is influenced by a culture, including clinicians (Surbone 2008, Wiener et al. 2013). Many beliefs which are attributed to non-Western cultures to mark them off as distinctive also apply to those from the highly developed world to Europe and the Americas. For example, reluctance to talk about death and dying is not unique to non-Western cultures. Feifel (1959) and Kubler-Ross (1969) and others promoted the idea that death denial is also widely practised, at least in the USA. Bluebond-Langner (1978) found widespread use of what Glaser and Strauss' termed mutual pretence in parents' discussions of the ill child. More recent observers have noted that "Frank discussions about death with children still remain relatively uncommon in most acute pediatric settings" (Evan and Cohen 2011). In 2009, French clinicians in a study of preference for place of death for children wrote "In France, as in most Western countries, death is a subject of taboo that is very rarely or never discussed with the family" (Montel et al. 2009).

Cultural variations on a variety of other issues have also been found within Western societies. In a study of parental participation in neonatal ethical decisions in 11 European cultures, significant differences in policies were found. The authors concluded that "Policies do vary widely across countries, and variations cannot be explained by differences in the unit level, size, resources, or extent of teaching and research activities: they are probably, in essence, culturally determined" (Cuttini et al. 1999).

The world of cancer treatment and the hospital is very much a subculture in which it is located and into which all lay persons—regardless of their country or culture of origin—must be socialized or enculturated. It has a language, customs and rituals. All families are at least initially foreigners in the world of the hospital. That world is a tightly knit social world. So we may say that to some extent "all families experience challenges in these areas, as the hospital environment is an unfamiliar and daunting world, demanding adaptability on the part of all whose lives become centered there" (Kupst and Patenaude 2016).

A concomitant of cultural difference is the issue of competence in the language of the clinicians providing treatment. Language, including medical jargon and shorthand, is the medium of the clinical consultation. It is the medium of all the explanations of procedures and investigations which children will undergo. It is the medium in which care and treatment options are presented and decisions made. Language in the fullest sense is clearly a point at which interventions are crucial and can make a substantial difference. In urban tertiary centres, this can be a daunting task in that the census of languages spoken can reach well over 100 languages. The task is compounded by not only the technical nature of the language but the sometimes fraught nature of the exchange. This is indeed a special form of translation and requires our close attention.

2.9 Conclusions

2.9.1 Summary

Cancer impacts children and their entire families. The stress which it causes rises and falls in relation to clinical events and the adaptations which children and families make. Children and families' understanding of the illness and of themselves changes with experience with the disease and with others whom they encounter in the course of treatment. Eventually children enter into survivorship or parents become bereaved. It is beyond the scope of this chapter but one can foresee that late effects for survivors and new life experiences will continue their interplay long into the future. Bereavement is a protracted process of change as well. Survivors and bereaved parents are forever changed by the cancer experience and it figures into their continuing growth or life course.

One often reads in studies quotations from parents saying that their response to living with cancer is to take 1 day at time, to focus on the present. The studies cited in this chapter help to flesh out this adage. Parents realize that in order to do this they have to put aspects of their own relation on hold. They realize that the well siblings in the family are receiving less than the attention which they need and deserve. In response parents think about making this up in the future. Grandparents conceal their own anxieties and feelings in order not to burden their children—the parents—and to carry on with the task of helping to maintain that sought after normality, the new normality. Parents and other family thus practise a sort of emotional, cognitive and practical triage in order to get on with life with cancer. Important issues are thus deferred, but they are not overlooked.

Remarkably the majority of children and families adapt to cancer and do not develop significant psychological problems as a direct result of the cancer experience. They are "ordinary people in exceptional circumstances" (Eiser 1990). Some find positive aspects of the experience. Those who do show clinically significant psychological symptoms do so, research suggests, because of issues and patterns of behaviour which existed before the onset of cancer. The cancer population resembles the wider population in this respect; 20–30% show clinical symptoms. These can be exacerbated by the experience of cancer, however, and so identifying and supporting such individuals are important tasks. All families facing cancer feel, at least at predictable times, and appropriately, increased stress, and it is always appropriate to strive to mitigate this.

2.9.2 Directions for Future Research

Prospective, longitudinal studies should be the norm going forward. Even multipoint cross-sectional studies are not adequate as what is needed is that a process be observed. Long and Marsland (2011) in reviewing the literature on family adjustment to cancer write that there is too much of a focus on outcomes at a point rather than attention to the process through which families adapt to cancer. They note the paucity of mixed method studies and find this unfortunate because this misses the utility of "combining process-oriented explanatory…qualitative approaches with the statistical benefits of quantitative methods". Methods and approaches are needed which are adapted to the dynamic, changing impact of cancer and the fact that individual and family adjustment is not a linear process.

Proxy reporting needs to be curtailed. This is especially true since these reports tend to come predominantly from mothers. Regardless of specific gender-based differences, mothers and fathers as a practical matter divide duties in the family and as a result likely have somewhat different experiences and points of view (Phares et al. 2005).

2.9.3 Recommendations for Clinical Practice

- In engaging with patients, parents and other family members, it is important to assess where individuals are on the biopsychosocial trajectory. Their views and constructions can differ from one another and from yours, the clinician's. Knowing this is a part of knowing to whom you are speaking in a consultation.
- When events occur which you perceive as significant for the management of the ill child, remember that parents (and children) need to

both understand what is happening and to internalize that knowledge. Time and experience facilitate this process for families. The views and understandings of different members of the family will not necessarily change for all members at the same time in relation to clinical events. With the first point above, one establishes a baseline. The task then becomes to track the progress of ill child and parents as they move along the illness trajectory.

- Keep in mind that knowledge and understanding of the prognosis is not a black-and-white issue of simply knowing or not knowing. Parents manage their awareness and keep foremost in it what is necessary to carry on in the day to day with care for the ill child in order to maintain family life. Recognizing that one's child is dying is not simply a matter of information; it is something that each parent must come to him- or herself.
- Parents want to leave no stone unturned. If a child reaches a point where no appropriate disease-directed options are available, parents may still want to continue looking for options. They may ask you the clinician to do this; they may do it themselves or both. They may want to keep open the possibility of scans or other investigative procedures if appropriate. Being open to engage in these discussions with parents allows them to maintain both aspects of their role.
- Hinds et al. (1996) write that knowing that they were doing their best to help their child survive helped parents consider the reality that treatment might fail and that their child would die. A parent in the study said that though they realized that the time *might* come when they would say "enough", "I may even have to help say that. But I don't want to be the one".
- Understanding by clinicians of parents' role and of what they are trying to balance can facilitate parents' participation in such decisions. Clinicians need to demonstrate their understanding in the interaction with parents by engaging with the parent as both advocate and protector. For some parents, this might mean supporting the desire to search for further therapy even up to the last weeks of the child's life.
- Resources of different kinds are critical to families' adaptation to the impact of cancer. Adult siblings of parents and grandparents often help with tasks of care for children in the family. Economic resources, flexibility with working arrangements and sufficient income to deal with increased expenses are also needed, when this lacking parental stress increases. Pelletier and Bona (2015) propose that parents be assessed for financial hardship and that appropriate referrals for counselling or support be provided.
- Ill children, even young children, will acquire a great deal of knowledge about their illness and its treatment whether they explicitly told this or not. This includes the fact that they might be dying. It is important that children and adolescents have informed people with whom they can talk in order that they have accurate information, comfort and support. It is best if the ill child or adolescent chooses when and with whom such conversations take place. It is not essential that ill children and adolescents be willing to speak openly with everyone involved in their care treatment even if that means they avoid certain issues with the attending or consultant physician or with one or both of their parents. What is important is that there is some informed person in their lives with whom they can discuss their illness and its ultimate outcome.
- Ill children, like their parents, value and strive for a sense of normality. Important components of this normality are relations with peers and, when feasible, return to school. Peer relationships and return to school can be facilitated by maintaining some contact when the ill child is under treatment or in hospital via written or video media.
- Return to school is best supported by preparing teachers and classmates with information about what to expect and trying to allay fears and address concerns. Information should be general. It should be up to the ill child or adolescent to disclose particular facts of their illness.
- Simple acts can help well siblings. Making it possible for parents to bring siblings with

them when consultations take place or for clinic visits is a positive step. Alderfer et al. (2010) suggest reminding us of the importance of speaking to well siblings about themselves and not just about their ill sibling. Talking to well siblings about their ill sibling's treatment or giving them a tour of parts of the facility can help to lessen well siblings' feelings of exclusion.

References

Alderfer MA, Long KA, Lown EA, Marsland AL, Ostrowski NL, Hock JM et al (2010) Psychosocial adjustment of siblings of children with cancer: a systematic review. Psycho-Oncology 19(8):789–805

Alderfer MA, Stanley C, Conroy R, Long KA, Fairclough DL, Kazak AE et al (2015) The social functioning of siblings of children with cancer: a multi-informant investigation. J Pediatr Psychol 40(3):309–319

Bleyer A (2008) Returning to work after parenting a child with the most curable chronic disease. Pediatr Blood Cancer 51(1):1–2

Bluebond-Langner M (1978) The private worlds of dying children. Princeton University Press, Princeton

Bluebond-Langner M (1998) In the shadow of illness. Princeton University Press, Princeton

Bluebond-Langner M, Perkel D, Goertzel T, Nelson K, McGeary J (1990) Children's knowledge of cancer and its treatment: impact of an oncology camp experience. J Pediatr 116(2):207–213

Bluebond-Langner M, Perkel D, Goertzel T (1991) Pediatric cancer patients' peer relationships. J Psychosoc Oncol 9(2):67–80

Bluebond-Langner M, Belasco JB, Goldman A, Belasco C (2007) Understanding parents' approaches to care and treatment of children with cancer when standard therapy has failed. J Clin Oncol 25(17):2414–2419

Bluebond-Langner M, Hargrave D, Henderson EM, Langner RW (2017) "I have to live with the decisions i make": laying a foundation for decision making for children with life-limiting conditions and life-threatening illnesses. Arch Dis Child 102:468–471

Bona K, Dussel V, Orellana L, Kang T, Geyer R, Feudtner C et al (2014) Economic impact of advanced pediatric cancer on families. J Pain Symptom Manag 47(3):594–603

Brown RT, Wiener L, Kupst MJ, Brennan T, Behrman R, Compas BE et al (2008) Single parents of children with chronic illness: an understudied phenomenon. J Pediatr Psychol 33(4):408–421

Carnevale FA, Macdonald ME, Bluebond-Langner M, McKeever P (2008) Using participant observation in pediatric health care settings: ethical challenges and solutions. J Child Health Care 12(1):18–32

Chekryn J, Deegan M, Reid J (1986) Normalizing the return to school of the child with cancer. J Assoc Pediatr Oncol Nurses 3(2):20–24

Chesler MA, Allswede J, Barbarin OO (1992) Voices from the margin of the family. J Psychosoc Oncol 9(4):19–42

Choquette AMRN, Rennick JEPMRN, Lee VPMRN (2016) Back to school after cancer treatment: Making sense of the adolescent experience. Cancer Nursing 39(5):393–401

Christiansen HL, Bingen K, Hoag JA, Karst JS, Velazquez-Martin B, Barakat LP (2015) Providing children and adolescents opportunities for social interaction as a standard of care in pediatric oncology. Pediatr Blood Cancer 62(5):25774

Creswell PD, Wisk LE, Litzelman K, Allchin A, Witt WP (2014) Parental depressive symptoms and childhood cancer: the importance of financial difficulties. Support Care Cancer 22(2):503–511

Cuttini M, Rebagliato M, Bortoli P, Hansen G, de Leeuw R, Lenoir S et al (1999) Parental visiting, communication, and participation in ethical decisions: a comparison of neonatal unit policies in Europe. Arch Dis Child Fetal Neonatal Ed 81(2):F84–F91

Day E, Jones L, Langner R, Bluebond-Langner M (2016) Current understanding of decision-making in adolescents with cancer: a narrative systematic review. Palliat Med 30(10):920–934

De Graves S, Aranda S (2008) Living with hope and fear—the uncertainty of childhood cancer after relapse. Cancer Nurs 31(4):292–301. Epub 2008/07/05

Dixon-Woods M, Young B, Heney D (2002) Childhood cancer and users' views: a critical perspective. Eur J Cancer Care 11(3):173–177. Epub 2002/09/26

Dixon-Woods M, Young B, Heney D (2005) Rethinking experiences of childhood cancer. Open University Press, Berkshire

Dussel V, Kreicbergs U, Hilden JM, Watterson J, Moore C, Turner BG et al (2009) Looking beyond where children die: determinants and effects of planning a child's location of death. J Pain Symptom Manag 37(1):33–43. Epub 2008/06/10

Dussel V, Bona K, Heath JA, Hilden JM, Weeks JC, Wolfe J (2011) Unmeasured costs of a child's death: perceived financial burden, work disruptions, and economic coping strategies used by American and Australian families who lost children to cancer. J Clin Oncol 29(8):1007–1013. https://doi.org/10.200/JCO.2009.27.8960. Epub 2011 Jan 4

Dussel V, Bilodeau M, Uzal L, Orellana L, Requena ML, Wolfe J. Normalization of symptoms: a leading barrier to symptom management in advanced cancer. Poster presented at: 3rd Congress on Paediatric Palliative Care-A Global Gathering. 2016 Nov 16–19; Rome, Italy.

Eilegard A, Kreicbergs U (2010) Risk of parental dissolution of partnership following the loss of a child to cancer: a population-based long-term follow-up. Arch Pediatr Adolesc Med 164(1):100–101. Epub 2010/01/06

Eiser C (1990) Psychological effects of chronic disease. J Child Psychol Psychiatry 31(1):85–98

Eiser C, Upton P (2007) Costs of caring for a child with cancer: a questionnaire survey. Child Care Health Dev 33(4):455–459
Eiser C, Parkyn T, Havermans T, McNinch A (1994) Parents' recall on the diagnosis of cancer in their child. Psycho-Oncology 3(3):197–203
Emond A, Edwards L, Peacock S, Norman C, Evangeli M (2016) Social competence in children and young people treated for a brain tumour. Support Care Cancer 24(11):4587–4595
Evan EA, Cohen H (2011) Child relationships. In: Wolfe J, Hinds P, Sourkes B (eds) Textbook of interdisciplinary palliative care. Elsevier, Philadelphia, pp 31–34
Feifel H (1959) The meaning of death. McGraw Hill, New York
Fluchel MN, Kirchhoff AC, Bodson J, Sweeney C, Edwards SL, Ding Q et al (2014) Geography and the burden of care in pediatric cancers. Pediatr Blood Cancer 61(11):1918–1924
Futterman EH, Hoffman I (1973) Crisis and adaptation in the families of fatally ill children. In: Anthony EJ, Koupernik C (eds) The child in his family. Wiley, New York, pp 127–143
Gerhard CA, Salley CG, Lehman V (2016) The impact of pediatric cancer on the family. In: Abrams AN, Muriel AC, Wiener L (eds) Pediatric psychosocial oncology: textbook for multidisciplinary care. Springer, Switzerland, pp 143–155
Gibson F, Mulhall AB, Richardson A, Edwards JL et al (2005) A phenomenologic study of fatigue in adolescents receiving treatment for cancer. Oncol Nurs Forum 32(3):651–660
Gibson F, Hibbins S, Grew T, Morgan S, Pearce S, Stark D et al (2016) How young people describe the impact of living with and beyond a cancer diagnosis: feasibility of using social media as a research method. Psychooncology 25:1317–1323
Gogan JL, Koocher GP, Foster DJ, O'Malley JE (1977a) Impact of childhood cancer on siblings. Health Soc Work 2(1):41–57. Epub 1977/02/01
Gogan JL, O'Malley JE, Foster DJ (1977b) Treating the pediatric cancer patient: a review. J Pediatr Psychol 2(2):42–48
Grootenhuis MA, Last BF (1997) Parents' emotional reactions related to different prospects for the survival of their children with cancer. J Psychosoc Oncol 15(1):43–62
Heath JA, Lintuuran RM, Rigguto G, Tokatlian N, McCarthy M (2006) Childhood cancer: its impact and financial costs for Australian families. Pediatr Hematol Oncol 23(5):439–448. Epub 2006/05/27
Hinds PS, Birenbaum LK, Clarke-Steffen L, Quargnenti A, Kreissman S, Kazak A et al (1996) Coming to terms: parents' response to a first cancer recurrence in their child. Nurs Res 45(3):148–153
Hinds PS, Birenbaum LK, Pedrosa AM, Pedrosa F (2002) Guidelines for the recurrence of pediatric cancer. Semin Oncol Nurs 18(1):50–59
Hinds PS, Drew D, Oakes LL, Fouladi M, Spunt SL, Church C et al (2005) End-of-life care preferences of pediatric patients with cancer. J Clin Oncol 23(36):9146–9154
Hinds PS, Oakes LL, Hicks J, Powell B, Srivastava DK, Spunt SL et al (2009) "Trying to be a good parent" as defined by interviews with parents who made phase I, terminal care, and resuscitation decisions for their children. J Clin Oncol 27(35):5979–5985
Hinds PS, Oakes LL, Hicks J, Powell B, Srivastava DK, Baker JN et al (2012) Parent-clinician communication intervention during end-of-life decision making for children with incurable cancer. J Palliat Med 15(8):916–922. Epub 2012/06/28
Hovén E, von Essen L, Norberg AL (2013) A longitudinal assessment of work situation, sick leave, and household income of mothers and fathers of children with cancer in Sweden. Acta Oncol 52(6):1076–1085
Iobst EA, Alderfer MA, Sahler OJZ, Askins MA, Fairclough DL, Katz ER et al (2009) Brief report: problem solving and maternal distress at the time of a child's diagnosis of cancer in two-parent versus lone-parent households. J Pediatr Psychol 34(8):817–821
Jones BL, Gilmer MJ, Parker-Raley J, Dokken DL, Freyer DR, Sydnor-Greenberg N (2011) Parent and sibling relationships and the family experience. In: Wolfe J, Hinds P, Sourkes B (eds) Textbook of interdisciplinary pediatric palliative care. Elsevier, Philadelphia, pp 135–147
Katz LF, Leary A, Breiger D, Friedman D (2011) Pediatric cancer and the quality of children's dyadic peer interactions. J Pediatr Psychol 36(2):237–247
Klassen AF, Dix D, Papsdorf M, Klaassen RJ, Yanofsky R, Sung L (2012) Impact of caring for a child with cancer on single parents compared with parents from two-parent families. Pediatr Blood Cancer 58(1):74–79. Epub 2011/01/22
Kleinman A (1988) The illness narratives: suffering, healing and the human condition. Basic Books, New York
Kubler-Ross E (1969) On death and dying. Macmillan, New York
Kupst MJ, Patenaude A (2016) Coping and adaptation in pediatric cancer: current perspectives. In: Abrams AN, Muriel AC, Wiener L (eds) Pediatric psychosocial oncology: textbook for multidisciplinary care. Springer, Switzerland, pp 67–79
Last BF, Grootenhuis MA (1998) Emotions, coping and the need for support in families of children with cancer: a model for psychosocial care. Patient Educ Couns 33(2):169–179
Levi RB, Marsick R, Drotar D, Kodish ED (2000) Diagnosis, disclosure, and informed consent: learning from parents of children with cancer. J Pediatr Hematol Oncol 22(1):3–12
Limburg H, Shaw AK, McBride ML (2008) Impact of childhood cancer on parental employment and sources of income: a Canadian pilot study. Pediatr Blood Cancer 51(1):93–98
Lindsay M, McCarthy D (1974) Caring for the brothers and sisters of a dying child. In: Burton L (ed) Care of the child facing death. Routledge and Kegan-Paul, London, pp 189–206
Long KA, Marsland AL (2011) Family adjustment to childhood cancer: a systematic review. Clin Child Fam Psychol Rev 14(1):57–88. Epub 2011/01/12

Lövgren M, Bylund-Grenklo T, Jalmsell L, Wallin AE, Kreicbergs U (2016) Bereaved siblings' advice to health care professionals working with children with cancer and their families. J Pediatr Oncol Nurs 33(4):297–305
Mack JW, Hilden JM, Watterson J, Moore C, Turner B, Grier HE et al (2005) Parent and physician perspectives on quality of care at the end of life in children with cancer. J Clin Oncol 23(36):9155–9161. Epub 2005/09/21
Mack J, Wolfe J, Grier HE, Cleary PD, Weeks J (2006) Communication about prognosis between parents and physicians of children with cancer: parent preferences and the impact of prognostic information. J Clin Oncol 24(33):5265–5270
Mack J, Cook EF, Wolfe J, Grier HE, Cleary PD, Weeks J (2007a) Understanding of prognosis among parents of children with cancer: parental optimism and the parent-physician interaction. J Clin Oncol 25(11):1357–1362
Mack JW, Wolfe J, Cook EF, Grier HE, Cleary PD, Weeks JC (2007b) Hope and prognostic disclosure. J Clin Oncol 25(35):5636–5642. Epub 2007/12/11
Mack JW, Joffe S, Hilden JM, Watterson J, Moore C, Weeks JC et al (2008) Parents' views of cancer-directed therapy for children with no realistic chance for cure. J Clin Oncol 26(29):4759–4764. Epub 2008/09/10
Martinson I, Cohen MH (1989) Themes from a longitudinal study of family reaction to childhood cancer. J Psychosoc Oncol 6(3–4):81–98
McGrath P (2001) Findings on the impact of treatment for childhood acute lymphoblastic leukaemia on family relationships. Child Fam Soc Work 6(3):229–237
Miedema B, Easley J, Fortin P, Hamilton R, Mathews M (2008) The economic impact on families when a child is diagnosed with cancer. Curr Oncol 15(4):6. Epub 2008-08-25
Montel S, Laurence V, Copel L, Pacquement H, Flahault C (2009) Place of death of adolescents and young adults with cancer: first study in a French population. Palliat Support Care 7(1):27–35
Moules NJ, Laing CM, McCaffrey G, Tapp DM, Strother D (2012a) Grandparents' experiences of childhood cancer, part 1: doubled and silenced. J Pediatr Oncol Nurs 29(3):119–132
Moules NJ, McCaffrey G, Laing CM, Tapp DM, Strother D (2012b) Grandparents' experiences of childhood cancer, part 2: the need for support. J Pediatr Oncol Nurs 29(3):133–140
Mullins LL, Wolfe-Christensen C, Chaney JM, Elkin TD, Wiener L, Hullmann SE et al (2011) The relationship between single-parent status and parenting capacities in mothers of youth with chronic health conditions: the mediating role of income. J Pediatr Psychol 36(3):249–257
Noll RB, Kupst MJ (2007) Commentary: the psychological impact of pediatric cancer hardiness, the exception or the rule? J Pediatr Psychol 32(9):1089–1098
Noll RB, Bukowski WM, Rogosch FA, LeRoy S, Kulkarni R (1990) Social interactions between children with cancer and their peers: teacher ratings. J Pediatr Psychol 15(1):43–56
Noll RB, Gartstein MA, Vannatta K, Correll J, Bukowski WM, Davies WH (1999) Social, emotional, and behavioral functioning of children with cancer. Pediatrics 103(1):71–78
Pai ALH, Greenley RN, Lewandowski A, Drotar D, Youngstrom E, Peterson CC (2007) A meta-analytic review of the influence of pediatric cancer on parent and family functioning. J Fam Psychol 21(3): 407–415
Patenaude AF, Kupst MJ (2005) Psychosocial functioning in pediatric cancer. J Pediatr Psychol 30(1):9–27. Epub 2004/12/22
Pelletier W, Bona K (2015) Assessment of financial burden as a standard of care in pediatric oncology. Pediatr Blood Cancer 62(S5):S619–SS31
Phares V, Lopez E, Fields S, Kamboukos D, Duhig AM (2005) Are fathers involved in pediatric psychology research and treatment? J Pediatr Psychol 30(8):631–643
Phipps S (2007) Adaptive style in children with cancer: implications for a positive psychology approach. J Pediatr Psychol 32(9):1055–1066
Rechner M (1990) Adolescents with cancer: getting on with life. J Pediatr Oncol Nurs 7(4):139–144
Rosenberg AR, Dussel V, Kang T et al (2013) Psychological distress in parents of children with advanced cancer. JAMA Pediatr 167(6):537–543
Salmon P, Hill J, Ward J, Gravenhorst K, Eden T, Young B (2012) Faith and protection: the construction of hope by parents of children with leukemia and their oncologists. Oncologist 17(3):398–404. Epub 2012/03/01
Schwab R (1998) A child's death and divorce: dispelling the myth. Death Stud 22(5):445–468
Silva-Rodrigues FM, Pan R, Pacciulio Sposito AM, de Andrade AW, Nascimento LC (2016) Childhood cancer: impact on parents' marital dynamics. Eur J Oncol Nurs 23:34–42
Sisk BA, Bluebond-Langner M, Wiener L, Mack J, Wolfe J (2016) Prognostic disclosures to children: a historical perspective. Pediatrics 138(3):e20161278
Stegenga K, Ward-Smith P (2009) On receiving the diagnosis of cancer: the adolescent perspective. J Pediatr Oncol Nurs 26(2):75–80
Stewart JL (2003) "Getting used to it": children finding the ordinary and routine in the uncertain context of cancer. Qual Health Res 13(3):394–407
Stewart JL, Pyke-Grimm KA, Kelly KP (2012) Making the right decision for my child with cancer: the parental imperative. Cancer Nurs 35(6):419–428. Epub 2012/02/02
Sullivan NA, Fulmer DL, Zigmond N (2001) School: the normalizing factor for children with childhood leukemia; perspectives of young survivors and their parents. Prevent School Fail 46(1):4–13
Surbone A (2008) Cultural aspects of communication in cancer care. Support Care Cancer 16(3):235–240
Suzuki LK, Kato PM (2003) Psychosocial support for patients in pediatric oncology: The influences of Parents, Schools, Peers, and Technology. J Pediatr Oncol Nurs 20(4):159–174

Syse A, Loge JH, Lyngstad TH (2010) Does childhood cancer affect parental divorce rates? A population-based study. J Clin Oncol 28(5):872–877

Taylor RM, Pearce S, Gibson F, Fern L, Whelan J (2013) Developing a conceptual model of teenage and young adult experiences of cancer through meta-synthesis. Int J Nurs Stud 50(6):832–846

Tsimicalis A, Stevens B, Ungar WJ, McKeever P, Greenberg M, Agha M et al (2013) A mixed method approach to describe the out-of-pocket expenses incurred by families of children with cancer. Pediatr Blood Cancer 60(3):438–445

U.S. Bureau of Labor Statistics (n.d.) Current Population Survey (CPS). N.p., Web. 2015

Valdimarsdottir U, Kreicbergs U, Hauksdottir A, Hunt H, Onelov E, Henter JI et al (2007) Parents' intellectual and emotional awareness of their child's impending death to cancer: a population-based long-term follow-up study. Lancet Oncol 8(8):706–714. Epub 2007/07/24

Van Schoors M, Caes L, Verhofstadt LL, Goubert L, Alderfer MA (2015) Systematic review: family resilience after pediatric cancer diagnosis. J Pediatr Psychol 40(9):856–868

Vance YH, Eiser C (2002) The school experience of the child with cancer. Child Care Health Dev 28(1):5–19

Wakefield CE, Drew D, Ellis SJ, Doolan EL, McLoone JK, Cohn RJ (2014) Grandparents of children with cancer: a controlled study of distress, support, and barriers to care. Psycho-Oncology 23(8):855–861

Wakefield CE, Fardell JE, Doolan EL, Drew D, De Abreu LR, Young AL et al (2016) Grandparents of children with cancer: quality of life, medication and hospitalizations. Pediatr Blood Cancer 21(10):26153

Wallander JL, Varni JW (1998) Effects of pediatric chronic physical disorders on child and family adjustment. J Child Psychol Psychiatry 39(1):29–46

Wallin AE, Steineck G, Nyberg T, Kreicbergs U (2015) Insufficient communication and anxiety in cancer-bereaved siblings: A nationwide long-term follow-up. Palliat Support Care First View:1–7

Wicks L, Mitchell A (2010) The adolescent cancer experience: loss of control and benefit finding. Eur J Cancer Care 19(6):778–785

Wiener L, McConnell DG, Latella L, Ludi E (2013) Cultural and religious considerations in pediatric palliative care. Palliat Support Care 11(01):47–67

Wilkins KL, Woodgate RL (2005) A review of qualitative research on the childhood cancer experience from the perspective of siblings: a need to give them a voice. J Pediatr Oncol Nurs 22(6):305–319

Woodgate RL (2006) Life is never the same: childhood cancer narratives. Eur J Cancer Care 15(1):8–18. Epub 2006/01/31

Woodgate RL, Degner LF (2002) "Nothing is carved in stone!": uncertainty in children with cancer and their families. Eur J Oncol Nurs 6(4):191–202

Woodgate RL, Degner LF (2004) Cancer symptom transition periods of children and families. J Adv Nurs 46(4):358–368

Woodgate RL, Degner LF, Yanofsky R (2003) A different perspective to approaching cancer symptoms in children. J Pain Symptom Manag 26(3):800–817

Yang H-C, Mu P-F, Sheng C-C, Chen Y-W, Hung G-Y (2016) A systematic review of the experiences of siblings of children with cancer. Cancer Nurs 39(3):E12–E21

Young B, Dixon-Woods M, Findlay M, Heney D (2002) Parenting in a crisis: conceptualising mothers of children with cancer. Soc Sci Med (1982) 55(10):1835–1847. Epub 2002/10/18

Zaider T, Kissane D (2007) Resilient families. In: Monroe B, Oliviere D (eds) Resilience in palliative care. Oxford University Press, New York, pp 67–81

The Interdisciplinary Oncology Team and the Role of Palliative Care Consultation

3

Jorge Mauricio Cervantes Blanco and Emma Jones

It takes a village to raise a child—Igbo Proverb

This well-known proverb demonstrates the role of the community in the healthy development of its members. For children with cancer, this saying could be paraphrased to "It takes a team." This group of clinicians must provide care, not only for the child and families but also for the parents, grandparents, siblings, peers, and teachers who are affected by the illness. Interdisciplinary care is a core element of cancer treatment and provides a firm foundation on which to incorporate additional palliative care elements into pediatric oncology. In this chapter, we focus on the development and structure of interdisciplinary oncology teams and discuss ways to enhance existing roles to allow for greater incorporation of palliative care concepts. We will also consider the role of specialty palliative care teams and discuss paradigms for incorporating consultation into the care of children with cancer.

J.M. Cervantes Blanco
Head of Division and attending Physycian, Pediatric Neurologist and Pediatric Palliative Care Specialist, Quality of Life Department/Palliative Care, Hospital Infantil Teletón de Oncología, Queretaro, Queretaro, Mexico

E. Jones (✉)
Pediatric Palliative Care, Boston Children's Hospital and Dana Farber Cancer Institute, Boston, MA, USA
e-mail: emma_jones@dfci.harvard.edu

Case 1

Jackie is a 16-year-old girl who is currently in her sophomore year in high school. She is an active soccer player and very involved in community service and volunteer work. She presented to the emergency room with a prolonged nosebleed and has just been diagnosed with acute myeloid leukemia. Jackie and her parents, Bill and Debbie, will now meet the **oncology consultant** who will give them some information about the diagnosis and order additional tests. She will then be admitted to the oncology ward where she will meet the **oncology ward nurse, resident, fellow, and attending oncologist**. As the medical team begins initial supportive care, Jackie's blood will be studied by **pathologists**, and **blood bank specialists** will prepare transfusions. Once the final diagnosis is confirmed, the oncologist will recommend a chemotherapy regimen based on **cooperative group** best practice. Jackie and her parents may be offered a clinical trial, in which they would also meet the **research team**. Chemotherapy orders are written by the oncologist and reviewed by a **chemotherapy nurse** and **pharmacist**. **Surgeons** are consulted for placement of a central line,

J. Wolfe et al. (eds.), *Palliative Care in Pediatric Oncology*, Pediatric Oncology,
https://doi.org/10.1007/978-3-319-61391-8_3

and Jackie receives care from an **anesthesiologist, surgical technicians, operating room nurses, and recovery room staff** before returning back to the oncology ward to begin her treatment.

The day after receiving the diagnosis, Jackie and her parents meet with the **social worker** to learn about available supports and discuss their hopes and worries. This initial meeting identifies that the family has a very deep faith and relies on prayer to get through difficult circumstances. A **chaplain** is consulted for additional spiritual support. A few days later, a **child life specialist** visits with Jackie and learns that Jackie is devastated that she will be unable to return to school this year due to the chemotherapy regimen. The social worker and child life specialist work together with **school counselor and principal** to establish in hospital schooling for Jackie and set up a Skype account for her to keep in touch with friends. Despite these interventions, Jackie has extreme anxiety about her ability to return to normal life, particularly sports, after her treatment. A **psychologist** is consulted to meet with her regularly and provide counseling, and the **attending psychiatrist** considers if pharmacologic management of anxiety is needed. A **physical therapist** works with Jackie every week to help her maintain strength as much as possible, and the **dietician** recommends meals and supplements to optimize nutrition. A biweekly meeting is established with Jackie, her parents, and the interdisciplinary team to discuss holistic care in an ongoing manner.

Two months later, Jackie's mood is becoming more depressed. She has been in the hospital since diagnosis and experienced significant nausea, pain, and fatigue with chemotherapy. During her first cycle of chemotherapy, she developed sepsis which required transfer to **intensive care unit** and consultation with **infectious disease specialists**. She is expressing fears about dying while also sometimes saying she wishes she would die to escape the misery of her symptoms. She is unable to sleep at night and has begun refusing physical therapy or child life activities during the day due to lack of energy. Debbie has been at Jackie's side throughout. She has not been home to visit her other two children. Bill has been home trying to work to support the family and care for the other children. The interdisciplinary team meets again and invites members of the **palliative care consultation service** to attend to lend their expertise to the ongoing care planning. This expanded team identifies additional symptom management strategies that may be of benefit and decide that a formal palliative care consultation to provide advanced symptom management is indicated. The **palliative care physician, fellow, and nurse practitioner** meet with the patient and family to make a more thorough symptom assessment and provide ongoing guidance on pharmacologic and non-pharmacologic management of pain, nausea, fatigue, anxiety, and sleep disturbance. As her physical symptoms improve, Jackie's mood also improves. She does continue to express concerns about dying, particularly worries about experiencing pain or being alone at the end of her life. This topic is specifically addressed at the next interdisciplinary meeting with the consensus of the group to introduce opportunities for Jackie to participate in age-appropriate advance care planning. The **palliative care social worker partners with oncology social worker and psychologist** to review available resources for advance care planning in adolescents and decide to utilize the "Voicing My Choices" conversation guide. The **palliative care interdisciplinary team** provides a brief training workshop for Jackie's providers on the use of this guide as well as other communication pearls to allow them to feel confident in undertaking such a conversation. Both teams agree that the **psychologist** with whom Jackie has become quite close over the past few months is the best person to initiate this discussion. The **oncology social worker** continues in the role of supporting Bill and Debbie and explores their desire to discuss advance care planning as well.

After a series of guided conversations utilizing the "Voicing My Choices" tool, Jackie's fears about end of life are diminished. She shares the contents of the discussion with her **oncologist** and **palliative care team** stating "Of course I hope I don't die, but it makes me feel better to know that my wishes will be honored if it does happen." The **palliative care team** remains involved to manage symptoms throughout the remainder of therapy. Jackie completes her treatment course and remains in remission. After discharge, the palliative care team collaborates with **child life** to reach out to **Jackie's school** to facilitate her re-enrollment. Jackie enjoys working with **physical therapist** and **dietician** to create a reconditioning plan to get her back to the soccer field soon. Jackie remains in the palliative care program for 1 year and then is discharged. She is thankful for the care the team provided and reflects during the final visit "I hope I don't have relapse, but if I do, I want you to be a part of my team. Thanks for helping me feel my best even when I was at my worst."

Case 1 demonstrates the potentially large number of clinicians that are involved in care delivery for a pediatric oncology patient. It also illustrates how pediatric palliative care team can seamlessly integrate into the existing oncology interdisciplinary teams. It is also an example of how regular use of care team meetings and recognition of each member's unique strengths and role can allow for more comprehensive and holistic care planning.

Pediatric oncology has always included multidisciplinary care. Patients often have ten or more clinicians or groups involved in provision of care as illustrated in case vignette 1. Most pediatric cancer centers have some structure in place to meet regularly to discuss such multidisciplinary care such as tumor boards or case conferences (Cantrell and Ruble 2011). Unfortunately, the psychosocial aspects of care are not typically included in such discussions. Tending to patient and family well-being and quality of life during therapy is no less complex than deciding which chemotherapeutic regimen or surgical approach to utilize. Important organizations as the American Academy of Pediatrics (AAP), Children's Oncology Group (COG), and the SIOPE (European Society for Paediatric Oncology) have standards for the minimum access to services and expertise within a pediatric cancer center, including palliative care, but little is written about how the team interaction can be (American Academy of Pediatrics 2004; Children's Oncology Group 2014; Kowalczyk et al. 2014; European Society for Paediatric Oncology). The model of care in most centers, however, is that patients interact with various members of the care team in parallel or serially with little attention to the interactions between team members that are necessary for true collaborative care. Models of team functioning which have been utilized within specialty palliative care teams can be utilized throughout the trajectory of illness to improve patient care and allow for more seamless integration of palliative care principles.

Relationship-centered focus: The palliative care approach to team functioning builds on the relationship-centered focus integral to patient care in this field. The human elements of caregiving cannot be ignored and are a vibrant part of each participant's value. Well-functioning teams recognize that there is always reciprocal influence in any encounter and that individual values, subjectivity, and past experiences shape decisions both for patients and professionals. Each clinician brings a unique set of experiences and skills which will enhance the overall care experience (Papadatou et al. 2011).

3.1 Members of a Comprehensive Care Team

In order to achieve the goal that all children with cancer receive access to palliative care, the primary oncology team must be the center. Within this model the oncology team should have sufficient collective expertise to address the range of physical, psychosocial, emotional, practical, and spiritual needs of the child and family. To achieve this goal most teams include physicians, nurses, social workers, psychologists, case managers, spiritual care providers, bereavement specialists, and child life specialists. Figure 3.1 shows how different disciplines assess all dimensions of care, and Table 3.1 describes distinctions in expertise that clinicians may provide. The team

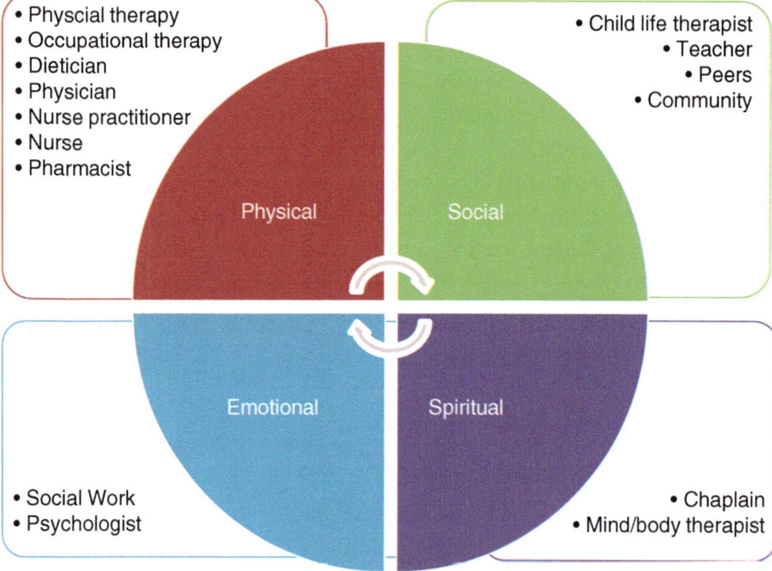

Fig. 3.1 The four domains of quality of life and the clinicians who most often work within each domain

Table 3.1 Distinctions of expertise between palliative care providers (adapted from Ogelby and Goldstein (2014)

Medicine	Address medical needs such as pain and symptom management
	Consider the implications of medical interventions
	Take the lead on framing the illness trajectory and prognosis
	Take on special role interacting with other medical specialties
Nursing	Clinical support and hands-on care
	Teaching families how to best provide care for their children
	Support other staff at bedside
Social work	Address broad spectrum of factors that influence families, such as housing, transportation, and family dynamics
	Provide psychosocial/emotional and bereavement supports
Psychologist	Helps patient to cope with disease, diagnostic or therapeutic procedures based on developmental stage, strengthen family coping strategies
	Provide psychosocial/emotional and bereavement supports
Child life	Provide psychosocially driven intervention that promotes coping through play, preparation, education, and self-expression activities for both patient and siblings
Pastoral care	Support spiritual needs of child and family
	Access supports specific to a family's religious belief and values
	Communicate spiritual needs of family to care team for considerations in care plan

should also have access to high-quality adjunct services including psychiatry, pharmacology, nutrition, expressive therapies (e.g., music or art therapy), and rehabilitation services (physical, occupational, and speech therapy).

3.2 Team Development

Moving toward true interdisciplinary care requires a process of team development. The major difference between a *multidisciplinary* team working in parallel and a true *interdisciplinary team* is the relational component between clinicians. The latter recognizes that each team member not only affects the patient and family but also the other team members as well (Fig. 3.2).

Growing from a group to be a team: Becoming a team requires commitment and common purpose. The members must recognize their mutual goal and value teamwork as a means to achieve more than could be accomplished alone. This transition from a group to a team may not always be easy and should be seen as a dynamic process. The movement from a loose collection of indi-

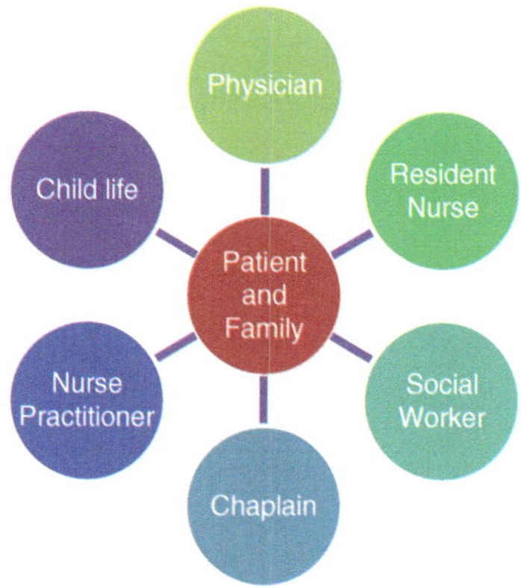

A multidisciplinary team has multiple members who all interact with the patient and family in a parallel fashion

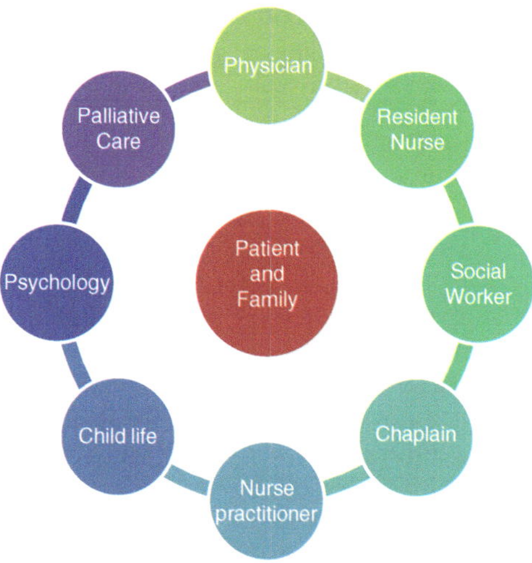

An interdisciplinary team relies on strong relationships between clinicians to provide optimal patient care

Fig. 3.2 Models of multi- and interdisciplinary care

viduals who coexist to an integrated team working in *collaborative alliance* is often a nonlinear process (Papadatou 2009). It may be characterized by periods of forward and regressive movement as well as times of disorganization, stagnation, and growth. For such an alliance to develop, care providers must spend time working together, sharing experiences, exploring different points of view, and developing a common language within a *holding environment* (Kahn 2001). Refer to Box 3.1 to learn more about these two concepts. Table 3.2 describes some essential principles of a good interdisciplinary team work.

Box 3.1 Essential elements for developing an interdisciplinary team

Holding environment
A psychological space that is both safe and challenging. For clinicians caring for children with serious illness, this space is one of understanding and support that allows for management of distress. An ideal holding environment allows clinicians to express feelings of sadness, anxiety, anger, or fear with others who can validate their feelings and at the same time emphasize their abilities to explore new horizons and manage challenges.

Collaborative Alliance
Emphasis is on open communication between clinicians. Team members learn from each other, broaden horizons of understanding, and thoughtfully review their work by assessing their strengths and limitations.

This team development process requires intentionality and will not occur without specific attention to create opportunities for clinicians to interact in a team-based way. Training on new skills as a team or working together on a quality improvement project to enhance integration of palliative care is an ideal mechanism to enhance team functioning in addition to knowledge and skill of each member (Weller et al. 2014). Table 3.3 details the phases a group goes through to become a team.

Table 3.2 Ten principles of a good interdisciplinary team work

Leadership and management	The team should identify a leader who establishes a clear direction and vision for the team while also listening and providing support to the team members
Clarity of vision	The team incorporates a set of values that clearly provide direction for the team's service
Climate	The team demonstrates a team culture and interdisciplinary atmosphere of trust where contributions are valued
Appropriate resources and procedures	The team ensures appropriate processes, and infrastructures are in place to uphold the vision of the service
Quality and outcomes of care	The team provides quality patient-focused services with documented outcomes and utilizes feedback to improve the quality of care
Communication	The team utilizes communication strategies that promote intra-team communication, collaborative decision-making, and effective team processes
Appropriate skill mix	The team integrates an appropriate mix of skills, competencies, and personalities to meet the needs of patients and enhance smooth functioning
Individual characteristics	The team recruits staff who demonstrate interdisciplinary competencies and assists individuals in developing additional competencies
Respecting and understanding roles	The team promotes interdependence among various team roles while also respecting individual autonomy
Personal rewards, training, and development	The team fosters the development of members through appropriate training, rewards, recognition, and opportunities for career development

Adapted from Nancarrow et al. (2013)

Table 3.3 Tuckman's stages of team development (Tuckman 1965)

These stages describe a process many teams go through. Team development is a nonlinear process and even the most high-performing teams will revert to earlier stages in certain circumstances. Many long-standing teams go through these cycles many times as they react to changing circumstances. For example, a change in leadership may cause the team to revert to *storming* as the new people challenge the existing norms and dynamics of the team	
Forming	The team meets to learn about the tasks and challenges and then agree on goals. Team members tend to behave quite independently. They may be motivated but are usually relatively uninformed of the issues and objectives of the team. Team members are usually on their best behavior but very focused on themselves
Storming	In this stage team members begin to form opinions about the work ethic of other members and may voice opinions if they are dissatisfied. Disagreements and personality clashes must be resolved before the team can progress out of this stage. Some groups may avoid the phase altogether; for others the duration, intensity, and destructiveness of the "storms" can be varied. Tolerance of each team member and their differences should be emphasized; without tolerance and patience the team will fail
Norming	As the team resolves disagreements and personality conflicts, a stronger alliance and spirit of cooperation emerge. In this stage, all team members take the responsibility and have the ambition to work for the success of the team's goals. The danger here is that members may be so focused on preventing conflict that they are reluctant to share controversial ideas
Performing	The team now has established roles and norms of function. They can begin to achieve common goals and often reach unexpectedly high level of success. Dissent is expected and allowed as long as it is channeled through means acceptable to the team

3.3 Procedures of the Interdisciplinary Care Team

3.3.1 Interdisciplinary Team Meeting

The core procedure to ensuring well-coordinated care for complex patients with serious illness is the interdisciplinary team meeting. The interdisciplinary team meeting is a convening of providers to discuss the care plan for one or multiple patients. Although such meetings may seem to be time-consuming and may be difficult to schedule, they are essential in creating an integrated, holistic care plan; they may facilitate shared decision-making that incorporates the patient and family perspective to a greater degree than standard practice. They could be understood as the "headquarter" where everyone in the team will know what their specific tasks will be and have a protective effect, as every clinician will know how to complement each others' goals without duplicating efforts and joining the essential information gathered from the family by each discipline. This will allow a more fluent and effective communication between family and the team by providing the whole team of the essential information that is going to be "on the air" while making the experience of the patient and family less painful by telling their story less times (Connor et al. 2002).

Literature on the best way to conduct such a meeting is lacking, but there is consensus on a few vital principles. Firstly, an interdisciplinary team meeting is a nonhierarchical affair. One team member may take the leadership role in keeping the discussion on track or asking key questions, but all members should have an equal voice. Secondly, all aspects of the care plan (physical, social, spiritual, and emotional) are considered with equal importance. Lastly, an agenda or routine structure to the meeting will improve the efficiency and effectiveness of these meetings and help the team to find value in this use of time (Fig. 3.3) (Demris et al. 2008).

3.3.2 Family Care Conference

The family care conference is a distinct type of interdisciplinary meeting in which the patient and family are the center of the interaction. This type of conference has been most well described in the intensive care unit setting, but can be used

Fig. 3.3 Sample agenda for an interdisciplinary team meeting

Interdisciplinary Team Sample Agenda
Process:

- Once weekly,one hour meeting
- Each patient will be discussed: new patients, readmitted/reconsulted patients, continuing patients, discharged patients with any updates
- Facilitator and time keeper assigned
- Each discipline presents their field followed by brief team discussion:
    - Medical (Physician/Nurse Practitioner)
    - Pain Management
    - Rehab
    - Child Life

Table 3.4 Framework for a family care conference

Timeframe	Procedures	Objectives	Logistical considerations
Premeeting	Clinician-only meeting	Preparing participants Identify key participants and set the agenda Identify key psychosocial issues Identify who will facilitate the meeting Gather family concerns (if known previously)	Identify someone to take notes Arrange interpreter if needed Set a location Determine the role of learners Discourage interruptions
Care conference	Introductions and overview Family engagement Shared decision-making	Information sharing Input from continuity providers Family advocacy Emotional connection	Allow ample time for family to speak
Post-meeting	Closure and follow-up	Thank participants Summarize what was discussed Highlight next steps	Document a summary of the meeting Share documentation with family and continuity providers Consider next meeting

Adapted from Fox et al. (2014)

successfully in inpatient and outpatient settings as well. The family care conference is an as-needed procedure and should be considered when delivering difficult news, discussing prognosis, considering major medical decisions, or considering end-of-life care. A family care conference may also be beneficial for patients with prolonged hospital stay, involvement of multiple subspecialists, or in preparation for discharge. While there are no standardized recommendations for how to conduct a family care conference, the model proposed by Fox et al. provides a nice framework for conducting such a meeting (Table 3.4) (Fox et al. 2014). Careful planning and skill should go in to all phases of the procedure. A clinician with in-depth knowledge of the family communication preferences and interpersonal dynamics should lead the meeting. This may be the attending oncologist, but could also be a social worker, nurse practitioner, or palliative care specialist. One of the tasks during the premeeting phase should be to determine who is most suited for this role.

Letting the family know that a conference will be held with the clinicians involved and encouraging them to think ahead and develop a list of questions could be really helpful. The team will be able to know in advance how the family thinks and which are its main concerns (physical, spiritual, social, or emotional), so the chance of having a meaningful family-centered conference and effective shared decision-making increases. The literature supports that interdisciplinary conferences including family caregiver are challenging because potential barriers must be considered: time constraints, communication skill deficits, unaddressed emotional needs, staff absences, and unclear role expectations. Nevertheless when studied in non-hospice settings, shared decision-making has been found to be associated with increased patient knowledge, more confidence in treatment decisions, and more active patient involvement in care (Washington et al. 2016).

3.3.3 Huddle

The idea of a quick huddle draws from sports teams who meet quickly and with a distinct purpose before the start of a play. In healthcare, the huddle can be used as a "just-in-time" review of the plan for a patient. Huddles have been utilized in the outpatient setting to begin each clinic session and optimize the patient flow and care coordination of the day (Dingley et al. 2008). The literature on the use of huddles in pediatric oncology or palliative care is lacking, but it is plausible that this tool may be very beneficial. Huddles enable teams to have frequent but short briefings so that they can stay informed, review work, make plans, and move ahead rapidly. The huddle is an ideal way to include team members who may not be included in interdisciplinary team meetings or family conferences such as residents, bedside nurses, or other unit staff that participate in the frontline patient care. For example, a huddle for a patient at end of life on the inpatient oncology unit could include attending oncologist, oncology fellow, on-call resident, nurse, palliative care physician, pharmacist, and social worker. This team could huddle at the start and end of each day (to allow for each shift to be included) to review the previous 12 h and make plans for the upcoming 12 h. This 5–10 min time investment is invaluable in avoiding the suffering associated with unanticipated complications and last minute, on-call care planning. The use of a checklist as a guide would further ensure that such meetings are conducted in the timeliest and efficient manner possible.

3.3.4 Debriefing

Debriefing is the process of spending a few minutes immediately after a procedure or encounter to assess what went well, what were the challenges, and what the team will do differently next time. This is a great opportunity for team learning while the events are fresh (Leonard et al. 2004). In palliative care, more in-depth debriefings are often needed to allow space for the team to process cognitive and emotional elements of complex patient encounters. A bereavement debriefing is a special type of debrief in which the focus is on team members' own experiences of grief following the death of a patient (Keene et al. 2010).

Case 2

Interdisciplinary care and excellent team function do not necessarily equate to universal consensus in every clinical scenario. Often team members have differing opinions, and disagreements can surface that lead to greater conflict without open communication and respect for the personal and professional contributions of other team members.

3.4 Integration of Palliative Care into Oncology

Palliative medicine is a rapidly growing subspecialty of medicine with a focus on assessment, evaluation, and treatment of the physical, psychological, social, and spiritual needs of patients and families with serious illnesses. In most places, palliative medicine physicians work within interdisciplinary care teams to provide holistic palliative care. The goal of palliative care is to optimize quality of life while living with a serious illness (Wolfe et al. 2008). As described by the World Health Organization (WHO), it is the "active total care of the child's body, mind, and spirit and also involves giving support to the family. It begins when illness is diagnosed and continues regard-

Jasmine was a 17-year-old girl with osteosarcoma. She had initially been diagnosed 5 years earlier and had experienced a relapse 9 months ago. Despite intensive chemotherapy and surgery, her tumors continued to progress including diffuse pulmonary metastases and pleural effusions. She was admitted for management of respiratory distress and also found to have a large pericardial effusion which was causing arrhythmias and decreased cardiac output. Attempts were made to drain the fluid collection and improve her cardiopulmonary status with marginal effect. One week after admission, Jasmine experienced a cardiac arrest due to acute arrhythmia. She was successfully resuscitated, stabilized, and transferred to intensive care unit. Following the cardiac arrest, she developed acute renal failure which required dialysis, and she remained in a coma with evidence of acute anoxic brain injury on magnetic resonance image.

Jasmine's family was devoutly religious and perceived this hospitalization as a test they must endure. They had faced many near death experiences in the past and saw their daughter as a strong-willed fighter. They displayed an unwavering belief that prayer and faith would heal her. They continued to hope for a miracle and requested that all medical interventions be continued to keep her alive.

Several physician members of the team acknowledged that Jasmine's survival was extremely unlikely and believed that the care plan should turn toward emphasis on comfort measures. Some felt burdened by the suffering caused by ongoing treatments to prolong her life. Others believed that the family wishes should be supported despite Jasmine's poor prognosis; the social worker held that the parents deserved to feel supported in their choices as they would reflect upon them for years after her death. The care team at this point included an oncologist, oncology nurse practitioner, intensivist, nephrologist, cardiologist, neurologist, palliative medicine specialist, psychologist, palliative care social work, and numerous intensive care unit nurses. Palliative care had been consulted at the time of relapse and had an established relationship prior to this admission. Recognizing that there may be differing opinions between this large care team and fearful that the family may receive mixed messages, the palliative care team scheduled a meeting to discuss the case. Through this discussion, the intensivist was able to share his perception that he was doing harm in the process of providing care that was no longer beneficial. The pain and suffering caused by the medical interventions was challenging for the nursing staff and others at the bedside. The psychologist and palliative care social worker were able to share their perspectives on the family, noting that unlike the physicians who have a large body of collective experience, this family is operating with only their singular experiences of their child. This allowed the team to gain a broader perspective for why the perceptions of the family may differ so greatly from that of the medical team. The psychologist also partnered with the hospital chaplain to caution the physicians against challenging the very strong faith which the family must draw on for strength now and throughout bereavement.

Though this meeting did not end with consensus of clear goals or a unanimous opinion regarding the appropriate treatment course, the discussion allowed for the team members to better appreciate the others perspectives. This process allowed for increased compassion within the team and enabled team members to have a little more patience to allow the natural course of illness to unfold. The team members were mindful of presenting themselves to the family as a cohesive and unified team and continued to interact with the family in a manner that encouraged ongoing dialogue. A few days later, Jasmine's dialysis catheter clotted, and a new one could not be placed. The family recognized that the end of life was near and elected to have Jasmine extubated to allow for death. The intensivist, oncologist, and palliative medicine specialist were present to provide symptomatic management and assure Jasmine's comfort. The palliative care team remained involved with the family to provide psychosocial support and bereavement follow-up.

less of whether or not a child receives treatment directed at the disease..." (World Health Organization 2016). This expertise and philosophy is increasingly being incorporated into standard oncologic care for both adults and children. Palliative care is appropriate at any age and at any stage in a serious illness and can be provided together with curative treatment (Meier 2011).

In a remarkable phase III random controlled study published in 2010, Temel et al. describe the benefits of early consultation to palliative care as part of the treatment of patients with metastatic non-small cell lung cancer (NSCLC) (Temel et al. 2010). They reported a significant improvement in mood and even survival in the group that received support by a palliative care team from the beginning. Inspired by these findings, the American Society of Clinical Oncology (ASCO) issued an expert consensus statement in 2012 stating "Substantial evidence demonstrates that palliative care—when combined with standard cancer care or as the main focus of care—leads to better patient and caregiver outcomes...While evidence clarifying optimal delivery of palliative care to improve patient outcomes is evolving, no trials to date have demonstrated harm to patients and caregivers, or excessive costs, from early involvement of palliative care... combined standard oncology care and palliative care should be considered early in the course of illness for any patient with metastatic cancer and/or high symptom burden." (Smith et al. 2012)

To achieve that noble goal, two major barriers must be addressed. One is the medical culture and attitudes that create a false dichotomy between curative therapy and palliative care. The other is the lack of access to palliative care teams and/or the inability of a specialty team to fully meet the patient care demands. Table 3.5 outlines some of the perceptions which may present barriers to early integration of palliative care (Dalberg et al. 2013).

Interestingly, in a study by Dalberg et al., physicians were more reluctant to integrate palliative care early, while nurses and social workers believed earlier integration of the palliative care team would benefit their patients care (Dalberg et al. 2013). This finding suggests that strong interdisciplinary care and team discussion about indications for referral may lead to a shift in these attitudes. Knowing how to utilize each team member to the fullest potential and draw from individual strengths while also leveraging team dynamics to accelerate therapeutic goals with patients and families is advanced "team-ness." In pediatric oncology, a patient's care team often

Table 3.5 Clinician perceptions of barriers to early integration of palliative care (Dalberg et al. 2013)

Overlapping roles	Physicians perceive that patients' palliative care needs are already adequately addressed by the primary oncology team
Conflicting philosophies	Physicians' belief that the purpose of palliative care is inconsistent with cure and only appropriate when cure is no longer the goal
Patient readiness	Clinicians worry that introducing the pediatric palliative care team early could lead to additional parental burden
Emotional issues	Primary care providers may influence patient care. Often nonphysician clinicians perceive that physicians' hope for cure, even when the prognosis is poor, may bias treatment decisions and how information regarding therapeutic options is relayed to patients and families. This emotional attachment and potential seems to intensify over time and may drive clinicians to be overly optimistic when it comes to their own patients (World Health Organization 2016)

expands greatly as the illness becomes more severe or complex. Admittedly, advanced team work skills are needed with increasing size and complexity. Oncology teams which have developed practices and behaviors to work as a seamless unit will be most well positioned to incorporate additional members, such as palliative care consultants. A team with common goals and shared vision is less susceptible to fears that new clinicians may swoop in and "steal" the patient. Similarly, consulting teams must recognize the value of the care team already in place and work diligently to enhance as opposed to replace that care.

In the traditional model, the oncology team provides care with primary focus on cure with psychosocial care primarily focused on concrete needs and helping the child and family cope with the stress of illness. The palliative care team is consulted once all therapeutic options have been exhausted. This transition is seen as a handoff in care with an abrupt shift in the composition of the team members involved. The palliative care team provides care through the end of life and into bereavement with little involvement from the oncology team. This model offers end-of-life care, which is noble, but also may create deficiencies in care. There may be missed opportunities for enhanced symptom management or quality of life support earlier in the disease course as well as missed opportunities for oncology clinicians to participate in end-of-life care. Patients and families may feel abandoned by their oncology teams if they become less involved as goals of care shift. The dichotomy between cancer-directed treatment and quality of life is emphasized in a model that implies each team only thinks about one of these. Regardless of this pitfall, this model is a frequent and valuable starting point when palliative care programs are newly implemented (i.e., developing countries).

A newer and better model is to think of the various roles as layers that all work together seamlessly to create a whole better than the sum of its parts. Patients do not need to choose between cancer treatments and supportive/palliative care. Everyone can work together to optimize both the quantity and quality of life. This is particularly important in the new era of targeted therapy, which has seen an explosion of novel therapeutic options that are less toxic than traditional chemotherapy, making it feasible for patients to receive cancer treatments closer to the end of life (Bruera and Hui 2010).

3.5 Conceptual Models of Integration

It may be beneficial to use a conceptual model to understand how palliative can integrate with standard oncologic care. Such models allow for the team to have a common understanding of what they are trying to achieve and have a common language when describing palliative care to patients and families. Bruera and Hui have described several helpful models including multilayered model of supportive care as illustrated in Fig. 3.4.

Additionally, they present an analogy of the illness trajectory as a road trip and the preparations for the car as advance care planning. A hopeful and unrealistic driver will set out on the road without any safety features (insurance, seat belts, airbags) or comfort measures (air-conditioning, seat cushions). The prepared driver will plan for uncertainty by having safety features in place while remaining hopeful that such preparations will not be needed. Additionally, the

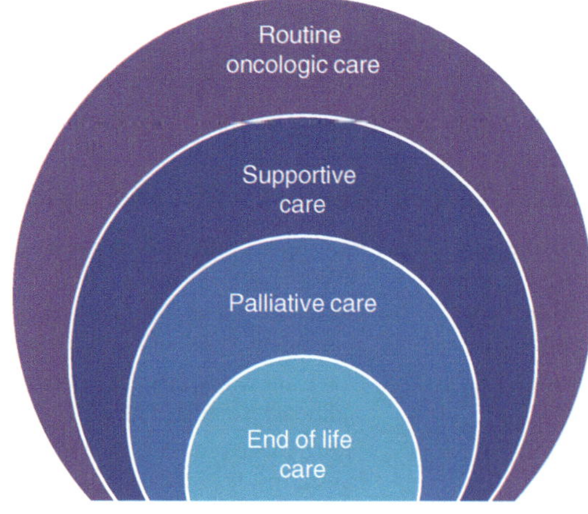

Fig. 3.4 Multilayered model of supportive care. Adapted from Bruera and Hui (2010)

prepared driver recognizes that attention to comfort measures does not impair the ability to reach the destination (Bruera and Hui 2010).

Even as we overcome philosophical barriers, access continues to be a major issue. Currently only 58% of Children's Oncology Group institutions in the United States report having a pediatric palliative care team (Dalberg et al. 2013; Kang et al. 2014; Johnston et al. 2008). This number is increasing every year, but innovative models are needed to insure all patients receive palliative care services.

3.6 Collaborative Generalist (Primary) and Specialized Palliative Care

Oncology teams are actively engaged in symptom control caused by the disease or by the treatments (i.e., fever, nausea, vomiting, constipation, with basic skills for managing pain) and often develop strong relationships with the patient and family through which they provide emotional support. This should be acknowledged as generalist palliative care. The partnership with specialized pediatric palliative care team evolves as the goals of care change based on clinical status making it necessary to bring clinicians trained in advanced palliative care to the picture (Johnston 2012; Quill 2013). Further study is needed to better understand the proportion of pediatric oncology patients who require this level of specialty palliative care consultation, and this will vary between institutions based on the primary team composition, competencies, number of clinicians, burden of clinical demand, and clinician skills in advanced symptom control. This frame of integration is effective in enhancing a quality-of-life driven institutional culture.

In many settings where pediatric palliative care trained providers and/or resources are not abundant, institutions can use existing resources to meet the needs of their patients, with an expert pediatric palliative care provider guiding coordination of care rather than personally delivering services (Wentlandt et al. 2014). A significant proportion of palliative cancer care can be provided by the primary cancer care team; and consultation with palliative cancer care specialists may range from a single consultation about a specific issue to several encounters or ongoing involvement until death and into the period of bereavement. Actually, this is considered a more sustainable model as the demand of palliative care services increases (Quill 2013; Levin et al. 2016).

3.7 Other Potential Models for Innovation in Incorporating Palliative Care into Routine Oncology Care

3.7.1 Multispecialty Clinics

The concept of multidisciplinary clinics has gained great momentum in pediatric centers. Any disease for which the management requires multiple specialists from multiple fields may benefit from creation of such a model including the care of patients with sickle cell disease, osteosarcoma, or brain tumors. Such clinics are preferred from a patient/family perspective as

Clinical case 3

This case illustrates a successful complementary interaction between primary oncology team, strong psychosocial support, palliative care, and pain medicine clinicians from the moment of diagnoses through death. Palliative care and psychosocial teams helped to assess goals of care along the illness trajectory, and having a strong relationship from the beginning was very helpful for future interventions, including end-of-life care. Decisions were shared and negotiated, and the patient's wishes were supported and successfully accomplished. This case highlights the value of shared knowledge and skills between members of an interdisciplinary team and the networking needed to extend the best care possible to the patient/family preferred care setting.

Mariana, a 17-year-old female that is admitted with an abdominal mass, with multiple associated symptoms and signs: abdominal and back pain, cachexia, anorexia, severe nausea, vomiting and altered mental status (somnolence), dyspnea, and difficulty breathing. Initial Karnofsky Performance Scale score was 40. She was referred with a biopsy preliminary report of abdominal alveolar rhabdomyosarcoma. The primary oncology team started treatment with intravenous fluids, antiemetics, a nasogastric tube, and oxygen by mask; pain medicine was started including intravenous opioids. Based on clinical findings and hypercalcemia, the diagnosis of malignant hypercalcemia was made, and bisphosphonates were administered. Further work-up revealed she had metastases in her lungs, vertebrae, and bone marrow. Her oncologist gave a very poor prognosis and recommended chemotherapy with the intention of alleviating symptoms and prolonging life. Palliative care was consulted and recommended advanced management of nausea and vomiting (i.e., antipsychotics) and began building a relationship with her and her mother. They lived in a poor area of rural Mexico. Mariana had been independent for 2 years having moved to a bigger town to study high school. She had a 13-year-old sister with trisomy 21 and developmental delay.

After treating the hypercalcemia, Mariana recovered her mental status and participated, along with her mother, in a discussion about her diagnosis and prognosis. She accepted treatment with chemotherapy understanding that cure was not a goal, but expecting to live longer with good quality of life. The palliative care physician and psychologist assessed goals of care and offered emotional support. Even before starting chemotherapy, the team was able to have conversations about resuscitation status, which she understood and agreed to have a do not resuscitate order entered on her behalf.

Mariana's cancer-directed treatment lasted live 10 months and resulted in good quality of life and performance (Karnofsky 90). She and her family were followed by psychology, social work, pain medicine, nutrition, physical therapy, and frequent informal but meaningful encounters with the palliative care physician. Each member of the interdisciplinary team built strong relationships with her and her mother.

When the tumor was small for surgical resection, she went to the operating room where the surgeons discovered peritoneal carcinomatosis; palliative care was called to help in discussing the difficult news and facilitate the goals of care discussion. At the moment of delivering the news, Mariana experienced a panic attack which palliative care physician successfully managed with deep breathing and guided imagery. From goals of care conversations, Mariana expressed her wishes to be at home as her primary goal. Since she lived very far from any medical service, this was a challenging goal to accomplish, and some suggested that the best place for her to die was hospital or hospice. The interdisciplinary team worked diligently to support Mariana's wishes and guarantee availability of medical services. She and her family made the decision to stay at her aunt's home, in the town were her school was. She was ultimately discharged there and "24 × 7" telephone support was available. She and a community-based nurse received emotional support as well as guidance about opioids, steroids, laxatives, and antiemetic. She died peacefully 1 month later. The local nurses, who had no training in palliative care, were very grateful for being part of a compassionate and professional end-of-life care team.

they offer "one stop shopping" but have also been shown to improve the quality of care outcomes. Incorporation of palliative care specialists into such as model would allow for normalization by demonstrating that this is a core part of care for this complex patient population. The model for delivery of service in this case would be for the palliative care team to see all of the patients in a given clinic session. The "team" should be comprised of at least two interdisciplinary clinicians, and there could be standardized battery of assessments and guidance that is provided at each visit. These visits would need to be kept relatively brief to keep the flow of the clinic but could also be paired with additional pediatric palliative care interventions for those with more complex needs. An additional advantage of this model is allowing the pediatric palliative care team to discuss care with the multidisciplinary group during the briefing period before the clinic. Similar to the embedded expert, the pediatric palliative care team can encourage "team-ness" and help other members see themselves as a unified team as opposed to a series of providers. This model may be difficult to implement due to scheduling conflicts if the palliative care team is also covering inpatients and other outpatient services. Creation of a multispecialty clinic is a complex task which requires rigorous coordination and administrative support as well as buy-in from all the parties involved.

3.7.2 Embedded Expert Model

As noted previously, ideally all children with cancer should be introduced to palliative care early in the disease process; it may make sense to have a dedicated clinician (most likely nurse practitioner) with advanced training in palliative care embedded in the core oncology teams. The number and distribution of such specialists would depend on the size and structure of the cancer center. In large centers with specific disease groups (solid tumor, brain tumor, hematologic malignancies, stem cell transplant), a palliative expert could be assigned to each group. This palliative "expert" could meet with patients at the start of treatment and regularly throughout their course and collaborate with other team members to create the most holistic treatment plan possible. The embedded expert would also serve as a "team enhancer" encouraging physicians, nurses, social workers, child life specialists, psychologists, and pharmacists to work more closely more often. The advantage of this system is that the palliative clinician is woven into the core care teams and does not have any competing clinical duties outside of the cancer patient population. Expertise would be consistently available to the other team members, and strong team bonds could form. The disadvantage is that the palliative care delivered itself is only unidimensional. This model may limit the quality of the palliative care provided unless the embedded expert has access to and interfaces regularly with a larger consult-based interdisciplinary pediatric palliative care team. Theoretically both the embedded expert model and pediatric palliative care consultative model could be used together. The embedded expert would provide much of the generalist level care with specialist consultation reserved for the more complex cases.

3.7.3 Embedded Psychosocial Expert

This model is based on a strong and continuous psychosocial support to every patient and family starting at the time of diagnosis and following the patient until survivorship or death. The focus of the support would emphasize hope but would help the patients and their families to have realistic goals of care, favoring functional coping of losses (health, home, stability). Each child would have his/her psychologist and social worker that work together with the treating oncologist but who are also part of a larger team that focuses on quality of life regardless the probabilities of illness outcome and could make additional recommendations in a multidimensional way, including considering emotional, spiritual, and social aspects that may influence in the intensity of symptoms. The psychosocial expert may also recommend useful complementary (non-pharmacologic) treatments such as aromatherapy, acupressure, massage therapy, and music.

This model requires that the whole team has an understanding of palliative care principles and has the capacity to be flexible in order to speak the same language and adjust to the patient needs at any time in the illness trajectory, a team for whom there is no dichotomy between curative or palliative intentions, for whom palliative means *better quality of life*.

3.8 Community Palliative Care and Hospice

As clinical case 3 illustrates, involvement of a community agency will be an integral part of a comprehensive palliative care plan. Community-based palliative care refers to any service that is primarily provided in the patient's own home. In the United States, these services are increasingly being provided for children through state funded palliative care initiatives. These programs provide interdisciplinary support for children with serious illness and do not have any life expectancy regulations (Kaye et al. 2015). Many hospital-based palliative care teams also provide support in the community via home visits, telephone case management, and telemedicine. Strong partnerships with community providers are essential to ensure that all children receive the care they need, particularly in areas where patients may live hundreds of miles from the cancer center or children's hospital.

Hospice care is a subset of palliative care. The hospice philosophy of care focusing the person, not the disease, is consistent throughout the world, although with varying application. In the United States, hospice is primarily defined by a Medicare benefit available to patients with life expectancy of 6 month or less. Hospice agencies provide interdisciplinary care focused on symptom management and quality of life; most commonly this care is provided in the patient's home. The Affordable Care Act of 2010 provides concurrent care for all patients less than 21 years old (National Hospice and Palliative Care Organization). This means that patients may receive hospice services even while continuing usual medical care (including transfusions, chemotherapy, or phase I trials). Outside the United States, hospice primarily refers to a facility that provides palliative care. These facilities are often philanthropically supported and offer respite care, urgent symptom management, and complimentary therapies in a home-like setting. Hospice care for children remains an area of development throughout the world (Worldwide Hospice Palliative Care Alliance). The core hospice skills of symptomatic assessment, individualized care planning, and psychosocial support for the family are readily applied to pediatric patients. This is a complimentary expertise to an existing oncology or palliative care team. Regular check-ins with the hospice team can assure a well-coordinated care plan and allows the hospital-based team to serve as a resource for medication dosing or other pediatric-specific concerns.

3.9 Education and System-Wide Improvement

Regardless of the other models utilized, some attention should be given to elevating the standard of care for all children within the hospital or health system. Ongoing education on communication skills, symptom assessment and management, discussing and documenting goals of care, and bereavement care should be provided to all clinicians on a routine basis. This education can be provided through the health system via didactic sessions or newsletters. Education resources are also available through national and international organizations, ELNEC (End-of-Life Nursing Education Consortium), ASPHO (American Society of Pediatric Hematology/Oncology), APON (Association of Pediatric Oncology Nurses), and SIOP (the International Society of Paediatric Oncology). Clinicians can access education content directly through online or attending national and international conferences. EPEC®-Pediatrics

(Education in Palliative and End of Life Care) utilizes a train the trainer model designed to help with widespread dissemination of palliative care knowledge. Palliative care specialist and oncology teams should partner in planning such educational offerings. Elevating the baseline level of care will decrease the background level of suffering and allow consultant services to be focused on those with more complex needs. Leadership should support staff in accessing ongoing education and could encourage providers to dedicate time to palliative topics. Palliative care should be part of every pediatric oncology fellowship curricula.

Policies and procedures are also needed to improve the baseline level of care. Palliative medicine specialists should be responsible for remaining up to date on most current practices and working with oncologists, nurses, and hospital administrators to create policy accordingly. Policies are often utilized to ensure patient safety or to standardize access and utilization of certain medications. Broadening the view to include policies and procedures that enhance the patient and family voice or encourage more attention to comfort and quality of life could be transformative.

3.10 Considerations from Global Health Data

The resources for pediatric oncology around the world are heterogeneous, just as the development of pediatric palliative care (Rodriguez-Galindo et al. 2013). North America and Europe have the greatest percentage of countries with a major level of development in pediatric palliative care. On the other hand, outstandingly successful programs have been created in more limited resources settings (Knapp et al. 2011).

Creative and collaborative strategies have been established in order to provide care for seriously ill children with cancer. Sometimes, oncologists will serve as palliative care providers if there is no pediatric palliative care clinician; or experts on adult palliative care will take care of these children, and their skills will be different but always valuable. Recommended strategies to standardize the knowledge about pediatric palliative care are partnering with more experienced institutions and mentorship (Rodriguez-Galindo et al. 2013; Knapp et al. 2011).

3.11 Summary and Take-Home Points

- Palliative care is appropriate at any age and at any stage in a serious illness and can be provided together with disease-directed treatment.
- Neither clinicians nor patients need to choose between cancer treatments and palliative care. Rather, they can take advantage of the expertise of both the oncology and the palliative care teams in optimizing quantity and quality of life under a simultaneous care model.
- To achieve the aim of granting all children with cancer or other serious illness access to palliative care, it is essential to have strong interdisciplinary team work at all levels. Oncology clinicians and palliative care clinicians must develop a model in which all are working together as part of a well-integrated team serving the patient and family.
- Moving toward true interdisciplinary care requires a process of team development in which the various roles are understood as different layers working together seamlessly to create a whole better than the sum of its parts.

References

American Academy of Pediatrics (2004) Guidelines for pediatric cancer centers: section on hematology/oncology policy statement on guidelines for pediatric cancer centers. Pediatrics 113(6):1833–1835

Bruera E, Hui D (2010) Integrating supportive and palliative care in the trajectory of cancer: establishing goals and models of care. J Clin Oncol 28(25):4013–4017

Cantrell MA, Ruble K (2011) Multidisciplinary care in pediatric oncology. J Multidiscip Healthc 4:171–181

Children's Oncology Group (2014) https://www.childrensoncologygroup.org/downloads/MI_

PersonServiceRequirementsFINAL.PDF. Accessed 18 Jun 2016
Connor SR, Eagan KA, Kwilosz D, Larson DG, Reese DL (2002) Interdisciplinary approaches in assisting with end-of-life care and decision making. Am Behav Sci 46(3):340–356
Dalberg T, Jacob-Files E, Carney PA, Meyrowitz J, Fromme E, Thomas G (2013) Pediatric oncology providers perceptions of barriers and facilitators to early integration of pediatric palliative care. Pediatr Blood Cancer 60(11):1875–1881
Demris G et al (2008) A study of informaiton flow in hospice interdisciplinary team meetings. J Interprof Care 22(6):621–629
Dingley C, Daugherty K, Derieg MK et al (2008) Improving patient safety through provider communication strategy enhancements. In: Henriksen K, Battles JB, Keyes MA et al (eds) Advances in patient safety: new directions and alternative approaches, vol. 3: performance and tools. Agency for Healthcare Research and Quality (US), Rockville, MD
European Society for Paediatric Oncology (2011) Standards of care for children with cancer. https://www.siope.eu/european-research-and-standards/standards-of-care-in-paediatric-oncology. Accessed 10 Aug 2016
Fox D, Brittan M, Stille C (2014) The pediatric inpatient family care conference: a proposed structure toward shared decision-making. Hosp Pedatri 4:305
Johnston DL, Vadeboncoeur C (2012) Palliative care consultation in pediatric oncology. Support Care Cancer 20:799–803
Johnston DL, Nagel K, Friedman DL, Meza JL, Hurwitz CA, Friebert S (2008) Availability and use of palliative care and end-of-life services for pediatric oncology patients. J Clin Oncol 26:4646–4650
Kahn WA (2001) Holding environments at work. J Appl Behav Sci 37(3):260–279
Kang TI, Munson D, Hwang J, Feudtner C (2014) Integration of palliative care into the care of children with serious illness. Pediatr Rev 35:318–326
Kaye EC, Rubenstein J, Levine D, Baker JN, Dabbs D, Friebert SE (2015) Pediatric palliative care in the community. CA Cancer J Clin 65(4):316–333
Keene EA, Hutton N, Hall B, Rushton C (2010) Bereavement debriefing sessions: an intervention to support health care professionals in managing their grief after the death of a patient. Pediatr Nurs 36(4):185–189
Knapp C, Woodworth L, Wright M, Downing J, Drake R, Fowler-Kerry S, Hain R, Marston J (2011) Pediatric palliative care provision around the world: a systematic review. Pediatr Blood Cancer 57:361–368
Kowalczyk JR, Samardakiewicz M, Fitzgerald E, Essiaf S, Ladenstein R, Vassal G, Kienesberger A, Pritchard-Jones K (2014) Towards reducing inequalities: European standards of care for children with cancer. Eur J Cancer 50:481–485
Leonard M, Graham S, Bonacum D (2004) The human factor: the critical importance of effective teamwork and communication in providing safe care. Qual Saf Health Care 13(Suppl 1):i85–i90
Levin DR, Johnson LM, Snyder A, Wiser RK, Gibson D, Kane JR, Baker JN (2016) Integrating palliative care in pediatric oncology: evidence for an evolving paradigm for comprehensive cancer care. J Natl Compr Cancer Netw 14(6):741–748
Meier DE, Brawley OW (2011) Palliative care and the quality of life. J Clin Oncol 29:2750–2752
Nancarrow S et al (2013) Ten principles of good interdisciplinary team work. Hum Resour Health 11:19
National Hospice and Palliative Care Organization (2013) Section 2302 of the Affordable Care Act (ACA), titled "Concurrent Care for Children", amended sections 1905(o)(1) and 2210(a)(23) of the Social Security Act. http://www.nhpco.org/sites/default/files/public/ChiPPS/CCCR_Appendix1.pdf. Accessed 29 Sept 2016. (The complete Social Security Act can be found at https://www.ssa.gov/OP_Home/ssact/ssact-toc.htm)
Ogelby M, Goldstein RD (2014) Interdisciplinary care: using your team. Pediatr Clin N Am 61:823–834
Papadatou D, Bluebond-Langner M, Ann G (2011) The team. In: Wolfe J, Hinds PS, Sourkes BM (eds) Textbook of interdisciplinary pediatric palliative care. Elsevier/Saunders, Philadelphia, pp 55–63
Papdatou D (2009) In the face of death: professionals who care for the dying and bereaved. Spring, New York
Quill TE, Abernethy AP (2013) Generalist plus specialist palliative care — creating a more sustainable model. N Engl J Med 368(13):1173–1175
Rodriguez-Galindo C, Friedrich P, Morrissey L, Frazier L (2013) Global challenges in pediatric oncology. Curr Opin Pediatr 25:3–15
Smith TJ, Temin S, Alesi ER, Abernethy AP, Balboni TA, Basch EM, Ferrell BR, Loscalzo M, Meier DE, Paice JA, Peppercorn JM, Somerfield M, Stovall E, Von Roenn JH (2012) American Society of Clinical Oncology provisional clinical opinion: the integration of palliative care into standard oncology care. J Clin Oncol 30:1–9
Temel JS, Greer JA, Muzikansky A et al (2010) Early palliative care for patients with metastatic non-small-cell lung cancer. N Engl J Med 363:733–742
Tuckman B (1965) Developmental sequence in small groups. Psychol Bull 63(6):384–399
Washington KT, Oliver DP, Gage LA, Albright DL, Demiris G (2016) Palliat Med 30(3):270–278
Weller J, Boyd M, Cumin D (2014) Teams, tribes and patient safety: overcoming barriers to effective teamwork in healthcare. Postgrad Med J 90:149–154
Wentlandt K, Kryzyzanowska MK, Swami N, Rodin G, Le LW, Sung L, Zimmerman C (2014) Referral prac-

tices of pediatric oncologists to specialized palliative care. Support Care Cancer 22:2315–2322

Wolfe J, Hammel JF, Edwards KE, Duncan J, Comeau M, Breyer J, Aldridge SA, Grier HE, Berde C, Dussel V, Weeks J (2008) Easing of suffering in children with cancer at the end of life: is care changing? J Clin Oncol 26:1717–1723

World Health Organization (2016) http://www.who.int/cancer/palliative/definition/en. Accessed 18 Jun 2016

Worldwide Hospice Palliative Care Alliance (2014) Global atlas of palliative care at the end of life. http://www.thewhpca.org/resources/global-atlas-on-end-of-life-care. Accessed 9 Sept 2016

4 Communication with Children with Cancer and Their Families Throughout the Illness Journey and at the End of Life

Erica C. Kaye, Jennifer M. Snaman, Liza Johnson, Deena Levine, Brent Powell, Amy Love, Jennifer Smith, Jennifer H. Ehrentraut, Joanna Lyman, Melody Cunningham, and Justin N. Baker

"Speak clearly, if you speak at all; carve every word before you let it fall."

Oliver Wendall Holmes

"The way you tell the truth to families makes a huge difference…if you know the person that's coming in there and they're telling the truth, as hard as it is, but you know they care about you and they love your child, it's okay. As hard as it is, it's okay and it makes all the difference."

Bereaved parent

E.C. Kaye, M.D. (✉)
Department of Oncology, St. Jude Children's Research Hospital,
262 Danny Thomas Place, Mail Stop 260, Memphis, TN 38105-3678, USA

Department of Oncology, St. Jude Children's Research Hospital, Memphis, TN, USA

Division of Quality of Life and Palliative Care, St. Jude Children's Research Hospital, Memphis, TN, USA
e-mail: erica.kaye@stjude.org

J.M. Snaman
Division of Pediatric Palliative Care, Boston Childrens Hospital, Boston, MA, USA

Department of Psychosocial Oncology, Dana-Farber Cancer Institute, Boston, MA, USA

L. Johnson • D. Levine • J.N. Baker
Department of Oncology, St. Jude Children's Research Hospital, Memphis, TN, USA

Division of Quality of Life and Palliative Care, St. Jude Children's Research Hospital, Memphis, TN, USA

B. Powell
Spiritual Care Services, Patient Care Services, St. Jude Children's Research Hospital, Memphis, TN, USA

A. Love • J. Smith
Child Life Program, Patient Care Services, St. Jude Children's Research Hospital, Memphis, TN, USA

J.H. Ehrentraut
Department of Psychology, St. Jude Children's Research Hospital, Memphis, TN, USA

J. Lyman • M. Cunningham
Threads of Care Program, Division of Hospice and Palliative Care, Le Bonheur Children's Hospital, University of Tennessee Health Science Center, Memphis, TN, USA

J. Wolfe et al. (eds.), *Palliative Care in Pediatric Oncology*, Pediatric Oncology,
https://doi.org/10.1007/978-3-319-61391-8_4

4.1 What Is "Good Communication" in the Context of Pediatric Oncology and Palliative Care?

Skillful communication has long been considered a key pillar in the "art" of practicing medicine (Feudtner 2007; Kaye et al. 2015). "Good communication" is integral to the development of meaningful connections between individuals and is a critical aspect of the therapeutic alliance (Mack and Hinds 2011). Yet the practical definition and real-life application of "good communication" can vary among individuals. What exactly does "good communication" mean? And how do we interpret and further uncover the nuanced meaning of this phrase within the context of pediatric oncology and palliative care?

Communication is defined both as "a process by which information is exchanged between individuals" and as "personal rapport" (Merriam-Webster Dictionary). Effective transmission of information is necessary, but not sufficient, to achieve good communication; forging and nurturing human connection and trust are also essential (Mack and Hinds 2011). Simply stated, good communication in the medical setting requires a synergy of effective information sharing and trust building, with the ultimate goal of developing meaningful relationships that inform and guide the illness experience for patients, families, and healthcare providers (HCPs).

Although skillful communication is important across all fields of medicine, it becomes particularly critical at the intersection of pediatric oncology and palliative care. In many settings, conversation might be the primary way (and, at times, one of the only ways) for HCPs to alleviate the suffering of children with cancer and their families (Mack and Grier 2004). Moreover, effective communication is required to build trust and relationships not only among children, families, and HCPs but also among members of the interdisciplinary team (Feudtner 2007; Kaye et al. 2015). Sharing information in an honest, clear, and compassionate manner facilitates the building of relationships and trust among HCPs, patients, and families, which in turn promotes optimal holistic continuity of care that transcends illness stage or care location (Kaye et al. 2015). Through the establishment of relationships and rapport, transparent and empathic communication also creates a framework for successful family-centered identification of goals as a means by which to guide difficult decision-making (Feudtner 2007; Kaye et al. 2015).

In recent years, the importance of communication has been increasingly recognized as a key aspect of providing optimal care to children with high-risk cancer and other life-threatening illnesses. The American Academy of Pediatrics (AAP) and the Institute of Medicine have published statements advocating for the promotion of effective communication among HCPs, patients, and families in pediatrics and palliative care (American Academy of Pediatrics 2000; Fallat and Glover 2007; Institute of Medicine 2003, 2014). A similar consensus regarding the need for good communication has been seen in the oncology setting, with the American Society of Clinical Oncology, the American Society of Pediatric Hematology-Oncology, and the International Society of Pediatric Oncology all highlighting the importance of improving communication among HCPs, patients with high-risk cancer, and families (Peppercorn et al. 2011; Arceci et al. 1998; Spinetta et al. 2009; Jankovic et al. 2008; Masera et al. 1999; Masera et al. 1997). Recently, experts in pediatric oncology and palliative care identified communication as both a standard of care and a top research priority within both fields (Weaver et al. 2015; Baker et al. 2015), further solidifying the critical importance of good communication in caring for children with high-risk cancer and their families.

In the context of this call to action, the following chapter will review the literature on the practical benefits of effective communication for HCPs working in the fields of pediatric oncology and palliative care. We also will discuss domains, models, and strategies for achieving good communication among HCPs, children with high-risk cancer, and their families as well as among members of the interdisciplinary medical team. Using a patient's story, we will review common communication scenarios ranging from sharing a difficult diagnosis and prognosis to discussing goals of care at the end of life (EOL). We also will discuss barriers and pitfalls to effective communication and offer strategies to overcome these issues. Finally, we will offer interdisciplinary recommendations for effective communication from the valuable perspectives of a psychologist, chaplain, child life specialist, and music therapist who specialize in the care of children with high-risk cancer and their families.

4.2 Why Is Communication so Important in Pediatric Oncology and Palliative Care?

> "The right word may be effective, but no word was ever as effective as a rightly timed pause."—Mark Twain

Clear, honest, and empathic communication is the cornerstone of collaborative decision-making in both pediatric oncology and palliative care. Caregivers who make decisions for children with high-risk cancer consistently express the need for compassionate delivery of truthful information that uses nontechnical language; this type of communication builds trust and deepens the therapeutic alliance (Feudtner 2007; Kaye et al. 2015; Masera et al. 1998; Levetown 2008; Mack et al. 2006, 2007a, 2009a), while enabling families to make informed decisions about treatment preferences and goals of care (Mack et al. 2006; Wolfe et al. 2000; Weeks et al. 1998; Wright et al. 2008; Apatira et al. 2008). In addition, clear and open communication helps promote the child's participation in decision-making (Levetown 2008).

At the intersection of pediatric oncology and palliative care, the integration of excellent communication principles and practices not only fulfills the legal and ethical mandates regarding informed consent and assent, but it also augments hope and improves coping for children with high-risk cancer and their families (Apatira et al. 2008; Ranmal et al. 2008; Kaye and Mack 2013; Mack et al. 2009b; Hagerty et al. 2005; Davison and Simpson 2006). In addition, skillful communication alleviates suffering (Mack and Grier 2004; Mack et al. 2009a), including anxiety and depression related to the illness and treatment (Last and van Veldhuizen 1996), while improving quality of life (QOL) (Hays et al. 2006) and the overall EOL experience for patients and families (Mack et al. 2009a; Apatira et al. 2008; Davison and Simpson 2006; Hechler et al. 2008). Furthermore, effective communication facilitates collaboration among members of the interdisciplinary team (Feudtner 2007) and reduces administrative barriers to providing holistic care (Vollenbroich et al. 2012), which often leads to improved satisfaction with care for patients and families (Schaefer and Block 2009). Interestingly, the effects of excellent communication are not limited to the illness trajectory of the child: effective communication is also an essential component of grief management and may even mitigate complicated bereavement (Wright et al. 2008; Schaefer and Block 2009; Garrido and Prigerson 2014; Meert et al. 2001). Conversely, ineffective communication often leads to increased distress for patients and families (Contro et al. 2002, 2004; Wallin et al. 2016; Eilertsen et al. 2013; Rosenberg et al. 2015) as well as additional uncertainty, which can adversely impact hope (Hsu et al. 2003).

4.3 What Are the Elements of "Good Communication" in Pediatric Oncology?

> "The difference between the right word and the almost right word is the difference between lightening and a lightening bug."
> – *Mark Twain*

> "It is more fun to talk with someone who doesn't use long, difficult words but rather short, easy words like 'What about lunch?'"
> – *A.A. Milne*

Effective communication involves more than just providing information: it entails the exchange of information in an open, compassionate manner that is responsive to the needs of the patient and family. The AAP has identified three important domains in the communication among the physician, child, and parent: informativeness, interpersonal sensitivity, and partnership building (Levetown 2008) (Table 4.1). A HCP who tailors his or her communication strategy to meet these three domains is encouraging a shared decision-making process, ensuring that difficult conversations about diagnosis, prognoses, treatment, and EOL issues align with the goals of care of the patient and family. Table 4.2 provides the reader with several high-yield models that have been developed to promote effective communication between HCPs, patients, and families, which may be used in conjunction with the fundamental elements of communication outlined by the AAP.

The literature is ripe with strategies for achieving effective communication (Feudtner 2007; Levetown 2008; Eden et al. 1994; Ahmann 1998; Mahany 1990), from which emerge several core tenets pertinent to pediatric oncology and palliative care. First, HCPs should be cognizant that good communication always takes place within the context of a specific patient/family (Clarke et al. 2005; Young et al. 2011; Hinds et al. 2002). Second, HCPs should acknowledge that the patient and family are highly knowledgeable about the patient's experiences and needs, respecting them as "experts" on these issues during difficult conversations (Zwaanswijk et al. 2007). Third, child and adolescent patients should be included in discussions in age-appropriate ways (Parsons et al. 2007; Oshea et al. 2007; Snethen et al. 2006; Young et al. 2003; Hinds 2004; Ruhe et al. 2016; Zwaanswijk et al. 2011; Coyne et al. 2014). Fourth, good communication necessitates conversations about both medical and psychosocial issues, recognizing these spheres as overlapping and inextricably linked (Hinds et al. 2002; De Trill and Kovalcik 1997). Fifth, cultural competency is a fundamental aspect of effective relationship building and communication (Parsons et al. 2007; De Trill and Kovalcik 1997; Surbone 2008; Mystakidou et al. 2004). Perhaps most importantly, when striving to communicate well with young patients, HCPs should remember one simple principle: listen to the child and talk to the child; but listen more than you talk (Zwaanswijk et al. 2007; Beale et al. 2005; Ishibashi 2001).

Table 4.1 Important communication elements for HCPs, children, and parents (Levetown 2008)

Informativeness	The quantity and quality of health information provided by the physician to the patient or family
Interpersonal sensitivity	The relational behaviors that reflect an HCP's interest in eliciting and understanding the feelings and concerns of the family; these behaviors can be verbal or nonverbal and allow the child's or family member's concern to be heard
Partnership building	The extent to which the HCP invites the parents and child to share their concerns, ideas, and expectations; when this is conducted with empathy and a desire to build rapport, the patient and family might be more comfortable sharing their questions, fears, beliefs, and values with the HCP

4.4 Communication Topics Specific to Pediatric Oncology

4.4.1 Sharing a Difficult Diagnosis

Carly is a 9-year-old girl who is energetic, playful, and active in sports. While playing basketball, she injured her left leg, and her pediatrician obtained an x-ray to evaluate for possible occult fracture. The x-ray revealed a large lesion in her left femur, and she was referred to your oncology clinic. She underwent biopsy of the lesion that established a diagnosis of Ewing sarcoma, and an initial staging evaluation revealed multiple bilateral metastatic pulmonary nodules. As her primary oncologist, you sit down with Carly and her parents to inform them of the diagnosis and recommend treatment with standard chemotherapy, limb salvage surgery, and bilateral lung irradiation. Even with the use of these intensive combined treatment modalities, however, you know that Carly's prognosis for long-term survival is around 30%, and if the disease recurs she will be incurable.

Patients with cancer and their families experience high levels of psychosocial stress, and they need HCPs to provide them with accurate timely

Table 4.2 Models to promote "Good Communication"

Communication elements	SPIKES	PACE	SEGUE	Six E's of communication
Preparation	• *S*et up the interview • Assess *p*erceptions of the patient/family • Obtain an *i*nvitation from the patient/family	• *P*lan the setting • *A*ssess the knowledge and needs of the patient/family	• *S*et the stage • *El*icit information	• *E*stablish an agreement about communication • *E*xplore what the patient/family already knows
Informativeness	• Give *k*nowledge and information	• *C*hoose appropriate strategies for information delivery	• *G*ive information	• *E*xplain information according to patient's developmental status and needs
Interpersonal sensitivity	• Address *e*motion with *e*mpathic responses	• *Ev*aluate the understanding of the patient/family	• *U*nderstand the perspective of the patient/family	• *E*ngage the patient/family at the opportune time • *E*mpathize with the emotions of the patient/family
Partnership building and decision-making	• Offer a *s*trategy and *s*ummarize		• *E*nd the encounter	• *E*ncourage the patient/family that you will be there when needed

Adapted from Mack JW, Hinds PS. Practical Aspects of Communication. In: *Textbook of Interdisciplinary Pediatric Palliative Care*; 2011:179–189

information as well as emotional and social support throughout the illness trajectory (Sanson-Fisher et al. 2000; Stark et al. 2002; Zabora et al. 2001). Ideally, optimal communication should begin at the time of a cancer diagnosis, thereby setting the stage for subsequent high-quality communication about future sensitive topics such as prognosis and treatment options. In this way, HCPs can alleviate some of the distress associated with the illness experience (Hack et al. 2012; Zachariae et al. 2003) and improve QOL for patients and families (Girgis et al. 2009).

The period of time when a child receives an initial cancer diagnosis is highly stressful and full of uncertainty, often resulting in significant emotional anguish for patients and families. Compounding these early stressors are other illness-related issues, such as pain related to the underlying pathology and/or the need for invasive procedures to confirm the cancer diagnosis. Tremendous variation exists among patients and families regarding their level of understanding about current health status, diagnosis, prognosis, and treatment options. Therefore, these issues must be communicated in a way that is respectful and responsive to the specific needs of the patient and family. Communication should begin by eliciting the current knowledge, questions, and concerns about the diagnosis from the patient and family. Table 4.3 summarizes several key points to sharing a difficult diagnosis with a child and family.

4.4.1.1 Including Children and Young Adults in Conversations About High-Risk Diagnoses

Decisions about how or when to involve children in discussions about diagnosis and prognosis must be made in consultation with the child's family, recognizing that they know their child best (Young et al. 2003). Whenever possible and reasonable, HCPs should encourage a family to include the child in these conversations. Children who receive upfront, clear, and age-appropriate information about their diagnosis are likely to be better equipped to cope with their illness experience, adhere to medications, communicate openly with their families about fears and concerns, and place trust in their HCPs (Clarke et al. 2005). In a study

Table 4.3 Sharing an initial cancer diagnosis with the child and family

Who	Ask the child and family whom they would like to have present during this conversation
	Encourage parents to include young children in the discussion in an age-appropriate manner
	Advocate for adolescent patients to be present and have a voice in the discussion
	Invite ancillary staff (e.g., nurse, nurse practitioner, social worker, child life specialist, chaplain) to be present for the conversation to provide additional support
Where	Select a quiet, private space. Ideally, the space should have a door that can be closed, sufficient seating for all participants, and tissues positioned for easy access on a side table
	Allow family members to choose their seats; if possible, try not to block their route to the door
When	Initiate the conversation as soon as you have results to share; delaying the communication of bad news only makes the process more difficult
How	Turn your pager and phone to silent before starting the conversation
	Begin with a "warning shot" (e.g., "I am so sorry to tell you this…" or "unfortunately, I have some difficult news to share…")
	Share the news in one to two concise sentences. Speak clearly and slowly. Avoid medical jargon. Use the word "cancer" in your explanation; avoid euphemisms or phrases such as "the C word." Naming the illness is an important step in mitigating uncertainty and fear for both the child and family
	Pause to allow the patient and family space and time to process the information. Allow for silence. Allow for emotions. Resist the urge to fill the silence
	After the patient and family has had a chance to express their emotions, provide 1–2 min of additional information about the next steps
	Reassure the patient and family that this diagnosis is not anyone's fault. Emphasize the fact that they could not have done anything to prevent it
	Ask for questions. Try to encourage questions by asking, "What questions do you have?" (instead of asking, "Do you have questions?"). Validate all questions as excellent. Use simple and clear language in answering questions. Resist the temptation to share additional information if the family has not asked for it. Often, the family is so overwhelmed after receiving a cancer diagnosis that it will remember little of the information that you present in this first meeting
	Sharing a cancer diagnosis is not a "onetime" conversation. Most patients and families will need multiple discussions to help them process this difficult news. Set up a time to meet again in the near future at the convenience of the patient and family. Provide your contact information and encourage the family to be in touch if it has additional questions or concerns before the next meeting

examining the effect of open communication about diagnosis and treatment options, children who received a high level of information experienced less anxiety about undergoing treatment, being in the hospital, and interacting with physicians (Sato et al. 2015). Research on long-term survivors of childhood malignancies likewise indicates that early knowledge of the cancer diagnosis results in improved psychosocial adjustment. In addition, the majority of cancer survivors, parents, and siblings report that they believe a cancer diagnosis should be shared with young patients early on in the disease course (Slavin et al. 1982).

Understandably, some families might still hesitate to include children in difficult conversations at the time of diagnosis, particularly if the child is young and/or the diagnosis carries a poor prognosis. Interestingly, the literature demonstrates that even young children can possess a nuanced, albeit age-appropriate, understanding of their serious illness in a way that enables them to participate in discussions about future treatment options and EOL decisions (Hinds et al. 1999; Weir and Peters 1997; Nitschke et al. 1986).

Despite this data, some parents still struggle to balance their desire to maintain open communication with their child with the desire to protect their child from hearing bad news. In these circumstances, HCPs can ask parents what they think their child already knows. Often times, children are highly perceptive and in tune with their immediate environment, and HCPs can help parents recognize the degree to which the child is already cognizant of his or her illness and encourage honest, age-appropriate conversations to help the child better understand and cope with the new challenges that lie ahead. Some parents also report that involving children in difficult discussions about diagnosis and prognosis is easier if they have an opportunity to first discuss the information with the physician when the child is not present (Young et al. 2011). At the discretion of the family, HCPs can consider offering antecedent separate meetings to parents before including the child, with the goal of helping parents convey honest, age-appropriate information to their child at their preferred time and location and in a manner that aligns with their family's values. Most importantly, however, HCPs should individualize their approach to communication, respecting the cultural and personal preferences of the patient and family unit as much as possible.

In the context of adolescent patients, the literature demonstrates that the vast majority of chronically ill teenagers wish to be involved in the medical decision-making process, with most adolescents preferring to discuss their wishes earlier in the disease course (Lyon et al. 2004). Thus, we strongly recommend that HCPs invite adolescent patients to participate in all medical discussions. This recommendation is consistent with recent literature supporting that adolescents should be enabled and empowered in the medical decision-making process (Weaver et al. 2016). That said, it is also important to recognize that the communication preferences and needs of adolescent and young adult patients are unique (Essig et al. 2016); despite lacking the legal authority for decision-making, they may strive for autonomy and wish to have a voice distinct from their parents during difficult conversations. Depending on developmental stage, individual personality and preferences, and family culture and dynamics, it may be helpful to offer adolescents an opportunity to meet with clinicians without their family present to allow them a safe space to ask questions or express worries that they otherwise might not have expressed.

We also recommend that HCPs encourage an interdisciplinary team approach when communicating a difficult diagnosis in order to provide additional layers of support for the child and family. If the child or family has already bonded with a particular HCP, it can be helpful to invite that clinician to be a part of the conversation; if not, then consider including a clinician who will be providing future care to the patient and family. In addition to inviting physicians, advance practice nurses, and nurses to join the discussion, HCPs should strive to include the patient's social worker, child life specialist, chaplain, or other psychosocial providers to offer additional support to the child and family whenever possible. However, it is essential that HCPs ask permission from the patient and parents before inviting others to participate in these and other sensitive conversations.

4.4.1.2 How Is a Cancer Diagnosis Best Communicated?

Communicating difficult information to patients and families, often in the context of high levels of distress, is among the most challenging and meaningful aspects of an HCP's role within the therapeutic alliance (Arnold and Koczwara 2006). The initial delivery of information can have significant effects, both positive (Ptacek and Ptacek 2001) and negative (Essex 2001; Ablon 2000; Strauss et al. 1995), on a patient's adjustment to the diagnosis. Importantly, patient and family understanding of prognosis also affects future choices for therapy (Fried et al. 2002), and understanding of the burden and likely outcome of treatment may significantly influence goals of care (Fried et al. 2002).

Given the recognized importance of communicating difficult information and the complexity of this information exchange, established guidelines exist to help HCPs navigate the sensitive process of communicating a cancer diagnosis. Table 4.4 highlights key points from two commonly used guidelines related to communicating a diagnosis of cancer to pediatric patients and their families. Additional guidelines to help HCPs provide difficult information to patients and families are detailed in the previous section and in Tables 4.2 and 4.3; each of these strategies may be readily applied to the pediatric oncology context. In particular, the PACE paradigm (*P*lan

Table 4.4 Guidelines for communicating a pediatric cancer diagnosis

SIOP guidelines for communication of the diagnosis[a]	The day one talk[b]
1. Establish a protocol for communication 2. Communicate immediately at diagnosis and follow up later 3. Communicate in a private and comfortable space 4. Communication with both parents and other family members if desired 5. Hold a separate session with the child 6. Solicit questions from parents and child 7. Communicate in ways that are sensitive to cultural differences 8. Share information about the diagnosis and the treatment plan 9. Share information on lifestyle and psychosocial issues 10. Encourage the entire family to talk together	1. Plan the meeting: select a quiet location, minimize interruptions, include important family members or staff 2. Determine if the pediatric patient should be included in the conversation; discuss this with the patient and family ahead of time 3. Ask the patient/family about their understanding of the illness 4. Give the diagnosis; explain certainty or uncertainty; use the word "cancer" to avoid future confusion 5. Discuss treatment options and goals of treatment, assess preferences for receiving information, and provide prognostic information in accordance with these preferences 6. Address causation; offer reassurance (if appropriate) that no one is to "blame."

[a]Masera G, Chesler MA, Jankovic M, et al. SIOP Working Committee on Psychosocial Issues in Pediatric Oncology: Guidelines for Communication of the Diagnosis. Medical and Pediatric Oncology. 1997;28:382–385
[b]Adapted from Mack JW and Greer HE. The Day One Talk. *J Clin Oncol.* 2004;22(3):563–566

the setting, *A*ssess the family's background knowledge and experience, *C*hoose the strategy that best fits the family's particular situation, and *E*valuate the family's understanding of the information) is particularly applicable to communicating a cancer diagnosis to pediatric patients and their family (Garwick et al. 1995). Several iterations of the PACE model exist, incorporating helpful techniques such as the use of a "warning shot" (Fox et al. 2005), which are readily translatable to the pediatric oncology setting.

Regardless of which specific communication guide is used, HCPs who relay difficult diagnostic information to patients and families might consider the following several simple steps. First, HCPs should select a quiet location that allows for a private conversation to occur with minimal interruptions or distractions. Once the patient, family, and HCPs are seated comfortably, one clinician should take the lead in beginning the conversation. Beginning with a "warning shot" can be helpful to allow the patient and family to prepare themselves for hearing bad news. For example, a HCP might open with, "Unfortunately the labs results show us something concerning" or "I am afraid I have some bad news to share."

When conveying a diagnosis of cancer, the actual word "cancer" should be said aloud at the beginning of the conversation to ensure that patients and families understand the situation. The use of euphemisms (e.g., "the monster inside of you") or abbreviations (e.g., "the C word") can be confusing to children and lead to increased stress and fear. Likewise, children and families might not understand that medical words such as mass, tumor, or leukemia are synonymous with cancer, and they might be shocked or upset to learn it at a later time. To preempt this issue, HCPs should avoid medical jargon and technical terms as much as possible. It is common for patients and families to express disbelief of a devastating diagnosis; HCPs should respond with a gentle and consistent message that reiterates the certainty of the diagnosis with a clear explanation of the evidence supporting the diagnosis. After sharing difficult information, HCPs must give patients and families adequate time and space to digest the news. HCPs should be physically and emotionally present for the patient and family and respond to whatever emotions (e.g., tears, anger, frustration, questioning, denial) that arise during this difficult time:

After asking Carly whether she would like to be a part of the discussion, you and your clinic nurse sit down with Carly and her parents. You open by saying, "Tell me about what you think is going on," speaking directly to Carly. You validate Carly's concern that something serious is happening, and then you say gently, "Carly, I am sorry to tell you this, but we have found that you have cancer." Then you stop speaking, and you sit quietly with the family and allow them time and space to express their thoughts and feelings.

After sharing a cancer diagnosis, the discussion should move toward specifics of medical treatments, including the goal of the treatments. For the majority of pediatric patients with a new cancer diagnoses, the goal of treatment is curative. However, for some cancers that have extremely poor prognoses, the goal of any treatment (including upfront cancer treatment) may not be curative, and this information should be honestly and gently disclosed. Some patients and families wish to know comprehensive details regarding diagnosis and prognosis, whereas others prefer to learn information in generalities. HCPs cannot assume to know the preferences of patients and families; for optimal communication, they must ask what type of information the patients and families wish to hear. This can vary from vague statements such as "Overall, most children with this type of cancer do well with treatment" to more specific prognostic statements such as "About 80% of patients with this type of cancer will survive." How much of this information the patient and family absorbed should be reassessed by the team at a later time by asking the family to summarize their understanding of the diagnosis, prognosis, and treatment plan:

"Carly, the biopsy of your leg tells us that you have Ewing sarcoma, which is a type bone cancer." You again pause and allow for silence. "We have good treatments available, but we also know that when the cancer spreads to other places in the body, such as the lung in your case, it is more difficult to treat. I can share with you more specific information, including numbers or percentages, if this is something that you feel might be helpful."

As HCPs take cues from the patient and family regarding information preferences, they should be flexible and adapt to the conversation as necessary. Some patients and families might desire more abstract discussion or analogies (e.g., the weed in the flower garden analogy (Jankovic et al. 1994)), whereas others might prefer to receive more technical information with details regarding pathophysiology and therapeutic options.

After discussing the diagnosis and treatment plan, HCPs should address unspoken issues such as the possible cause of cancer and/or parental guilt associated with delayed diagnosis. Patients and families seeking meaning for the devastating event of a new diagnosis might blame themselves or others for the shocking news (Strauss et al. 1995; Weaver 2014). HCPs can help mitigate guilt and shame by providing reassurance (when appropriate) that no one could have predicted or prevented the cancer from occurring. This reassurance is particularly important for young children (and their siblings) who might experience age-appropriate "magical thinking" and fear that they caused the illness to strike. The unfairness of the situation should also be validated at this time: "I wish I knew what to say…you are right, this is so unfair." Such statements may open the door to further discussions about how the patient and family are feeling and processing the news, thereby offering HCPs insights into how best to offer additional support:

You say, "Carly, sometimes children worry that they might have done something to bring on cancer. I want you know that although we do not know exactly why you developed cancer, we do know that it was not because of anything that you did or did not do. There is nothing that you could have done to prevent this from happening." You pause, and then look at Carly's parents. "The same is true for the rest of the family. We are still learning more about what causes cancer in children, but I want to assure you that there is nothing that you missed or could have prevented. You did exactly the right thing by going to the hospital when you did, and you have brought your child to the right place for her to receive the treatment that she needs."

It is important to remember that communication of a cancer diagnosis is not a one-time event; it is an ongoing communicative process involving multiple conversations, often with various members of the medical team. Commonly, the stress surrounding the diagnosis of a serious medical condition is associated with poor retention of information by both patients and families (Mack and Grier 2004; Kodish et al. 2004), affirming the need for ongoing and iterative exchanges of information among HCPs, patients, and families.

In fact, the majority of parents who receive difficult information about their child's diagnosis understand less than half of the information provided to them at the initial consultation (Mack and Grier 2004; Kodish et al. 2004). Even after iterative discussions with HCPs, parents might continue to misunderstand their child's treatment regimen (Greenley et al. 2006), which underscores the need for information to be conveyed consistently across serial time points.

Given these potential road blocks to clear communication of a diagnosis, HCPs must balance their desire to provide comprehensive medical information during the initial visit with patients' and families' need for adequate time to absorb, understand, and process the provided information. After receiving difficult news, patients and families should be allowed time apart from the medical team and each other to process the information at their own pace (Hinds et al. 2002). In the interim, HCPs may provide a variety of information delivery formats (e.g., written pamphlets or links to accurate and vetted online resources) to help increase the absorption and retention of information, giving families an opportunity to review information after the initial conversation. In our experience, multiple short meetings bolstered by the inclusion of multimedia information offer an effective strategy for communicating an initial cancer diagnosis, prognosis, and treatment plan.

"Carly, I want to pause here to see what question you have," you say. Carly looks at the wall without answering. After about 20 seconds of silence, she shrugs and says, "I don't know." You reply, "That's perfectly ok. Whenever you have a question, you can always ask it at any time." You then turn to her parents and ask, "What questions do you have?" They silently shake their heads, clearly overwhelmed. "There will be plenty of opportunities to ask questions as we move forward," you say. "With your permission, I would like to share with you some information about Ewing sarcoma from our hospital's website, as well as a copy of the treatment plan that we briefly discussed today. There is no rush to start right now, and I want you to take some time to look over everything. We will talk more about it after you have had a chance to talk with one another. I would like to meet with you again tomorrow morning, and I will be happy to answer any questions and talk more about the treatment at that time. In the meantime, please write down any questions or thoughts that occur to you in this notebook, so I can be sure to answer all of your questions. The phone number for our clinic is written on the front of this notebook, in case you need to reach us before tomorrow."

In summary, sharing the difficult news of a new cancer diagnosis with children and families is a challenging process. Key themes to ensure good communication and relationship building during this first conversation include providing clear, individualized communication of information, avoiding euphemisms or medical jargon, paying attention to the emotional aspects of communication, letting the patients and families guide the flow of conversation, and ensuring that HCPs are available to answer questions and concerns raised by patients and families (Ahmann 1998).

4.4.2 Discussing Prognosis in the Context of Disease Progression or Relapse

Carly begins treatment, and she tolerates the chemotherapy and radiation therapy well. She undergoes limb salvage surgery without complications, and she and her parents feel optimistic that she will "beat this cancer." Unfortunately, repeat imaging for disease reevaluation reveals multiple new metastatic lesions in her lungs. You sit down with Carly and her parents to discuss the results of the scans.

Communication with patients and families about devastating information such as disease progression or relapse is distressing for all involved, including HCPs who might delay or "sugar coat" the information (Eggly et al. 2006). Unsurprisingly, parents of children with progressive cancer report that disease progression triggers feelings of uncertainty and fear, further compounding their distress. Patients and families are anxious and overwhelmed when trying to receive, comprehend, and integrate information about prognosis, treatment options, palliative care, EOL care, and hospice near their child's death (Hinds et al. 1997). Unfortunately, parents of children with cancer often feel that they do not receive high-quality information about prognosis at diagnosis or during disease progression (Kaye and Mack 2013; Singh et al. 2015). In the context of disease progression, parent–provider concordance about prognosis and goals is often poor, such that parental understanding that their child will die from the cancer occurs many months after it has become clear to the medical team (Wolfe et al. 2000; Rosenberg et al. 2014; Gordon and Daugherty 2003; Lamont and Christakis 2003). This discordance is exacerbated, at least in part, by the frequent delay of prognosis-related conversations until late in the disease trajectory (Morita et al. 2005; Thompson et al. 2009).

For these reasons, prognosis-related conversations and parental integration of the information early in the disease course are essential to the provision of optimal medical care to children with cancer and their families. Parents who have these conversations and come to an earlier understanding that their child will die report better ability to balance cancer-directed treatment and QOL-focused care, improved satisfaction with care, and opting for less "intensive" EOL care and more hospice care (Mack et al. 2005, 2006, 2007a, b, 2008, 2009b; Hinds et al. 1997; Valdez-Martinez et al. 2014; Mack and Smith 2012; Hill et al. 2014; Feudtner and Morrison 2012; Hinds et al. 2000; Bluebond-Langner et al. 2007). However, it is important to note that "more" is not necessarily better in the context of difficult conversations; excessive discussions about a poor prognosis might be as harmful to patients and families as avoidance of the issue. Many of the strategies for communicating a difficult diagnosis discussed in the previous section can and should be applied in this context as well. Tables 4.5 and 4.6 offer advice for additional communication strategies to use when discussing disease relapse or progression with patients and families and recommendations for language to facilitate a "goals of care" conversation, respectively.

Table 4.5 Communication strategies at the time of disease relapse or progression

Avoid saying…	Try saying…
There is nothing more that we can do	There is no chemotherapy that can cure your cancer. But there is always more that we can do to help you live as well as possible for as long as possible. We will never give up on you, and we will walk with you every step of the way during this difficult journey
It is up to you to decide; I can't make this decision for you	There is no right or wrong answer; the right answer is the one that is best for you and your family. I am here to help you talk through the different options and figure out which one is best for you
Most families choose this option	Different families make different choices. Loving families sometimes choose to receive cancer-directed treatment in the hospital, or to receive outpatient treatment, or to go home with no further cancer-directed treatment. Based on your goals and values, we will work with you to determine which choice is the right one for your child and your family. Any decision that we make together will be rooted in a place of love and wanting the best for your child, and this is how we will know that it is the "right" decision. Regardless of which path we take, our goal will be for your child to live as well as possible for as long as possible
I think that you need to do this option	I am here to help you decide which option is right for you and your family, and I will support and honor your decision to the best of my ability

Table 4.6 Language to "open the door" into a conversation about goals of care

In light of what we have discussed, what is most important to you and your family?
What are your worries?
What are you hoping for? *Validate and share in their hopes, and then ask a follow-up question:* And what else are you hoping for?
Where do you find strength in times of difficulty?
How can we best support you? What would be most helpful to you right now?

During these difficult conversations, HCPs should emphasize that, even if treatment is not working, there is always more that we can do to help the child and family. "More" may refer to further cancer-directed therapy, intensive supportive care, and/or interdisciplinary palliative care. HCPs should never tell a patient of family that "there is nothing more that we can do," as this may be interpreted as abandonment by the patient and family at their time of greatest distress. Instead, HCPs should truthfully acknowledge that there is no intervention that can cure the cancer, but there is always more that can be done to help the patient live as well as possible for as long as possible. HCPs also should inform patients and families that, when faced with difficult decisions, there is not one "right" choice; rather the "right" option is the one that best aligns with the values and goals of care of the patient and family. Additionally, HCPs should be prepared that patients and families might express two seemingly conflicting emotions: understanding of incurability and simultaneous hope for a miracle (Hagerty et al. 2005). This is a normal reaction and does not necessarily imply that the patient or family is in denial or lacks comprehension of the gravity of the situation; rather, it simply demonstrates how hope can serve as a powerful coping mechanism in the process of confronting a painful reality. HCPs should strive to provide honest information while still affirming the right of the patient and family to maintain hope.

You bring Carly and her parents into a private room, and you silence your pager and phone to minimize interruptions. You have invited Carly's primary clinic nurse and her child life specialist to join the conversation, and you wait until everyone is comfortably seated in a circle and then thank everyone for coming. You anticipate that Carly and her parents are very anxious to receive the scan results, so you skip the small talk and open the conversation with a warning shot: "I know that you are anxious to hear the results, and I am so sorry to tell you that the scans show bad news." You pause and allow this information to sink in.

After a few moments, Carly says, "But I did everything right, and you said that my treatments were going well." You nod and affirm her comment: "Yes, you did everything right. Your body handled the medications, radiation, and surgery well, and we were glad that you felt well during the treatments. But sometimes, even when everyone does everything right, the cancer still grows. It is nobody's fault. But it means that we need to talk about what choices we have going forward." Carly's father quickly says, "We want to keep going with the treatment, to beat the cancer once and for all!" You pause and wait to see if anyone else wishes to speak. After a few moments, Carly's mother whispers, "What good will more chemotherapy do, if it didn't stop the cancer from growing?"

You say, "These are both important points for us to talk about. With Carly's type of cancer, once the disease progresses our chances of curing the cancer become very small." You pause again to allow everyone time to process this bad news. No one speaks, and you continue: "I wish that we had better treatments that could cure the cancer. But the truth is that Carly's cancer has progressed despite our best interventions, and we do not have a medication that can cure her disease. But there are still many things that we can do to help her live as well as possible for as long as possible. We are not giving up on Carly, and we will continue to walk with all of you along every step of this difficult journey."

After a moment, Carly's father asks, "So, what are our options now?" You explain that there are 4 possible paths: experimental chemotherapy on a study, with the understanding that the goal of the study is not cure; standard intravenous chemotherapy with the goal of life prolongation, which may entail more severe side effects and more time spent in the hospital; outpatient oral or intravenous chemotherapy administered in the clinic, with the goal of minimizing side effects while still prolonging life; going home with no further cancer-directed care, but with a great deal of supportive care and resources to maximize quality of life. You emphasize that there is no right or wrong answer; loving families chose different paths, and the right choice is the one that best aligns with the goals and needs of Carly and her family.

You pause again, and no one speaks. You sit in silence for several minutes. Then Carly asks, "So, I can go home?" Her mother says tearfully, "I don't know what to do." Her father interrupts, "No! We are going to try an experimental therapy, and pray for a miracle!" You allow for another moment of silence, and then say, "We do not need to decide anything today. Let's plan to meet tomorrow to talk more about the different options. No matter what you choose, I will support and honor your decisions to the best of my ability. And regardless of the path you take, I will hope and pray for a miracle every step of the way along with you."

4.4.3 Discussing Enrollment in Phase I Trials

Clinical research in pediatric oncology often involves the enrollment of children with cancer in clinical trials to study new treatment plans. If the cancer is refractory to available curative therapies, the option to enroll the child in a phase I clinical trial may be presented to the family. By definition, a phase I clinical trial is a dose-finding study conducted to identify the maximum tolerated dose of an investigational therapy; it is not intended or expected to provide a direct benefit to participants, and few phase I clinical trial participants receive any disease-directed benefit (Levine et al. 2015). Unfortunately, often parents (along with HCPs and researchers) possess an overly optimistic view about their child's chance of benefit and believe that participation in a phase I trial will afford their child a disease-directed benefit (de Vries et al. 2011). Parental comprehension of the primary intent of phase I research is reported to be quite low (Cousino et al. 2012; Simon et al. 2004), with little improvement in this understanding over time despite high-quality communication (Marshall et al. 2012). Despite widespread misconceptions about the therapeutic benefit of phase I trials, the majority of parents who attend a consent conference for a phase I trial ultimately enroll their child in the trial (Baker et al. 2013).

Multiple reasons contribute toward the desire of a patient or parent to enroll on a phase I trial, including a wish to prolong life and improve quality of life, altruism, and legacy building (Hinds et al. 2009; Miller et al. 2013). Participation in a phase I trial often aligns with the goals of a patient and family, particularly when the treatments are fairly well tolerated and readily facilitated in an outpatient setting. However, given the potential for iatrogenic harm secondary to participation in a phase I study, HCPs should explain the voluntary nature of phase I trials, the primary intention behind the research, and the low likelihood of direct benefit to participants. Unfortunately, HCPs who discuss phase I protocols with parents often inadequately convey the distinction between medical care and research, as well as frequently incorporate hopeful and persuasive messages when explaining the trial, which encourages enrollment (Miller et al. 2014a). HCPs should ensure that patients and families understand that participation in a phase I trial is unlikely to alter the trajectory of a poor prognosis. Moreover, patients who opt to participate in a phase I trial should be offered concomitant cancer-directed therapy as part of their holistic care (Miller et al. 2014a).

Interestingly, HCPs communicate about phase I trial enrollment more often with parents than with patients. However, direct communication between HCPs and patients is associated with greater levels of patient understanding regarding disease and prognosis (Miller et al. 2014b), which may alleviate some of the stress and uncertainty that plagues the illness experience. We strongly encourage that HCPs engage in an age-appropriate dialogue with children and adolescents with cancer and advocate that informed assent be obtained from all underage patients before participation in phase I trials (Spinetta et al. 2003). A phase I communication model that integrates recommendations from both HCPs and families has been described in the literature; it entails a two-part educational process, including the provision of an informative phase I fact sheet to patients and families prior to the formal informed consent discussion (Johnson et al. 2015).

Communication about enrollment in phase I clinical trials often involves complex interpersonal, psychosocial, and ethical issues (Oppenheim et al. 2005), which fall beyond the scope of this chapter. Open communication and age-appropriate participation of children with cancer in the decision-making process prior to enrollment in a phase I trial, as well as assent to participate, should be prerequisites to their participation.

4.4.4 Communication Around Advance Care Planning

Following Carly's disease progression, you led Carly and her family in multiple conversations about their goals. Carly expressed a desire to go home, but her father remained adamant that she enroll on a Phase I trial in the hopes that she might still be cured. Unfortunately, Carly's pulmonary metastases progress rapidly, making her ineligible for enrollment in a Phase I trial. Over several long conversations, you help the family reach a compromise: since Carly's greatest goals are to visit Disney World and spend time with her friends at home, you coordinate a regimen of chemotherapy with the goals of prolonging her life, minimizing her time spent in the hospital, and allowing her to take short trips in between treatment cycles. Carly and her family use her Make-a-Wish to visit Disney World, and they have a wonderful time.

Carly's father initially declines a palliative care consult, as he equates palliative care with "giving up." You continue to encourage the family to consider consultation, describing the team as "a group of experts whose job is to improve Carly's quality of life and provide support to your family, in whatever way is most helpful to Carly and your family." Eventually, Carly's parents agree to meet with the palliative care team, and they are pleased to learn that they are eligible for a number of home services and resources through a local hospice. Carly's father frequently reminds you, "We are only using hospice because they help us at home, not because Carly is dying." You tell him that you are glad to hear that the services are helpful and that Carly is doing well and enjoying her time at home.

Unfortunately, several days later, Carly acutely develops respiratory distress, and she is admitted to the hospital. Once she is placed on supplemental oxygen, she feels more comfortable. Repeat scans show significant disease progression throughout her lungs, and you share this bad news with Carly and her parents. "What treatment am I going to get next?" Carly asks. You gently reply, "I am so sorry, Carly, but your chemotherapy is not working, and I worry that it may be causing you more harm than good. But we have many different treatments to help your breathing and to make you feel as comfortable as possible." Carly thinks about this for a moment. "Does this mean that I going to die?" she asks you. Her parents are silent, waiting for your response.

Clear, empathic communication from HCPs, while always important, is particularly essential as patients experience further illness progression. Unfortunately, many oncology clinicians self-report a lack of formalized training in communication around difficult topics including advance care planning (Hebert et al. 2009; Buss et al. 2011), leading to a lack of comfort and proficiency in communicating with patients and families during this exceedingly stressful time.

It is important for HCPs to recognize that effective communication about advance care planning does not spring out of a vacuum; it requires a certain degree of preemptive legwork. When HCPs have relationships with patients and families that are built upon trust and mutual respect, communication about prognosis and goals of care can gradually metamorphose into conversations about the EOL in an organic and nonthreatening way (Baker et al. 2007). However, before jumping into a conversation about advance care planning, HCPs should ensure that the right people are present for the conversation, that an appropriate environment is selected, and that all participating HCPs have a comprehensive understanding of the current medical situation (von Gunten et al. 2000) (Table 4.7).

HCPs should begin a conversation about advance care planning by establishing what the patient and family understand. Open-ended questions are valuable for achieving this goal. HCPs

Table 4.7 Steps to follow prior to initiating a conversation about EOL goals

Invite the right people	Whenever possible, the HCP leading a conversation about EOL goals should be someone whom the patient and/or family trust. If this is not feasible due to extenuating circumstances, every effort should be made to include in the discussion other providers (e.g., social worker, child life specialist, chaplain, psychologist) with whom the patient or family have an established rapport
	Ask the patient and family ahead of time about whom they would like to have present in the discussion. Encourage patient participation as much as possible. If the family expresses hesitation about including the patient, explore their feelings and rationale. Invite child life specialists and other psychosocial support providers to help parents and HCPs present information in the most age-appropriate way possible
Plan your time and setting	Select a private, quiet space with minimal distractions. For hospitalized patients, offer to hold the conversation at a location that is separate from the "safe space" of their hospital room, if preferred
	Choose a time at which HCPs will not be rushed or interrupted; ensure that this time is convenient for the patient and family
Do your research	HCPs who plan to attend the conversation need to ensure that they have a good understanding of the patient's medical history, current clinical status, and future potential treatment options
	HCPs need to discuss and resolve any differences of opinion before meeting with the patient and family

should deliver information in a sensitive and straightforward manner, responding empathically to any emotions expressed by the patient and family, validating their shared values and experiences, and affirming the HCP's role as their advocate (Levine et al. 2013). If the HCP feels unsure about what a patient or family member means during a conversation, they should always ask for clarification. For example, a child who asks, "Am I dying?" might be asking a number of different things. She might be experiencing a new or worsening symptom, which she believes to be a harbinger of imminent death. Alternatively, she might be worrying about who will take care of her beloved pet or how her family will get along when she is gone. She might be wondering whether death will hurt or whether she will meet her grandparents in heaven. If we do not ask for clarification, we might miss an opportunity to explore the EOL issues that are most important to the patient and family:

You feel startled when Carly bluntly asks, "Am I dying?" You want to respond honestly to her question, but you feel unsure about exactly what information she is hoping to receive. You gently ask her, "What makes you ask this question?" Carly thinks quietly for a few moments, and then she responds, "I felt like I could not breathe this morning. If I cannot breathe, then does this mean that I am dying today?"

You reply, "I am very glad that you asked this question. You are right that the cancer in your lungs can make it feel hard to breathe. This does not mean that you are dying right now, but it does mean that your lungs are very sick." You pause, and then ask Carly if this makes sense, and she nods "yes." You continue, "We will give you medicines so that your breathing feels more comfortable. Hopefully this will allow you to do the things that you have told me are important to you, like playing with your friends and watching Disney movies." You pause again, and Carly smiles and nods emphatically in agreement.

You turn towards Carly's parents, who have been sitting silently during this exchange. "Carly is so smart, and she is asking such important questions," you tell them. Carly's father looks down at the ground, while her mother nods and begins to cry. "These are such difficult things to talk about," you say. "But perhaps we should begin talking about what might happen when Carly's lungs get sicker. I think it is important for us to discuss what goals you and Carly share, and how we can make sure that our treatments match your goals moving forward."

Initiating and facilitating conversations about advance care planning can be challenging for many reasons. The patient and family might have conflicting goals, or they might share the same goals yet face disagreement from HCPs. To complicate things further, the patient (or parent) might express multiple goals at the same time, some of which might appear contradictory to HCPs, making it difficult to create management plans in alignment with fluctuating goals of care. However, it is important to remember that hoping for cure does not necessarily preclude the recognition of incurable disease and a wish for prolonging a life with quality. HCPs should validate both of these hopes, even if they seem contradictory, and help guide the patient and family toward making decisions that best match their values and goals:

Carly's father says, "I know that she is very sick. I just want Carly to be cured. I feel like she can be cured, if we just pray hard enough." You notice that Carly is watching her mother cry. You tell Carly, "Sometimes your mom cries because she loves you so much, and she wants you to feel better." Carly nods, squeezes her mother's hand, and then goes back to watching her Disney video.

You turn to Carly's parents and say, "I also hope and pray with you that Carly will be cured." You pause for several moments, and then say, "What other things are you hoping for?" There is a long silence. Finally, Carly's father whispers, "I hope that Carly can have as much good time as possible. I pray that she will be comfortable and not suffer." You reply, "I also share this hope with you. We have excellent treatments for Carly's symptoms, and we will do everything possible to ensure that Carly feels comfortable and has as much good time as possible."

You then turn to Carly and ask, "What are you hoping for?" Carly looks at her father and says, "I want to be at home. I hope that I never have to stay overnight in the hospital again." Her mother slowly nods in agreement, while her father remains quiet. "Thank you for sharing this with me," you tell Carly. "Why don't you talk about this with your parents more tonight, and then we can make a plan tomorrow. If this is what your family decides, then we can certainly make arrangements for you to be at home as much as possible. Based on everything that you'd told me, I think that this is very much aligned with your hopes and goals. And as we've discussed before, I recommend that we ask our hospice team to continue helping us achieve these goals. They can bring medications and supplies directly to your home, as well as help you manage symptoms so that you do not have to come into the hospital as frequently. I will work closely with them, and I will continue to walk with you through every step of this journey."

As a patient's illness progresses, it is critical to assess and address the physical, spiritual, and emotional needs of the patient and family (Baker et al. 2008). Including other providers such as psychologists or chaplains in the discussion can ensure additional layers of support as HCPs broach difficult topics such as advance care planning, preferred location of death, limitation or discontinuation of life-sustaining support, and anticipatory grief and bereavement (Rabow et al. 2004). Table 4.8 offers high-yield communication topics to address during a discussion about advance care planning, while Table 4.9 provides examples of statements to avoid and alternative statements to use while communicating with patients and families about EOL issues.

Timely communication about EOL preferences is critical to ensure that care plans honor

Table 4.8 High-yield topics to cover during advance directive discussions over time

Resuscitation status (including ways to ensure that their wishes are followed in the community)
Use of antibiotics, intravenous hydration, parenteral nutrition, and other life-prolonging interventions
Preferred location of care/location of death
Which individuals should be present or called during the dying process (or after death)
Rituals/family traditions/legacy-building wishes at (or after) the time of death
Autopsy

Table 4.9 Communicating with patients and families about EOL issues

Statements to avoid	Alternative statements	Clinical pearls
"Do you understand what I have just told you? Do you have any questions?"	"I have a tendency to use big words and medical language. I have given you a lot of information today. Can you summarize where you think we are right now?"	The term "understand" can be loaded. Consider asking what the family has heard from the medical team instead
"What do you want us to do in case your child's heart stops?"	"Other families have found it helpful to hear recommendations from the team. Would this be helpful to you?"	Always ask permission before giving opinions or recommendations Reference previous discussions about goals of care
"It is time to pull back."	"Let us think about discontinuing treatments that are not helping and may be causing discomfort or harm."	Echo language or phrases that the family has used previously. For example, "You told me that you do not want your daughter to suffer any longer. Let us talk about ways that we can do that."
"There is nothing more that we can do."	"I wish there was more that we could do that would halt the progression of this disease, but none of the treatments we have are able to do this. We are still devoted to taking care of your child and will do everything in our power to keep pain and discomfort away."	Doing everything includes recognizing when the limits of medicine have been reached
"I know/understand how you feel."	"What might be helpful to you at this time? Would you like me to talk with other family members or be with you when you talk to them?"	Bring in a multidisciplinary team and consultants and allow team members to be useful to the family
"This will make you a better/stronger person."	May I sit here with you?	Be present physically and emotionally. Avoid distractions; feel free to respond to the situation with emotions

the wishes of the patient and family, particularly in the context of advance care planning and limitation of life-sustaining treatments that are not in alignment with the goals of the patient and family (Freyer 1992). Parents' choices regarding limitation or discontinuation of medical therapies can be influenced by their past experience, intrinsic personality, emotional state, religious affiliation, or opinions of other family or community members (Sharman et al. 2005). Parents value the recommendations of their child's HCPs (Meert et al. 2000; Carnevale et al. 2006), particularly if they have previously established a trusting relationship with them (Meert et al. 2000). In this way, HCPs can empower patients and families to make decisions that align with their values and represent the best interest of their child and family:

You work with the palliative care and hospice team to allow Carly and her family to leave the hospital and remain at home on supplemental oxygen with close home-based supportive services. Carly continues to come to the outpatient clinic once a week to receive blood products and discuss her symptom management. At her visit today, Carly appears quite comfortable. She tells you, "It is awesome to be at home, since I have all of my toys and my friends come over to play with me." Carly then leaves the room to meet with her child life specialist, who has been working with Carly to explore her hopes and questions about going to heaven through play therapy.

After Carly exits, her parents share that the hospice team has been very helpful in ensuring that Carly has sufficient supplies and medications at home to control her shortness of breath. Carly has grown attached to her hospice nurse, who visits them 2–3 times a week to provide ongoing symptom assessment and management. You tell Carly's parents how glad you are that Carly is feeling well and enjoying quality time at home. You then say, "I wonder if now might be a good time for us to plan ahead, like we discussed at our last visit. Just as we made a plan to control Carly's shortness of breath, we always want to prepare for the worst while still hoping for the best."

You pause, and sit in silence for several moments as Carly's mother nods and her father stares at the floor. You then say, "I am so sorry that we are having this conversation. It is so difficult to talk about this. But in my experience, it is better to have these discussions while Carly is doing well, as opposed to waiting until a time when she is very sick. Would it be okay if we talked about what you and Carly would want, in the event that her lungs become very sick and she was unable to breathe on her own?" Carly's mother begins to cry, and she takes her husband's hand and nods again, inviting you to speak.

You briefly summarize Carly's current medical situation: "We know that the cancer is in Carly's lungs, and our treatments are not able to stop it from growing. I think it is likely that Carly's lungs will continue to worsen over the next few weeks. We will give her medications and do everything possible to keep her comfortable so that she does not feel shortness of breath. But unfortunately, we do not have treatments that can make her lungs healthy again." You pause, and then ask Carly's parents what questions they have; both parents shake their heads and remain silent.

You continue, "Eventually, Carly's lungs will become so sick that she will stop breathing, and this will cause her heart to stop beating. We could put a breathing tube into her lungs and connect her to a machine that breathes for her, and push on her chest and shock her with electricity to try to make her heart beat again. But I worry that these interventions would cause harm to Carly, without offering her any benefit or changing the progression of her disease. Even if we were able to keep Carly alive, she would not be able to breathe without the machine, and she would need to be very sedated to prevent her from suffering." You pause again to allow Carly's parents time to process this information.

After a minute, you say, "Based on what Carly and you both have told me in the past, it sounds like your goals are for Carly to be able to spend as much quality time as possible at home and to avoid being in the hospital. Given your goals, my recommendation would be for Carly to remain at home and to receive medications to ensure that she is comfortable at the end of her life." Her mother quietly says, "I do not want Carly to go through any more suffering. I want her to stay at home." Her father does not speak, but eventually he nods. You tell her parents that this is a loving decision and that the team will do everything possible to prevent Carly from suffering. You then provide Carly's parents with state-specific paperwork that delineates your mutually-agreed upon recommendation for "Do not attempt resuscitation," explaining that this form will ensure that all healthcare providers respect these wishes in the community.

4.4.4.1 Involving Pediatric Patients in End-of-Life Discussions

HCPs should encourage families to include children and adolescents in EOL discussions in age-appropriate ways in order to address fears, answer questions, and provide anticipatory guidance (Levine et al. 2013). The use of open-ended

Table 4.10 Recommendations for responding to the question, "Am I dying?"

Strategy	Example language
Begin with reassurance that you will answer the child's question	"I promise to answer your question…"
Obtain more information about the child's motivation for asking the question	"…but first it would be helpful for me to know why you are asking this question." "Are you willing to share with me what you are thinking about?"
Elicit information about the child's concerns	"What are you most worried about?"
Validate the child's questions and worries	"You are asking very important questions." "What a good question. I can see that you are worried about [x] and/or feeling [y]."
Ask the child to share his/her preference for receiving information	"What would be most helpful for you to know right now?"

questions is a valuable strategy for eliciting what the patient believes about his or her condition, addressing misconceptions, and providing reassurance. Children with life-threatening conditions often possess a more advanced understanding of death and dying than do their healthy peers, and they may benefit greatly from having opportunities to communicate openly about their thoughts and feelings regarding their illness experience (Masera et al. 1999). Table 4.10 offers several recommendations for language to consider using in response to a child's question, "Am I dying?"

Adolescents similarly benefit from having an invitation to express their EOL preferences by using communication and advance care planning tools such as *Voicing My Choices* (Wiener et al. 2012). Unfortunately, adolescents often feel marginalized during medical discussions (Young et al. 2003); including them in important conversations and allowing them to participate in decision-making is an important strategy to empower them, increase hopefulness, and overall impact their care in a positive way (Hinds 2004).

Despite the data to support the need for open communication with pediatric patients about EOL issues, many families struggle to discuss such difficult topics with their children. This is understandable, and HCPs should meet families where they are and help them begin to work toward improving communication in a way that feels right for their family. For certain families, HCP might consider sharing the results of a study that found that none of the bereaved parents who communicated with their children about death regretted this decision (Kreicbergs et al. 2004). HCPs should also share with families that many children and adolescents at the EOL are cognizant of their imminent death, encouraging them that addressing the "elephant in the room" may actually alleviate stress for both the patient and family (Wolfe 2004). We recommend that HCPs use an interdisciplinary approach, involving child life specialists, chaplains, psychologists, social workers, and any other supportive clinicians to work with parents who are reticent to communicate with their dying child, encouraging them to consider how open communication might benefit the patient and family as a whole. Further recommendations about including siblings in these important conversations are discussed in a following section.

4.4.5 Communication During the Bereavement Period

Over the next 2 weeks, Carly's shortness of breath and pleuritic chest pain acutely worsen. With help from the palliative care team and the local hospice group, you are able to ensure that her symptoms remain well-controlled at home. During this time, multiple members from Carly's interdisciplinary care team remain closely involved in her care, speaking daily with her parents to provide them with support, manage her evolving symptoms, and offer information about what to expect at the EOL. Ultimately, Carly dies peacefully at home surrounded by her family. Over the following months, her parents struggle to regain a sense of normalcy. They later reflect that losing their daughter was made more difficult by the simultaneous loss of the community of HCPs who had become like family to them during their difficult journey.

The death of a child is an unimaginable and devastating event that results in profound grief for parents. Bereaved parents frequently experience debilitating feelings of shock, helplessness, and guilt (Higgs et al. 2015), and for many the grief journey can be intense and prolonged (Michon et al. 2003; Snaman et al. 2016a). These grief reactions may be compounded by other losses, such as the loss of support from the child's medical team (Back et al. 2009). Parents might experience the loss of this bond as a type of abandonment, thereby exacerbating the bereavement journey (Contro et al. 2004).

In addition, intrinsic factors such as language barriers can interfere with adjustment during the bereavement process (Koop and Strang 1997). Situational factors surrounding the death and bereavement period can also influence the grief response. Some situational factors, such as the suddenness of an unexpected death, cannot be changed; however, other factors, such as the availability, emotional attitudes, and communication skills of HCPs, can be optimized (Steele et al. 2013). Parents' cognitive coping resources, emotional attitudes of staff, and adequacy of the information provided to parents can predict the intensity of long-term grief (Koop and Strang 1997). As expected, parental perception of an uncaring emotional attitude of staff has a detrimental effect on coping with short- and long-term bereavement, whereas a caring attitude by staff has beneficial effects on coping with short- and long-term bereavement (Meert et al. 2001).

As we have discussed above, a HCP's ability to provide transparent and empathetic information to families is a critical aspect of holistic care (Weaver et al. 2016), and this includes delivery of compassionate, honest, complete, and caring information (Contro et al. 2004; Mack et al. 2005; Meert et al. 2008a, 2009; Neidig and Dalgas-Pelish 1991). Empathetic delivery of difficult news or discussion of EOL topics, including prognostication delivered in the context of a caring relationship, is associated with lower levels of long-term parental grief (Mack et al. 2007b; Zelcer et al. 2010). Specifically, discussions held near the EOL that center on goals of care are associated with the use of less aggressive medical care near death, which in turn is associated with better adjustment to bereavement (Wright et al. 2008). In one study, more than 50% of caregivers of pediatric cancer patients reported regret about their EOL care; however, communication about advance care planning helped caregivers adjust better to bereavement (Garrido and Prigerson 2014).

Communication with families of children who are managed in the intensive care unit (ICU) is particularly important to mitigate complicated bereavement. Empathic communication skills with families of patients in the ICU can improve family satisfaction and reduce adverse bereavement outcomes (Schaefer and Block 2009). Parents whose children died in the pediatric ICU have highlighted the critical importance of the communication style of the physician who gave the "bad news." (Meert et al. 2008b) The most common communication issue identified by parents is physician availability and attentiveness to their informational needs. Other communication issues are honesty and comprehensiveness of information, affect with which the information was provided, withholding of information, providing false hope, complexity of vocabulary, pace of providing information, contradictory information, and physicians' body language.

The significant sequelae experienced by grieving parents highlight the need for ongoing care and resources targeted specifically to this bereaved population (Michon et al. 2003). A multidisciplinary approach is needed to provide optimal bereavement care to parents (Higgs et al. 2015). Pediatric palliative care emphasizes the provision of holistic care designed to address the physical, psychological, social, and spiritual needs of patients and families throughout the illness course and into the bereavement period (Kaye et al. 2015). Importantly, parents were more likely to have received EOL anticipatory guidance and bereavement support if their child was referred to a palliative care team (Kassam et al. 2015), which highlights the important role of pediatric palliative care providers in the holistic care of children with cancer and their families.

Unsurprisingly, bereaved parents identify communication as a top priority during both the EOL and bereavement periods (Hinds et al. 2005) and highlight the importance of continuity of care extending beyond death (Steele et al. 2013). Specifically, families express a desire to remain connected to their child's HCPs even after the child's death (Steele et al. 2013; Snaman et al. 2016b). Unfortunately, the bulk of supportive services are offered during illness and at the EOL, with limited resources available to families after a child's death. Thus, many families receive little or no bereavement follow-up (Bradshaw et al. 2005). Yet parents who lose a child to cancer specifically express a desire to talk with those HCPs who cared for their child as an important aspect of their grief process (Snaman et al. 2016a, b; Jankovic et al. 1989; Lichtenthal et al. 2015). Even a simple phone call from a member of a deceased child's healthcare team to a bereaved parent affords an opportunity to remind a family that their child is not forgotten, screen bereaved relatives at risk for complicated grief for potential adverse outcomes, and link families to helpful resources in their local communities (Jankovic et al. 1989; Lichtenthal et al. 2015). Whether formal or informal, contact between HCPs and families during the bereavement period offers valuable meaning-making opportunities for parents, including making sense of their child's death, exploring positive outcomes such as volunteering or giving back to other families going through similar hardships, and promoting legacy-building opportunities to strengthen bonds with the decreased child (Snaman et al. 2016a; Meert et al. 2015).

The fact that bereaved families often wish to continue relationships with their child's HCPs suggests the importance of developing an institutionally based bereavement program to support families throughout their grief journey (Mullen et al. 2015). Table 4.11 offers a list of recommendations for HCPs to consider when providing support for bereaved parents (Snaman et al. 2016a).

4.4.6 Communication About Spirituality

Spiritual conversations are a significant and vital avenue for HCPs to explore in an effort to improve QOL for cancer patients and their families (Peteet and Balboni 2013). Communication about spirituality influences goal-directed decision-making and may reduce the use of intensive interventions in patients with advanced cancer at the EOL (Peteet and Balboni 2013; Balboni et al. 2013). Acknowledging the spiritual needs of children and adolescents with cancer, in particular, can help them cope with their illness (Proserpio et al. 2014). Because the concerns of

Table 4.11 Directives for providing grief support to bereaved parents

Communicate with patients and families clearly and honestly, providing accurate and timely information to allow them to participate in shared medical decision-making while taking into account goals of care and working to support decisions made by families
Involve bereaved parents in the design and implementation of communication training for healthcare staff
Show empathy as a part of a continuing and strong bond between HCPs and the patient and family. Find ways to continue to be involved with the family after the child's death, and work to continue the established therapeutic alliance
Acknowledge that the HCP identify might shift from a cure-focused medical provider to a companion on the parent's grief journey. Do not try to "fix" the hole in the heart of bereaved parents. Instead, recognize, acknowledge, and bear witness to its presence
Embrace the opportunity and challenge of initiating difficult conversations with patients and families throughout the disease process. Avoid giving false hope or offering unrealistic treatment choices. Enhance efforts at communication and ensure continuity of care around times of transition (e.g., between different care settings)

Adapted from Snaman JM et al. Helping parents live with the hole in their heart: The role of healthcare providers and institutions in the bereaved parents' grief journeys. *Cancer* 2016;122(17):2757–65 children and adolescents are primarily relational, spiritual chats with a trusted HCP can help them examine significant relationships with others, the sacred, and the self (Kamper et al. 2010). Spiritual conversations enable children and adolescents to deepen their feelings of personal value, personal empowerment, and overall peacefulness (Hart and Schneider 1997).

Although HCPs acknowledge that spiritual care is an important part of holistic care, cancer patients report that HCPs do not frequently provide spiritual care (Peteet and Balboni 2013). Even clinicians who recognize the benefits of spiritual care and are attentive to patient cues face professional and personal barriers that might prevent them from engaging in spiritual communication. Professional barriers include lack of professional training in spiritual care, time constraints, role uncertainty, and lack of administrative support (Rassouli et al. 2015). Personal barriers include fear and ambiguity about how they can talk with their patients about things they personally do not believe in or do not understand.

Let us consider a scenario in which our patient Carly, during a routine clinic, visit suddenly asks, "Why does God let kids get sick, and some die?" This question might feel unsettling, but it offers a great opportunity to promote positive spiritual well-being and enhance Carly's overall care. Before responding, it is important to recognize that children react to difficult circumstances according to their personal developmental trajectories (Hart and Schneider 1997). Key spiritual needs for a 9-year-old child include acceptance, love, recognition, security, compassion, and trust. Important spiritual concerns for a 9-year-old child include abandonment, chaos, guilt, fear, isolation, lack of trust, feelings of being punished, shame, and violation.

Carly's question might make us speculate that she feels any or all of the above spiritual concerns. However, we do not want to operate on speculation or come across as if we have an answer or "easy fix" for her difficult question. Our goal should be to frame the conversation in an age-appropriate way that allows Carly to define what is most important to her (Lima 2013).

Our first instinct might be to respond to Carly's difficult question with a spiritual cliché, such as "We must trust in God's will." Offering one of these comments might make us feel better, but it will likely not address Carly's specific concerns nor assuage her spiritual distress. Carly may be contemplating the impossible to answer such as mystery, justice, meaning, and mortality. Rather than wanting an answer, she wants someone to listen. She might even be testing you to see how honest, open, and nonjudgmental you are. She is seeking compassion, someone to suffer with her, and someone with the courage to hear her pain (Hart and Schneider 1997). She needs someone willing to be flexible, honor her pace, and not push an agenda onto her.

We also must remember that children process large issues in small bites. They typically do not spend hours having complex, nuanced discussions. They might talk for a few minutes, self-distract, and then return to the conversation later. When responding to a child's spiritual inquiry, it is best to provide short responses and then pause to see if he or she wishes to continue the conversation. Table 4.12 details those spiritual clichés that HCPs should try to avoid and potential responses to use instead during spiritual conversations. The responses in Table 4.12 help us model our human vulnerability for children. Professional competency is not compromised by vulnerability; rather, relationships are enhanced by it. Such responses invite the child to explore spiritual needs and help us identify potential concerns that reflect negative religious coping (Balboni et al. 2010). Soothing appropriate responses also help create a safe place for trust and leave the door open for future communication.

Often, prayer is an appropriate and welcome response to a spiritual concern (Hart and Schneider 1997). It is not, however, a magic bullet or a tool to pull out of our bag every time we feel uncomfortable. Prayer should be used sparingly and potently, and it needs to reflect the content of the conversation. Before praying, it is important to ask the patient or family if there is anything specific that they wish to include in the prayer. Table 4.13 describes the steps in introducing the idea of prayer to the child and

Table 4.12 Communicating with children about spiritual issues

Spiritual clichés to avoid	Possible responses to try
"You know, Carly, we have to accept God's will. He knows best."	"I struggle with the same questions. It does not seem fair does it?"
"You do not have to worry about dying. You are going to be okay."	"I can see that you feel worried. These are very normal feelings to have. Can you share with me what things are worrying you the most right now?" "It must make God very sad when a child gets cancer or dies. Do you think it makes God sad?"
"God knows more than we know. Perhaps it is best not to question."	"It can be hard to have questions or worries, and not know the answers. Is there something specific that is keeping you up at night?" "Sometimes when I have questions for God I ask God. Do you talk to God when you have questions? Are there other people you talk with when you have questions or worries?"
"Sometimes God needs to bring a child to heaven for a special mission."	"I'm very sorry you are sick. I really love (or like) you and I believe that there are many other people who love you, too." "I also believe that God loves you. Do you believe God loves you?" "What does heaven mean to you?"

Table 4.13 Strategies to introduce the idea of prayer to children with cancer: specifically for use by chaplains or other clinicians who feel comfortable with prayer

Steps to introduce the idea of prayer	Example language to use
If appropriate in the context, offer an invitation for prayer	"Carly, sometimes it helps people feel better when someone prays for them. Would you like me to pray with you?"
If the patient (or family) says "No," do not try and talk them into it or proceed without their assent	"Not everyone likes to pray, and that is okay. If you change your mind, you can let me know."
If the patient says "Yes," ask her to help you shape the prayer	"Carly, is there anything special you would like for us to pray about together?"
Before praying, position yourself at eye level, or close proximity, of the child	–
Some people like to hold hands or place a hand on the patient. Use your best clinical judgment in doing so; some people appreciate touch whereas others do not	–
Make the prayer short and to the point	"Dear God, Carly and I do not understand why children have to be sick and die sometimes. It seems unfair and makes us feel sad. Carly is a sweet and special girl. Everyone at our hospital loves her. We pray that she will not be in pain. We pray that when she feels afraid she will know we are here for her. And we pray that she will know that both you and I care about her. Amen."

family. Lastly, HCPs should not offer or accept an invitation to pray if they do not feel comfortable doing so. Particularly for patients with religious and cultural traditions different from those of the HCP, professional assistance from a chaplain or clergy person familiar with the patient's faith might be helpful.

In summary, children and adolescents have unique spiritual needs. As they deepen their relationships with their loved ones, their caregivers, and with God, they can derive personal value and empowerment (Hart and Schneider 1997). As practitioners, we have the responsibility and privilege to assist in nurturing the spiritual lives of children and adolescents with serious illnesses. Being alert, present, competent, and self-aware can help us identify the right moment—the sacred moment—at which to participate in the spiritual conversations that lead to optimal holistic care and deepen our patients' and our own humanity.

4.5 Communication Barriers in Pediatric Oncology and Palliative Care

"The most important thing in communication is hearing what isn't said."
– Peter Drucker

Although most HCPs strive to communicate effectively with patients and families, several barriers can hinder the best of intentions. Oncologists self-report that fear of causing distress and fear of abrogating hope are impediments to clear and honest communication of difficult prognostic information (The et al. 2000; Kodish and Post 1995; Miyaji 1993). Prognostic uncertainty (Lamont and Christakis 2003; Christakis and Iwashyna 1998) and paternalism involving a perception that the patient or family will be unable or unwilling to hear bad news (Parsons et al. 2007; Singh et al. 2015; Goldie et al. 2005) also contribute to ineffective or misleading communication. Oncologists acknowledge that poor communication secondary to avoidance of difficult information can stem from feelings of failure born from a realization that the patient might die (Thompson et al. 2009; Davies et al. 2008; Knapp and Thompson 2012; Knapp et al. 2008; Hilden et al. 2001). In addition, effective communication with children carries a unique set of challenges and requires specialized training in age-appropriate communication styles and strategies, which many oncologists do not receive. Non-physician providers who care for children with cancer face similar challenges as do their physician colleagues, which can result in self-reported feelings of anxiety during discussions about prognosis and goals of care with seriously ill children and their families (Masera et al. 1997; Contro et al. 2004; Feudtner et al. 2007).

Many of the above barriers are exacerbated by insufficient training in communication skills (Contro et al. 2004; Singh et al. 2015; Sanderson et al. 2015; Collins 2002) and lack of adequate communication role modeling (Hilden et al. 2001) for trainees and clinicians early in their career. In pediatric oncology, the lack of formalized palliative care education is increasingly recognized as a critical deficit in training (Fowler et al. 2006). In a 1998 survey, 90% of pediatric oncologists reported that they learned to manage dying children on the job and did not receive structured didactics or role modeling (Hilden et al. 2001). Although this percentage has decreased over the past decade, a 2014 Institute of Medicine report highlights the insufficient attention given to palliative care training and the failure to equip physicians with adequate communication skills (Institute of Medicine 2014). At the end of this chapter, we discuss the current status of communication-based training specific to pediatric oncologists and offer strategies for overcoming some of the barriers described above through formalized educational paradigms.

However, not all barriers to communication arise from HCPs; patients and parents can also contribute to the obstruction or delay of effective communication. The emotional state and receptiveness of patients or families to receiving difficult news can affect an HCP's ability to successfully transmit information or build rapport (Eden et al. 1994). Providers must be sensitive to the emotional fragility of patients and families. Good communication is a marathon and not a sprint: if the child or family cannot participate in an in-depth conversation for emotional reasons, the HCP should consider rescheduling the meeting to allow the patient and family time to collect themselves prior to engaging in the conversation.

The preferences, beliefs, and past experiences of the patient or family can also influence their ability to share or receive information from HCPs. For instance, depending on the patient's or family's frame of mind and prior circumstances, communication about goals of care can be mistaken for "giving up," which can result in fracturing of the therapeutic alliance (Jünger et al. 2010; Friedman et al. 2002; Claxton-Oldfield and Marrison-Shaw 2014). It is imperative that HCPs make careful language choices that facilitate reframing goals of care (Hill et al. 2014), as opposed to engendering feelings of abandonment. Patients and families might also have differing opinions about which topics are the most important to discuss. In one study, HCPs placed a higher importance on having conversations about death and dying whereas parents prioritized discussions about spiritual support and having the option for their child to receive cancer-directed therapy during the last month of life (Kassam et al. 2013). As such, even the most honest and empathic communication is only effective if it offers content valuable to the listener. Effective communication begins with the HCP asking what the child and family hopes to learn and in what way they wish to receive the desired information.

Parents might also choose to withhold difficult information from children in an effort to protect them, thereby compromising open lines of communication and placing the HCP in a difficult position (Last and van Veldhuizen 1996; Parsons et al. 2007; Singh et al. 2015; Gupta et al. 2010; Case Conference 1985). Balancing clinician respect for both the autonomy of the patient and the values of the family unit can be challenging (Young et al. 2003; Hinds 2004). We discuss strategies to overcome this barrier in the next section.

4.6 When Communication Does Not Go Well

Although honest communication with children about EOL care has been shown to be beneficial for both children and families (Kreicbergs et al. 2004), initiating these conversations can be challenging. A particularly difficult scenario for HCPs occurs when parents wish to withhold information from an ill child. In this section, we will discuss the difficulties inherent to this situation and offer strategies to help open the lines of communication while fortifying the therapeutic relationship among the HCP, patient, and family:

> *Imagine a scenario in which Carly's parents refused to discuss her cancer with her. Perhaps they felt that they needed to shield Carly from the truth about her illness in order to fulfill their roles as "good parents." Or perhaps they worried that if Carly knew that she was dying, she would "give up." Alternatively, her parents might have felt that telling Carly the truth would cause anxiety or be too much for her to bear. For whatever reason, consider a situation in which Carly's parents ask you not to tell Carly that her disease is progressing.*

Children, like adults, need information to help them prepare for the future and cope with receiving a potentially life-altering diagnosis such as cancer (Clarke et al. 2005). If they do not receive clear information about their illness, children may generate their own ideas about what is wrong by imagining a scenario worse than the truth, seeking out information from friends, or looking on the internet for answers. Very young children also employ "magical thinking," in which they harbor the misconception that their illness is a form of punishment for something that they thought, said, or did. Despite the fact that children who receive honest information about their diagnosis have less anxiety than those who are not told, some parents still prefer not to disclose diagnostic or prognostic information in an effort to protect their child (Clarke et al. 2005). This act of withholding information often results in discomfort and ethical consternation for HCPs (Slavin et al. 1982; Claflin and Barbarin 1991).

It is important for HCPs to remember that parents who wish to withhold information from their children do so because that they believe that it is in the child's best interest. Parents might feel that their child is too young to fully understand the complexities of a diagnosis such as cancer, and they might wish to shield their child from abstract concepts such as illness and death (Zwaanswijk et al. 2011). However, even children who are too young to understand the implications of disease are capable of perceiving changes in their environment and routine and may act out as they try to make sense of unpredictable deviations from the daily norm. Changes in behavior, however subtle, suggest that the child feels the need to communicate a question or fear. Children might not understand the medical language used by physicians to discuss illness and treatment; however, children come to understand their diagnosis and prognosis over time by reading the expressions on the faces of people they love, the body language of their medical teams, the tone and pace of speech used to talk about them, the urgency with which they receive treatment, and the signals they receive from their own bodies. HCPs need to help parents understand that these collective experiences often culminate into a sophisticated understanding of death and dying that can be expressed by children as young as 3 years of age (Bluebond-Langer 1980).

When parents express concerns about their child's ability to understand, it can be helpful to involve the services of a certified child life specialist (CCLS). CCLSs are trained to assess a child's individual informational needs and break down complex medical information into language appropriate to the child's cognitive and social-emotional stage of development. CCLSs are also trained to provide play-based interventions to assist children in assimilating new information about their changing world and to help them share thoughts, worries, and wishes that they might not be able to express with words alone. Children often reveal much of what they understand through their art or dramatic play. These moments can serve as evidence to resistant parents that their child does indeed comprehend far more about his or her condition than the parents believe. Thus, the child's play becomes an avenue for continued discussion between the parent and specialist about the importance of disclosing developmentally appropriate information. Working directly with a CCLS often allays the common parental fear of saying the wrong thing or saying too much.

For some parents, objections might not be related to the child's age or development, but rather stem from a fundamental parental instinct to protect the patient from an ugly reality. In an attempt to shelter the patient, some parents might refuse to engage their children in conversation or refuse to allow others to share information with them (Young et al. 2003). In these extreme cases, a well-intentioned desire to protect the child may result in considerable harm by damaging the trust between parents and the child. Conversely, children and adolescents who have a better understanding of their illness and mortality possess a sense of autonomy and control that enables coping and resiliency (Bates and Kearney 2015).

HCPs shoulder the responsibility of informing hesitant parents of the benefits of involving children and adolescents in conversations about their illness. Ideally, a child's early involvement will enhance his or her skills in the process of participating in future decision-making (Levetown 2008). Some families might require an extended period of time to adjust to receiving a cancer diagnosis; for these parents, a stepwise approach to including their child in conversations can be beneficial. Explaining that diagnostic disclosure is a process and that prognosis needs to be treated as a separate issue can also help parents to accept diagnostic disclosure (Cole and Kodish 2013).

If parents explicitly state that they do not wish for anyone to speak with their child about diagnosis or prognosis, it is important to recognize that this is where conversations *begin* and not where they end. HCPs need to approach this situation with respectful curiosity and use the inherent opportunity to learn more about the family's values and concerns. Refusal to talk is often a reflection of fear, and HCPs need to better understand the nature of this fear before attempting to address it. This often involves talking with parents about who they believe their child to be and listening with a willingness to be influenced by what the parents share. HCPs can approach these conversations in different ways; the ultimate goal is not to change the parents' mind but to communicate a genuine desire to see the child through the parents' eyes.

Misconceptions about the child's illness and treatment, previous negative medical experiences, and worry that the truth will depress or steal hope away from the child also may adversely impact a parent's willingness to disclose information to their child. It is important to explore these themes when there is parental resistance against open communication with the child. Table 4.14 offers open-ended questions to help guide a difficult conversation between HCPs and resistant parents.

In the worst-case scenario, parents might not waver from their intention to conceal the truth from their child. In this case, it is the ethical responsibility of the medical team to set clear boundaries with the parents going forward. HCPs should explain in a frank but compassionate manner that they will not lie overtly to the child. If the patient asks a direct question, it is the HCP's obligation to answer it truthfully and in a manner appropriate to the child's

Table 4.14 Open-ended questions or statements to guide difficult conversations between HCPs and resistant parents

"I hear how important this is to you. Can you please tell me more about your concerns?"
"How are you and your family talking about this illness at home?"
"What words are you comfortable with or not comfortable with?"
"What has this illness been like for you/your child/your family?"
"What questions do you think your child will ask?"
"What do you believe your child to understand about his/her illness?"
"What are your fears/hopes for your child?"
"What concerns you the most right now?"
"Does your family have a faith tradition that your child shares in?"
"I can't imagine what this must be like for you."

developmental level. However, HCPs can offer to compromise with parents by answering the child's questions in a language that aligns with the family's belief system or by providing parents with the language and skills to disclose the information themselves.

Methods for sharing medical information with children can vary significantly, depending on the child's social-emotional and cognitive developmental levels, the spirituality and culture of the family, and the individual preferences of the child and family. To effectively engage children in medical conversations in a meaningful way, all these factors need to be individually assessed and incorporated into the HCP's approach toward the patient and family. There is no one right way or answer for every child or parent; however, these considerations can help the HCP determine an appropriate starting point and identify the subsequent steps for facilitating honest communication about the life-threatening illness with the child and parents.

4.6.1 Practical Suggestions to Improve Communication in Difficult Situations

Traditional models of communication within the medical system generally involve asking direct questions to the patient and/or the family and receiving a series of "yes" or "no" responses. The nature of this design places the HCP in control of the exchange and creates little opportunity for the patient or family to identify areas of personal concern or ask the questions that are most relevant from their perspectives. Although this HCP-driven process was once thought to be time-efficient, it is effective only if the HCP asks the right questions. Otherwise, the HCP can spend the entire interaction asking about issues that the patient and family do not perceive as pertinent to their health or circumstance (Boyle et al. 2005). This strategy becomes particularly problematic in the context of a fractured therapeutic alliance.

When communicating with the patient and family in difficult situations, an open-ended approach to communication is often a more time-efficient method for gathering information, assessing the problem, and identifying potential solutions. As HCPs listen carefully to the patient and family, differences in perception and perspective are revealed: a "problem" can appear quite different from varying viewpoints. For example, the medical team might perceive the primary problem to be disease progression, while the family might perceive it to be the team's lack of faith that a miracle is possible. Asking the family to share its sense of the current situation and what it means to them can enable the medical team to compare and contrast the assessments of the situation. Promoting this inquiry might reveal that the discord between HCPs and the patient and family arises because each party focuses on different issues. In such cases, reframing the goals of HCPs and the patient and family into a mutually shared purpose can resolve the conflict (Feudtner 2007).

Although interview styles vary by HCP, certain standard questions can help HCPs and the patient and family resolve the differences in perception and perspective. Table 4.15 offers questions to assist HCPs in aligning the medical team's goals with those of the patient and family.

4.6.2 Interdisciplinary Communication: The Importance of Debriefing After Difficult Encounters

Regardless of a HCPs discipline or years of clinical experience, walking with a family at the time of the child's death can be physically and emotionally taxing. HCPs might experience disenfranchised grief, which is the grief one feels when he or she has suffered a loss that is not recognized as meaningful by society, such as the loss of a patient (Kaye 2015). Learning to manage grief responses to patient deaths is a crucial, yet underemphasized, skill for HCPs. HCPs who cannot manage their grief in healthy and constructive ways might find themselves avoiding patients who evoke heightened emotional responses or find their personal lives affected by unresolved feelings of angst or sadness (Keene et al. 2010).

In such instances, debriefings can serve as a high-yield tool for supporting staff as they experience emotional reactions to patient deaths and can also improve communication across disciplines. Team debriefings build emotional resiliency, strengthen team bonds, and reduce a sense of isolation in the workplace (Granek et al. 2015). Debriefings are frequently used to assist teams that might be dealing with physical or emotional signs of distress after the traumatic death of a patient or other challenging events within the hospital (Berg et al. 2014). Integrating debriefing sessions into the standard training of residents and fellows can provide opportunities for staff to learn effective strategies for dealing with patient deaths from experienced physicians (Granek et al. 2015; Eng et al. 2015). Offering debriefing sessions is one example of support that an institution can provide as part of a multifaceted approach to support staff. Table 4.16 offers basic guidelines for facilitating successful debriefing sessions within medical teams.

Table 4.15 Identifying the root of conflicts between HCPs and patients/families

"You have talked with multiple physicians about ___. Can you please share with me what you have heard so far and what you are most worried about?"
"A moment ago you mentioned___. It seems as though this is something that is very important to you. Can you please tell me more about that?"
"The last time we met we talked about several difficult and complicated things. Can you tell me which part of our conversation have you found yourself thinking about the most?"
"Can you please tell me what has been most difficult for you to hear so far? What has made this the most difficult piece of news to receive?"
"What do you worry will happen next?" Or, "Now that we know more about what your child is up against, what are you hoping to happen next?"
"___ seems quite important to me as we consider next steps. Is this something that you also see as important?"

Table 4.16 Basic guidelines for conducting debriefings sessions for the medical team

Participation is voluntary
Participants are invited to share their thoughts, feelings, and reactions freely
The facilitator makes every effort to clarify misconceptions about the event or patient death
The discussion remains staff-centered and focused on personal expression and support; suggestions for improving the process might be useful in some instances, but individual performance review should be reserved for a separate conversation

4.7 Facilitating Communication Within the Family Unit

Although communication with the patient and parent is a priority for HCPs, facilitating communication within the whole family unit is also highly important in both pediatric oncology and palliative care (Feudtner 2007; Levetown 2008; Contro et al. 2002; Snethen et al. 2006; Mullen et al. 2015). In particular, the inclusion of siblings in the communication process impacts the family unit's adjustment to the illness experience (Gaab et al. 2014). Bereaved parents of children with high-risk cancer report appreciation for HCPs who actively engaged their family in conversations about their child's care (Contro et al. 2002). Likewise, bereaved siblings of children who died from cancer who report receiving adequate preparation for their sibling's death and/or satisfaction with communication during the end of their sibling's life also report significantly lower levels of long-term maladjustment (Eilertsen et al. n.d.; Rosenberg et al. 2015).

Conversely, compared with siblings who report being satisfied with the extent or nature of communication at the end of their sibling's life, those who are dissatisfied have higher levels of anxiety 2–9 years later (Wallin et al. 2016). Further, siblings who recollect perceptions of inadequate social support during the last month of their sibling's life and at the time of the sibling's death often experience more anxiety later in life (Eilertsen et al. 2013). Correspondingly, the International Society of Pediatric Oncology highlights the importance of active back-and-forth communication with siblings of children with cancer (Spinetta et al. 1999). Nonetheless, many siblings recall poor knowledge and a lack of communication about their sibling's EOL experience and what to expect (Lövgren et al. 2016) and suggest that HCPs focus on improving communication with siblings and the family unit (Lövgren et al. 2015).

The Family Management Style Framework (FMSF) represents one possible framework for improving communication within the family unit (Knafl et al. 2008). This framework highlights the integral role of each family member, as well as the family unit as a whole, in caring for a child with a chronic and/or life-threatening condition. The FMSF posits that, when deciding about the most appropriate approach to use for family communication, one must consider how each family member defines the situation of having a child with a serious condition (definition of the situation), what each family member does to attempt to manage or address the condition (management of behaviors), how each family member perceives the effect of the child's condition on family life (perceived consequences), and unique thoughts about what affects family life and what affects the responses of family members to the child's condition (Knafl et al. 2008).

Knowledge about decision-making patterns within families is also useful for optimizing communication (Snethen et al. 2006). HCPs should devote time to acquiring a sufficiently complete understanding of the family's differing perspectives, as well as to recognizing and learning to manage their own heuristics, interaction styles, responses, automatic thoughts, and resultant intrapersonal and interpersonal processes; all of these factors significantly impact an HCP's ability to communicate with families (Feudtner 2007). In order to communicate effectively with the family unit, demonstration of respect and compassion for individual family members and the family unit as a whole is imperative (Feudtner 2007; Clarke et al. 2005; Meert et al. 2008b; Mullen et al. 2015). Tables 4.17 and 4.18 present strategies for parents and HCPs, respectively, for facilitating communication within and between the family unit.

4.8 Communicating Without Words

> "To communicate through silence is a link between the thoughts of man."
> – *Marcel Marceau*

> "The most basic and powerful way to connect to another person is to listen. Just listen. Perhaps the most important thing we ever give each other is our attention.... A loving silence often has far more power to heal and to connect than the most well-intentioned words."
> – *Rachel Naomi Remen*

Table 4.17 Strategies to help parents communicate with siblings of children with cancer

Consider family preferences and cultural norms during discussions with parents
Encourage parents to be open and honest with the patient's sibling(s); however, ensure that you remain respectful of the parents' preferences and wishes
Help parents find developmentally appropriate language. If appropriate, explain how children typically understand death at various developmental stages
Stress the importance of using clear language such as "death," "dying," "dead," "cancer," and "stopped working."
Suggest that parents follow the lead of the sibling(s). Some children ask many questions, whereas others do not ask any questions. Tell parents that there is not necessarily one "right way" to communicate and remind them that children will often tell what will work best for them
Reassure parents that it is okay for their children to see them sad and/or to see them cry. Parents can be encouraged to say something like "Mommy is crying because she is so sad that *[patient's name]* is sick/dying."
Encourage parents to actively listen to sibling(s) and remain sensitive to their feelings. Explain the benefit of allowing the sibling(s) to demonstrate strong emotions, but note that it is also okay if sibling(s) do not outwardly demonstrate feelings
Remind parents that they do not need to have all the answers. It is perfectly appropriate to say "I do not know the answer to that but we can ask the doctor" or "I wish I knew the answer to that."
Explain to parents that sibling(s) might ask questions about their own mortality or their parents' mortality

Table 4.18 Strategies to help HCPs communicate with siblings of children with cancer

Obtain parental permission and respect parental wishes
Avoid communication about the situation with a sibling when a parent/caregiver is not present or before parents/caregivers have initially communicated with the sibling(s) about the situation
Consider the sibling's age and developmental level
Use clear, specific, and concrete language; use correct words such as "death" or "dying." Avoid vague, unclear, and/or confusing language such as "passing away" or "will go be with the angels."
Be honest and encourage open communication
Remember it is okay to say "I do not know the answer to that but will try to find out," or "I wish we knew the answer to that."
Follow the lead of the sibling. Never force a child to discuss more than what is comfortable for him or her
Listen actively and be accepting of the sibling's feelings. You can say something like, "It is okay to feel any way you feel" or "Sometimes people cry when they hear something like this, but sometimes they do not." You might even find it appropriate to say something like "It is okay to cry" or "It is okay that you did not cry. It does not mean you do not love your sister."

Table 4.19 Strategies to achieve meaningful silent presence

Silence can feel uncomfortable, as we often want to feel like we are "doing something." Remind yourself that quietly bearing witness is, in fact, doing something very powerful for the child and family
If you feel compelled to fill the silence, consider counting slowly backward from 30 in order to give the child or family space to experience their emotions without interruption
If a child or family member is crying, you do not always need to speak in order to validate the emotions and offer support. Empathic listening can be reflected powerfully through your facial expressions and body language
If the child or family member is receptive to touch, consider offering your hand to hold. Another way to offer comfort through touch is to rest your hand on the forearm or shoulder of the child or parent; this type of physical contact is typically considered gender neutral and culturally and religiously acceptable for most individuals

4.8.1 Bearing Witness

While providing care to children with cancer and their families, HCPs sometimes face situations so difficult and painful that they struggle to find the words to express their empathy. At times, they feel the need to "fill the silence" with words, even if they are unsure of what to say. However, sometimes the most powerful way to communicate with patients and families is through silent presence (Himelstein et al. 2003). Table 4.19 gives suggestions on how HCPs can use silent presence with patients and families.

4.8.2 Communicating Through Play

Children often express themselves differently than do adults. Although children absorb information readily, they often need help with interpreting and applying this information to their lives. They might also struggle to find the right words to express their feelings. Nonverbal therapeutic modalities can help facilitate communication under these circumstances.

Psychosocial professionals such as CCLSs are trained to help children develop both verbal and nonverbal skills to identify emotions and improve communication with family members and HCPs. CCLSs meet children where they are and follow their lead, offering modalities such as therapeutic play and other creative activities to offer children an outlet to express their emotions about the illness experience (Rollins 2005).

Children play for several reasons, including normal development, entertainment, and normalization of stressful environments. CCLSs focus on age-appropriate play as a strategy for providing education and anticipatory guidance, facilitating therapeutic interventions, and offering emotional support. During therapeutic play, CCLSs can focus on sensory inputs (e.g., what can the child expect to hear, see, feel, smell, or taste) and cognitive skills (e.g., what is happening, why is it happening, where am I going, and how is it going to happen). Through play, CCLSs build trust and relationships with patients and families, with the goal of enabling the sharing of thoughts and feelings in order to enhance medical care and the overall illness experience.

Like adults, however, children require a non threatening environment to share their thoughts and emotions. HCPs need to listen with intention, offer sufficient space and silence to encourage sharing, and validate that the child's words and thoughts are valuable and worthy of their attention. HCPs can help children express their thoughts by supporting them in whatever activity they feel most comfortable doing, be it therapeutic play, role playing, drawing, or playing video games.

Even when children are able to express their opinions or emotions, they might still experience difficulty in answering direct verbal questions. In these cases, HCPs need to mobilize alternative strategies to communicate effectively and in an age-appropriate manner with patients (Sposito and de Montigny 2015). Various modalities of therapeutic play, including the use of medical dolls or puppets, have been extremely useful to communicate with hospitalized children with cancer and can encourage patients to share their illness experience in ways that improve their medical care (Sposito and de Montigny 2015). The use of drawing as a form of therapeutic play can also improve communication between children with cancer and medical providers (Rollins 2005). Likewise, dance or movement therapy is another nonconventional way to promote communication about the illness experience, and it can facilitate improved coping in children and adolescents with cancer (Cohen and Walco 1999).

4.8.3 Communicating Through Music

Music therapy is an effective supportive modality for children with cancer and their families (Tucquet and Leung 2014). Parents of children with cancer perceive music as a beneficial aspect of their child's holistic care (Kemper and McLean 2008). Music therapy can increase verbalization, interaction, independence, and cooperation in children with cancer as well as improve their relationships with their family and HCPs (Standley and Hanser 1995). Music therapy can be paired effectively with other psychosocial interventions to improve patient communication, adjustment, and coping (Standley and Hanser 1995).

Music therapy can also be a highly effective intervention and source of support for parents and siblings of children with cancer. In this context, the common goals of music therapy include (1) strengthening the attachment between the patient and family at the EOL, (2) creating memories and communicating important messages, (3) expressing fears and anxieties, (4) creating a space for the patient and family to be together in music of quiet contemplation or reflection, and (5) continuing the story of the patient with the family in bereavement (Wheeler 2015).

4.9 Educational Interventions to Improve Communication

As discussed in detail previously in this chapter, effective communication regarding prognosis and advance care planning leads to better QOL and EOL care for patients, as well as improved bereavement outcomes for families. While the delivery of good communication is an "art," it is also a fundamental skill that requires extensive instruction, role modeling, and practice in order to execute proficiently. Unfortunately, many HCPs do not receive adequate training in the provision of effective communication (Hilden et al. 2001; Sanderson et al. 2015; Boss et al. 2009). Moreover, educational interventions to train HCPs in communication about EOL issues are particularly lacking (Chung et al. 2016), highlighting an area in need of significant research and clinical intervention.

Pediatric oncologists in particular identify deficits in their communication training, with the vast majority (92%) reporting that they learned communication through trial and error (Hilden et al. 2001). Pediatric oncologists also report a lack of formalized instruction in palliative care principles and a need for strong role models to share communication strategies (Hilden et al. 2001). Yet while formalized training, rather than trial and error, is increasingly recognized as an essential aspect of medical communication education, little data or consensus exists regarding how best to achieve this training process (Bays et al. 2014; Curtis et al. 2013; Dickson et al. 2012; Moore et al. 2013).

In the context of this perceived deficit, the Institute of Medicine and the American Cancer Society have issued a call to action for the development of programs to improve clinical communication skills for HCPs (Kirch et al. 2016). Although the optimal method or combined methods to teach this critical skill remain undefined, a number of studies have investigated different strategies to enhance communication skill building for HCPs, including didactic lectures, small-group workshops, online modules, standardized patient simulations, and role-play with communication experts and bereaved parent educators (Moore et al. 2013; Downar et al. 2017; Fellowes et al. 2004; Szmuilowicz et al. 2012; Tulsky et al. 2011; Bragard et al. 2006; Delvaux et al. 2005; Razavi and Delvaux 1997; Snaman et al. 2017). A variety of creative sociodramatic techniques, including the use of theater, reflective writing, and Balint-type case discussion, have also been used to engage oncology trainees in the development of effective communication skills (Epner and Baile 2014). Additionally, a number of educational tools and opportunities exist with the goal of developing communication expertise in oncology clinicians, including Oncotalk (Fryer-Edwards et al. 2006), VitalTalk, EPEC (Widger et al. 2016), PCEP (Palliative Care Education and Practice (PCEP)), and The Conversation Project. These resources are summarized in Table 4.20 (Kaye et al. 2015).

However, although multiple training programs and resources have been developed to better prepare HCPs to sensitively and effectively communicate with children with cancer and their families, interventions to improve communication in pediatric oncology have not been widely or rigorously assessed (Ranmal et al. 2008). We advocate for formalized communication training to be a mandatory component of pediatric oncology training programs (Snaman et al. 2016c). Ongoing investigation is needed to better understand the optimal strategy for teaching effective communication skills to HCPs who care for children with cancer and their families.

Table 4.20 Resources to promote communication expertise in HCPs

Oncotalk (http://depts.washington.edu/oncotalk/): An online educational curriculum designed to improve the communication skills of oncologists
VitalTalk (http://www.vitaltalk.org): An educational forum with resources for HCPs about leading conversations about goals of care and oncology workshops designed for use in cancer centers. Resources are available in phone app format and online curricula are available for CME credit via the Center to Advance Palliative Care (CAPC: http://www.capc.org)
Education in Palliative and End-of-life Care Program (EPEC)—Pediatrics (epec.net/epec_pediatrics.php): A pediatric-specific conference that provides in-person training on effective teaching strategies, as well as access to comprehensive educational materials
Program in Palliative Care Education And Practice (PCEP)—Pediatric Track (http://www.hms.harvard.edu/pallcare/PCEP/PCEP.htm): An intensive conference on advanced topics in pediatric palliative care offered by Harvard Medical School's Center for Palliative Care
The conversation project (http://theconversationproject.org): A grass-roots movement dedicated to helping people talk about their wishes for end of life care, with access to pediatric "starter kits" to help clinicians, children, and families broach these difficult conversations

Adapted from Kaye EC, Rubinstein J, Levine D, et al. Pediatric palliative care in the community. CA Cancer J Clin 2015;65(4):316–33

4.10 Key Points

- Effective communication is a key pillar of optimal cancer care, espoused by the Institute of Medicine, American Academy of Pediatrics, and multiple national oncology societies.
- Good communication is necessary for building trust, promoting shared decision-making, and encouraging discussion of goals of care and quality of life.
- At times, conversation may serve as a therapeutic intervention itself, enabling clinicians to reframe hope, alleviate suffering, and mitigate complicated bereavement.
- Established guidelines exist to help clinicians navigate the challenging experience of communicating difficult news, whether about a new diagnosis, disease progression, relapse, goals of care, advance care planning, or anticipatory guidance toward the end of life.
- Conversations about prognosis early in the disease course establish a foundation of honesty and trust upon which to provide optimal medical care throughout the illness trajectory.
- Clinicians should strive to provide honest information while still affirming the right of the patient and family to maintain hope; hoping for cure does not preclude the recognition of incurable disease nor a wish for prolonging a life with quality.
- Communication is most effective when offered through an interdisciplinary approach, integrating expertise from physicians, nurses, child life specialists, chaplains, psychologists, social workers, and other supportive clinicians.
- Effective communication with children carries a unique set of challenges and requires specialized training in age-appropriate communication styles and strategies.
- Sometimes the most powerful way to communicate with patients and families is through silence, simply by offering one's presence and bearing witness.
- Formalized communication training should be an integral and mandatory part of pediatric oncology training programs.

References

Ablon J (2000) Parents' responses to their child's diagnosis of neurofibromatosis 1. Am J Med Genet 93(2):136–142

Ahmann E (1998) Review and commentary: two studies regarding giving "bad news". Pediatr Nurs 24(6):554–556

American Academy of Pediatrics (2000) Committee on bioethics and committee on hospital care. Palliative care for children. Pediatrics 106(2 Pt 1):351–357

Apatira L, Boyd EA, Malvar G et al (2008) Hope, truth, and preparing for death: perspectives of surrogate decision makers. Ann Intern Med 149(12):861–868

Arceci RJ, Reaman GH, Cohen AR, Lampkin BC (1998) Position statement for the need to define pediatric hematology/oncology programs: a model of subspecialty care for chronic childhood diseases. Health Care Policy and Public Issues Committee of the American Society of Pediatric Hematology/Oncology. J Pediatr Hematol Oncol 20(2):98–103

Arnold SJ, Koczwara B (2006) Breaking bad news: learning through experience. J Clin Oncol 24(31):5098–5100

Back AL, Young JP, McCown E et al (2009) Abandonment at the end of life from patient, caregiver, nurse, and physician perspectives: loss of continuity and lack of closure. Arch Intern Med 169(5):474–479

Baker JN, Barfield R, Hinds PS, Kane JR (2007) A process to facilitate decision making in pediatric stem cell transplantation: the individualized care planning and coordination model. Biol Blood Marrow Transplant 13(3):245–254

Baker JN, Hinds PS, Spunt SL et al (2008) Integration of palliative care practices into the ongoing care of children with cancer: individualized care planning and coordination. Pediatr Clin N Am 55(1):223–250, xii.

Baker JN, Leek AC, Salas HS et al (2013) Suggestions from adolescents, young adults, and parents for improving informed consent in phase 1 pediatric oncology trials. Cancer 119(23):4154–4161

Baker JN, Levine DR, Hinds PS et al (2015) Research priorities in pediatric palliative care. J Pediatr 167(2):467–470.e3

Balboni TA, Paulk ME, Balboni MJ et al (2010) Provision of spiritual care to patients with advanced cancer: associations with medical care and quality of life near death. J Clin Oncol 28(3):445–452

Balboni TA, Balboni M, Enzinger AC et al (2013) Provision of spiritual support to patients with advanced cancer by religious communities and associations with medical care at the end of life. JAMA Intern Med 173(12):1109–1117

Bates AT, Kearney JA (2015) Understanding death with limited experience in life: dying children's and adolescents' understanding of their own terminal illness and death. Curr Opin Support Palliat Care 9(1):40–45

Bays AM, Engelberg RA, Back AL et al (2014) Interprofessional communication skills training for serious illness: evaluation of a small-group, simulated patient intervention. J Palliat Med 17(2):159–166

Beale EA, Baile WF, Aaron J (2005) Silence is not golden: communicating with children dying from cancer. J Clin Oncol 23(15):3629–3631

Berg GM, Hervey AM, Basham-Saif A et al (2014) Acceptability and implementation of debriefings after trauma resuscitation. J Trauma Nurs 21(5):201–208

Bluebond-Langer M (1980) The private worlds of dying children. Princeton University Press, Princeton

Bluebond-Langner M, Belasco JB, Goldman A, Belasco C (2007) Understanding parents' approaches to care and treatment of children with cancer when standard therapy has failed. J Clin Oncol 25(17):2414–2419

Boss RD, Hutton N, Donohue PK, Arnold RM (2009) Neonatologist training to guide family decision making for critically ill infants. Arch Pediatr Adolesc Med 163(9):783–788

Boyle D, Dwinnell B, Platt F (2005) Invite, listen, and summarize: a patient-centered communication technique. Acad Med 80(1):29–32

Bradshaw G, Hinds PS, Lensing S et al (2005) Cancer-related deaths in children and adolescents. J Palliat Med 8(1):86–95

Bragard I, Razavi D, Marchal S et al (2006) Teaching communication and stress management skills to junior physicians dealing with cancer patients: a Belgian interuniversity curriculum. Support Care Cancer 14(5):454–461

Buss MK, Lessen DS, Sullivan AM et al (2011) Hematology/oncology fellows' training in palliative care: results of a national survey. Cancer 117(18):4304–4311

Carnevale FA, Canouï P, Hubert P et al (2006) The moral experience of parents regarding life-support decisions for their critically-ill children: a preliminary study in France. J Child Health Care 10(1):69–82

Conference C (1985) A father says, "Don't tell my son the truth". J Med Ethics 11(3):153–158

Christakis NA, Iwashyna TJ (1998) Attitude and self-reported practice regarding prognostication in a national sample of internists. Arch Intern Med 158(21):2389–2395

Chung H-O, Oczkowski SJW, Hanvey L et al (2016) Educational interventions to train healthcare professionals in end-of-life communication: a systematic review and meta-analysis. BMC Med Educ 16(1):131

Claflin CJ, Barbarin OA (1991) Does "telling" less protect more? Relationships among age, information disclosure, and what children with cancer see and feel. J Pediatr Psychol 16(2):169–191

Clarke S-A, Davies H, Jenney M et al (2005) Parental communication and children's behaviour following diagnosis of childhood leukaemia. Psychooncology 14(4):274–281

Claxton-Oldfield S, Marrison-Shaw H (2014) Perceived barriers and enablers to referrals to community-based hospice palliative care volunteer programs in Canada. Am J Hosp Palliat Care 31(8):836–844

Cohen SO, Walco GA (1999) Dance/Movement therapy for children and adolescents with cancer. Cancer Pract 7(1):34–42

Cole CM, Kodish E (2013) Minors' right to know and therapeutic privilege. Virtual Mentor 15(8):638–644

Collins JJ (2002) Palliative care and the child with cancer. Hematol Oncol Clin North Am 16(3):657–670

Contro N, Larson J, Scofield S et al (2002) Family perspectives on the quality of pediatric palliative care. Arch Pediatr Adolesc Med 156(1):14–19

Contro NA, Larson J, Scofield S et al (2004) Hospital staff and family perspectives regarding quality of pediatric palliative care. Pediatrics 114(5):1248–1252

Cousino MK, Zyzanski SJ, Yamokoski AD et al (2012) Communicating and understanding the purpose of pediatric phase I cancer trials. J Clin Oncol 30(35):4367–4372

Coyne I, Amory A, Kiernan G, Gibson F (2014) Children's participation in shared decision-making: children, adolescents, parents and healthcare professionals' perspectives and experiences. Eur J Oncol Nurs 18(3):273–280

Curtis JR, Back AL, Ford DW et al (2013) Effect of communication skills training for residents and nurse practitioners on quality of communication with patients with serious illness: a randomized trial. JAMA 310(21):2271–2281

Davies B, Sehring SA, Partridge JC et al (2008) Barriers to palliative care for children: perceptions of pediatric health care providers. Pediatrics 121(2):282–288

Davison SN, Simpson C (2006) Hope and advance care planning in patients with end stage renal disease: qualitative interview study. BMJ 333(7574):886

De Trill M, Kovalcik R (1997) The child with cancer. Influence of culture on truth-telling and patient care. Ann N Y Acad Sci 809:197–210

Delvaux N, Merckaert I, Marchal S et al (2005) Physicians' communication with a cancer patient and a relative: a randomized study assessing the efficacy of consolidation workshops. Cancer 103(11):2397–2411

Dickson RP, Engelberg RA, Back AL et al (2012) Internal medicine trainee self-assessments of end-of-life communication skills do not predict assessments of patients, families, or clinician-evaluators. J Palliat Med 15(4):418–426

Downar J, McNaughton N, Abdelhalim T et al (2017) Standardized patient simulation versus didactic teaching alone for improving residents' communication skills when discussing goals of care and resuscitation: a randomized controlled trial. Palliat Med 31(2):130–139

Eden OB, Black I, MacKinlay GA, Emery AE (1994) Communication with parents of children with cancer. Palliat Med 8(2):105–114

Eggly S, Penner L, Albrecht TL et al (2006) Discussing bad news in the outpatient oncology clinic: rethinking current communication guidelines. J Clin Oncol 24(4):716–719

Eilertsen M-EB, Eilegård A, Steineck G et al (2013) Impact of social support on bereaved siblings' anxiety: a nationwide follow-up. J Pediatr Oncol Nurs 30(6):301–310

Eng J, Schulman E, Jhanwar SM, Shah MK (2015) Patient death debriefing sessions to support residents' emotional reactions to patient deaths. J Grad Med Educ 7(3):430–436

Epner DE, Baile WF (2014) Difficult conversations: teaching medical oncology trainees communication skills one hour at a time. Acad Med 89(4):578–584

Essex C (2001) Delivering bad news. Receiving bad news will always be unpleasant. BMJ 322(7290):864–865

Essig S, Steiner C, Kuehni CE et al (2016) Improving communication in adolescent cancer care: a multiperspective study. Pediatr Blood Cancer 63(8):1423–1430

Fallat ME, Glover J (2007) Professionalism in pediatrics: statement of principles. Pediatrics 120(4):895–897

Fellowes D, Wilkinson S, Moore P (2004) Communication skills training for health care professionals working with cancer patients, their families and/or carers. Cochrane Database Syst Rev 2:CD003751

Feudtner C (2007) Collaborative communication in pediatric palliative care: a foundation for problem-solving and decision-making. Pediatr Clin N Am 54(5):583–607. ix

Feudtner C, Morrison W (2012) The darkening veil of "do everything". Arch Pediatr Adolesc Med 166(8):694–695

Feudtner C, Santucci G, Feinstein JA et al (2007) Hopeful thinking and level of comfort regarding providing pediatric palliative care: a survey of hospital nurses. Pediatrics 119(1):e186–e192

Fowler K, Poehling K, Billheimer D et al (2006) Hospice referral practices for children with cancer: a survey of pediatric oncologists. J Clin Oncol 24(7):1099–1104

Fox S, Platt FW, White MK, Hulac P (2005) Talking about the unthinkable: perinatal/neonatal communication issues and procedures. Clin Perinatol 32(1):157–170, vii–viii.

Freyer DR (1992) Children with cancer: special considerations in the discontinuation of life-sustaining treatment. Med Pediatr Oncol 20(2):136–142

Fried TR, Bradley EH, Towle VR, Allore H (2002) Understanding the treatment preferences of seriously ill patients. N Engl J Med 346(14):1061–1066

Friedman BT, Harwood MK, Shields M (2002) Barriers and enablers to hospice referrals: an expert overview. J Palliat Med 5(1):73–84

Fryer-Edwards K, Arnold RM, Baile W et al (2006) Reflective teaching practices: an approach to teaching communication skills in a small-group setting. Acad Med 81(7):638–644

Gaab EM, Owens GR, MacLeod RD (2014) Siblings caring for and about pediatric palliative care patients. J Palliat Med 17(1):62–67

Garrido MM, Prigerson HG (2014) The end-of-life experience: modifiable predictors of caregivers' bereavement adjustment. Cancer 120(6):918–925

Garwick AW, Patterson J, Bennett FC, Blum RW (1995) Breaking the news. How families first learn about their child's chronic condition. Arch Pediatr Adolesc Med 149(9):991–997

Girgis A, Breen S, Stacey F, Lecathelinais C (2009) Impact of two supportive care interventions on anxiety, depression, quality of life, and unmet needs in patients with nonlocalized breast and colorectal cancers. J Clin Oncol 27(36):6180–6190

Goldie J, Schwartz L, Morrison J (2005) Whose information is it anyway? Informing a 12-year-old patient of her terminal prognosis. J Med Ethics 31(7):427–434

Gordon EJ, Daugherty CK (2003) "Hitting you over the head": oncologists' disclosure of prognosis to advanced cancer patients. Bioethics 17(2):142–168
Granek L, Bartels U, Barrera M, Scheinemann K (2015) Challenges faced by pediatric oncology fellows when patients die during their training. J Oncol Pract 11(2):e182–e189
Greenley RN, Drotar D, Zyzanski SJ, Kodish E (2006) Stability of parental understanding of random assignment in childhood leukemia trials: an empirical examination of informed consent. J Clin Oncol 24(6):891–897
von Gunten CF, Ferris FD, Emanuel LL (2000) The patient-physician relationship. Ensuring competency in end-of-life care: communication and relational skills. JAMA 284(23):3051–3057
Gupta VB, Willert J, Pian M, Stein MT (2010) When disclosing a serious diagnosis to a minor conflicts with family values. J Dev Behav Pediatr 31(3 Suppl):S100–S102
Hack TF, Ruether JD, Pickles T et al (2012) Behind closed doors II: systematic analysis of prostate cancer patients' primary treatment consultations with radiation oncologists and predictors of satisfaction with communication. Psychooncology 21(8):809–817
Hagerty RG, Butow PN, Ellis PM et al (2005) Communicating with realism and hope: incurable cancer patients' views on the disclosure of prognosis. J Clin Oncol 23(6):1278–1288
Hart D, Schneider D (1997) Spiritual care for children with cancer. Semin Oncol Nurs 13(4):263–270
Hays RM, Valentine J, Haynes G et al (2006) The seattle pediatric palliative care project: effects on family satisfaction and health-related quality of life. J Palliat Med 9(3):716–728
Hebert HD, Butera JN, Castillo J, Mega AE (2009) Are we training our fellows adequately in delivering bad news to patients? A survey of hematology/oncology program directors. J Palliat Med 12(12):1119–1124
Hechler T, Blankenburg M, Friedrichsdorf SJ et al (2008) Parents' perspective on symptoms, quality of life, characteristics of death and end-of-life decisions for children dying from cancer. Klin Pädiatrie 220(3):166–174
Higgs EJ, McClaren BJ, Sahhar MA et al (2015) "A short time but a lovely little short time": Bereaved parents' experiences of having a child with spinal muscular atrophy type 1. J Paediatr Child Health 52:40–46
Hilden JM, Emanuel EJ, Fairclough DL et al (2001) Attitudes and practices among pediatric oncologists regarding end-of-life care: results of the 1998 American Society of Clinical Oncology survey. J Clin Oncol 19(1):205–212
Hill DL, Miller V, Walter JK et al (2014) Regoaling: a conceptual model of how parents of children with serious illness change medical care goals. BMC Palliat Care 13(1):9
Himelstein BP, Jackson NL, Pegram L (2003) The power of silence. J Clin Oncol 21(9 Suppl):41s
Hinds PS (2004) The hopes and wishes of adolescents with cancer and the nursing care that helps. Oncol Nurs Forum 31(5):927–934
Hinds PS, Oakes L, Furman W et al (1997) Decision making by parents and healthcare professionals when considering continued care for pediatric patients with cancer. Oncol Nurs Forum 24(9):1523–1528
Hinds PS, Quargnenti A, Fairclough D et al (1999) Hopefulness and its characteristics in adolescents with cancer. West J Nurs Res 21(5):600–620
Hinds PS, Oakes L, Quargnenti A et al (2000) An international feasibility study of parental decision making in pediatric oncology. Oncol Nurs Forum 27(8):1233–1243
Hinds PS, Birenbaum LK, Pedrosa AM, Pedrosa F (2002) Guidelines for the recurrence of pediatric cancer. Semin Oncol Nurs 18(1):50–59
Hinds PS, Drew D, Oakes LL et al (2005) End-of-life care preferences of pediatric patients with cancer. J Clin Oncol 23(36):9146–9154
Hinds PS, Oakes LL, Hicks J et al (2009) "Trying to be a good parent"; as defined by interviews with parents who made phase I, terminal care, and resuscitation decisions for their children. J Clin Oncol 27(35):5979–5985
Hsu T-H, M-S L, Tsou T-S, Lin C-C (2003) The relationship of pain, uncertainty, and hope in Taiwanese lung cancer patients. J Pain Symptom Manag 26(3):835–842
Institute of Medicine (2003) In: Field M, Behrman R (eds) When children die: improving palliative and end-of-life care for children and their families. National Academies Press, Washington, D.C.
Institute of Medicine (2014) Dying in America: improving quality and honoring individual preferences near the end of life. National Academies Press, Washington, D.C.
Ishibashi A (2001) The needs of children and adolescents with cancer for information and social support. Cancer Nurs 24(1):61–67
Jankovic M, Masera G, Uderzo C et al (1989) Meetings with parents after the death of their child from leukemia. Pediatr Hematol Oncol 6(2):155–160
Jankovic M, Loiacono NB, Spinetta JJ et al (1994) Telling young children with leukemia their diagnosis: the flower garden as analogy. Pediatr Hematol Oncol 11(1):75–81
Jankovic M, Spinetta JJ, Masera G et al (2008) Communicating with the dying child: an invitation to listening—a report of the SIOP Working Committee on psychosocial issues in pediatric oncology. Pediatr Blood Cancer 50(5):1087–1088
Johnson L-M, Leek AC, Drotar D et al (2015) Practical communication guidance to improve phase 1 informed consent conversations and decision-making in pediatric oncology. Cancer 121(14):2439–2448
Jünger S, Pastrana T, Pestinger M et al (2010) Barriers and needs in paediatric palliative home care in Germany: a

qualitative interview study with professional experts. BMC Palliat Care 9:10
Kamper R, Van Cleve L, Savedra M (2010) Children with advanced cancer: responses to a spiritual quality of life interview. J Spec Pediatr Nurs 15(4):301–306
Kassam A, Skiadaresis J, Habib S et al (2013) Moving toward quality palliative cancer care: parent and clinician perspectives on gaps between what matters and what is accessible. J Clin Oncol 31(7):910–915
Kassam A, Skiadaresis J, Alexander S, Wolfe J (2015) Differences in end-of-life communication for children with advanced cancer who were referred to a palliative care team. Pediatr Blood Cancer 62(8):1409–1413
Kaye EC (2015) Pieces of grief. J Clin Oncol 33(26):2923–2924
Kaye E, Mack JW (2013) Parent perceptions of the quality of information received about a child's cancer. Pediatr Blood Cancer 60(11):1896–1901
Kaye EC, Rubenstein J, Levine D et al (2015) Pediatric palliative care in the community. CA Cancer J Clin 65(4):315–333
Keene EA, Hutton N, Hall B, Rushton C (2010) Bereavement debriefing sessions: an intervention to support health care professionals in managing their grief after the death of a patient. Pediatr Nurs 36(4):185–189
Kemper KJ, McLean TW (2008) Parents' attitudes and expectations about music's impact on pediatric oncology patients. J Soc Integr Oncol 6(4):146–149
Kirch R, Reaman G, Feudtner C et al (2016) Advancing a comprehensive cancer care agenda for children and their families: Institute of Medicine Workshop highlights and next steps. CA Cancer J Clin 66(5):398–407
Knafl K, Deatrick JA, Gallo AM (2008) The interplay of concepts, data, and methods in the development of the family management style framework. J Fam Nurs 14(4):412–428
Knapp C, Thompson L (2012) Factors associated with perceived barriers to pediatric palliative care: a survey of pediatricians in Florida and California. Palliat Med 26(3):268–274
Knapp CA, Madden VL, Curtis CM et al (2008) Partners in care: together for kids: Florida's model of pediatric palliative care. J Palliat Med 11(9):1212–1220
Kodish E, Post SG (1995) Oncology and hope. J Clin Oncol 13(7):1817
Kodish E, Eder M, Noll RB et al (2004) Communication of randomization in childhood leukemia trials. JAMA 291(4):470–475
Koop PM, Strang V (1997) Predictors of bereavement outcomes in families of patients with cancer: a literature review. Can J Nurs Res 29(4):33–50
Kreicbergs U, Valdimarsdóttir U, Onelöv E et al (2004) Talking about death with children who have severe malignant disease. N Engl J Med 351(12):1175–1186
Lamont EB, Christakis NA (2003) Complexities in prognostication in advanced cancer: "to help them live their lives the way they want to". JAMA 290(1):98–104
Last BF, van Veldhuizen AM (1996) Information about diagnosis and prognosis related to anxiety and depression in children with cancer aged 8–16 years. Eur J Cancer 32A(2):290–294
Levetown M (2008) Communicating with children and families: from everyday interactions to skill in conveying distressing information. Pediatrics 121(5):e1441–e1460
Levine D, Lam CG, Cunningham MJ et al (2013) Best practices for pediatric palliative cancer care: a primer for clinical providers. J Support Oncol 11(3):114–125
Levine DR, Johnson L-M, Mandrell BN et al (2015) Does phase 1 trial enrollment preclude quality end-of-life care? Phase 1 trial enrollment and end-of-life care characteristics in children with cancer. Cancer 121(9):1508–1512
Lichtenthal WG, Sweeney CR, Roberts KE et al (2015) Bereavement follow-up after the death of a child as a standard of care in pediatric oncology. Pediatr Blood Cancer 62(Suppl 5):S834–S869
Lima NNR, do Nascimento VB, de Carvalho SMF et al (2013) Spirituality in childhood cancer care. Neuropsychiatr Dis Treat 9:1539–1544
Lövgren M, Jalmsell L, Eilegård Wallin A et al (2015) Siblings' experiences of their brother's or sister's cancer death: a nationwide follow-up 2-9 years later. Psychooncology 25(4):435–440
Lövgren M, Bylund-Grenklo T, Jalmsell L et al (2016) Bereaved siblings' advice to health care professionals working with children with cancer and their families. J Pediatr Oncol Nurs 33(4):297–305
Lyon ME, McCabe MA, Patel KM, D'Angelo LJ (2004) What do adolescents want? An exploratory study regarding end-of-life decision-making. J Adolesc Health 35(6):529.e1–529.e6
Mack JW, Grier HE (2004) The day one talk. J Clin Oncol 22(3):563–566
Mack JW, Hinds PS (2011) Practical aspects of communication. In: Wolfe J, Hinds P, Sourkes B (eds) Textbook of interdisciplinary pediatric palliative care. Elsevier Saunders, Philadelphia, PA, pp 179–189
Mack JW, Smith TJ (2012) Reasons why physicians do not have discussions about poor prognosis, why it matters, and what can be improved. J Clin Oncol 30(22):2715–2717
Mack JW, Hilden JM, Watterson J et al (2005) Parent and physician perspectives on quality of care at the end of life in children with cancer. J Clin Oncol 23(36):9155–9161
Mack JW, Wolfe J, Grier HE et al (2006) Communication about prognosis between parents and physicians of children with cancer: parent preferences and the impact of prognostic information. J Clin Oncol 24(33):5265–5270
Mack JW, Cook EF, Wolfe J et al (2007) Understanding of prognosis among parents of children with cancer: parental optimism and the parentphysician interaction. J Clin Oncol 25(11):1357–1362

Mack JW, Wolfe J, Cook EF et al (2007) Hope and prognostic disclosure. J Clin Oncol 25(35):5636–5642
Mack JW, Joffe S, Hilden JM et al (2008) Parents' views of cancer-directed therapy for children with no realistic chance for cure. J Clin Oncol 26(29):4759–4764
Mack JW, Block SD, Nilsson M et al (2009) Measuring therapeutic alliance between oncologists and patients with advanced cancer: the Human Connection Scale. Cancer 115(14):3302–3311
Mack JW, Wolfe J, Cook EF et al (2009) Peace of mind and sense of purpose as core existential issues among parents of children with cancer. Arch Pediatr Adolesc Med 163(6):519–524
Mahany B (1990) Working with kids who have cancer. Nursing (Lond) 20(8):44–49
Marshall PA, Magtanong RV, Leek AC et al (2012) Negotiating decisions during informed consent for pediatric Phase I oncology trials. J Empir Res Hum Res Ethics 7(2):51–59
Masera G, Chesler MA, Jankovic M et al (1997) SIOP Working Committee on psychosocial issues in pediatric oncology: guidelines for communication of the diagnosis. Med Pediatr Oncol 28(5):382–385
Masera G, Spinetta JJ, Jankovic M et al (1998) Guidelines for a therapeutic alliance between families and staff: a report of the SIOP working committee on psychosocial issues in pediatric oncology. Med Pediatr Oncol 30(3):183–186
Masera G, Spinetta JJ, Jankovic M et al (1999) Guidelines for assistance to terminally ill children with cancer: a report of the SIOP Working Committee on psychosocial issues in pediatric oncology. Med Pediatr Oncol 32(1):44–48
Meert KL, Thurston CS, Sarnaik AP (2000) End-of-life decision-making and satisfaction with care: parental perspectives. Pediatr Crit Care Med 1(2):179–185
Meert KL, Thurston CS, Thomas R (2001) Parental coping and bereavement outcome after the death of a child in the pediatric intensive care unit. Pediatr Crit Care Med 2(4):324–328
Meert KL, Briller SH, Schim SM, Thurston CS (2008) Exploring parents' environmental needs at the time of a child's death in the pediatric intensive care unit. Pediatr Crit Care Med 9(6):623–628
Meert KL, Eggly S, Pollack M et al (2008) Parents' perspectives on physician-parent communication near the time of a child's death in the pediatric intensive care unit. Pediatr Crit Care Med 9(1):2–7
Meert KL, Briller SH, Schim SM et al (2009) Examining the needs of bereaved parents in the pediatric intensive care unit: a qualitative study. Death Stud 33(8):712–740
Meert KL, Eggly S, Kavanaugh K et al (2015) Meaning making during parent-physician bereavement meetings after a child's death. Health Psychol 34(4):453–461
Merriam-Webster Dictionary. http://www.merriam-webster.com/dictionary/communication. Accessed 22 Jan 2016
Michon B, Balkou S, Hivon R, Cyr C (2003) Death of a child: parental perception of grief intensity—end-of-life and bereavement care. Paediatr Child Health 8(6):363–366
Miller VA, Baker JN, Leek AC et al (2013) Adolescent perspectives on phase I cancer research. Pediatr Blood Cancer 60(5):873–878
Miller VA, Cousino M, Leek AC, Kodish ED (2014) Hope and persuasion by physicians during informed consent. J Clin Oncol 32:3229–3235
Miller VA, Baker JN, Leek AC et al (2014) Patient involvement in informed consent for pediatric phase I cancer research. J Pediatr Hematol Oncol 36(8):635–640
Miyaji NT (1993) The power of compassion: truth-telling among American doctors in the care of dying patients. Soc Sci Med 36(3):249–264
Moore PM, Rivera Mercado S, Grez Artigues M, Lawrie TA (2013) Communication skills training for healthcare professionals working with people who have cancer. Cochrane Database Syst Rev 3:CD003751
Morita T, Akechi T, Ikenaga M et al (2005) Late referrals to specialized palliative care service in Japan. J Clin Oncol 23(12):2637–2644
Mullen JE, Reynolds MR, Larson JS (2015) Caring for pediatric patients' families at the child's end of life. Crit Care Nurse 35(6):46–56
Mystakidou K, Parpa E, Tsilila E et al (2004) Cancer information disclosure in different cultural contexts. Support Care Cancer 12(3):147–154
Neidig JR, Dalgas-Pelish P (1991) Parental grieving and perceptions regarding health care professionals' interventions. Issues Compr Pediatr Nurs 14(3):179–191
Nitschke R, Caldwell S, Jay S (1986) Therapeutic choices in end-stage cancer. J Pediatr 108(2):330–331
Oppenheim D, Geoerger B, Hartmann O (2005) Ethical issues in pediatric oncology phase I–II trials based on a mother's point of view. Bull Cancer 92(11):E57–E60
Oshea J, Smith O, O'Marcaigh A, McMahon C, Geoghegan R, Cotter M (2007) Breaking bad news—parents' experience of learning that their child has leukaemia. Ir Med J 100(9):588–590
Palliative Care Education and Practice (PCEP). http://www.hms.harvard.edu/pallcare/PCEP/PCEP.htm. Accessed 28 June 2016
Parsons SK, Saiki-Craighill S, Mayer DK et al (2007) Telling children and adolescents about their cancer diagnosis: cross-cultural comparisons between pediatric oncologists in the US and Japan. Psychooncology 16(1):60–68
Peppercorn JM, Smith TJ, Helft PR et al (2011) American society of clinical oncology statement: toward individualized care for patients with advanced cancer. J Clin Oncol 29(6):755–760
Peteet JR, Balboni MJ (2013) Spirituality and religion in oncology. CA Cancer J Clin 63(4):280–289
Proserpio T, Ferrari A, Veneroni L et al (2014) Spiritual aspects of care for adolescents with cancer. Tumori 100(4):130e–135e

Ptacek JT, Ptacek JJ (2001) Patients' perceptions of receiving bad news about cancer. J Clin Oncol 19(21):4160–4164
Rabow MW, Hauser JM, Adams J (2004) Supporting family caregivers at the end of life: "they don't know what they don't know". JAMA 291(4):483–491
Ranmal R, Prictor M, Scott JT (2008) Interventions for improving communication with children and adolescents about their cancer. Cochrane Database Syst Rev 4:CD002969
Rassouli M, Zamanzadeh V, Ghahramanian A et al (2015) Experiences of patients with cancer and their nurses on the conditions of spiritual care and spiritual interventions in oncology units. Iran J Nurs Midwifery Res 20(1):25–33
Razavi D, Delvaux N (1997) Communication skills and psychological training in oncology. Eur J Cancer 33(Suppl 6):S15–S21
Rollins JA (2005) Tell me about it: drawing as a communication tool for children with cancer. J Pediatr Oncol Nurs 22(4):203–221
Rosenberg AR, Orellana L, Kang TI et al (2014) Differences in parent-provider concordance regarding prognosis and goals of care among children with advanced cancer. J Clin Oncol 32:3005–3011
Rosenberg AR, Postier A, Osenga K et al (2015) Long-term psychosocial outcomes among bereaved siblings of children with cancer. J Pain Symptom Manag 49:55–65
Ruhe KM, Badarau DO, Brazzola P et al (2016) Participation in pediatric oncology: views of child and adolescent patients. Psychooncology 25:1036–1042
Sanderson A, Hall AM, Wolfe J (2015) Advance care discussions: pediatric clinician preparedness and practices. J Pain Symptom Manag 51:520–528
Sanson-Fisher R, Girgis A, Boyes A et al (2000) The unmet supportive care needs of patients with cancer. Supportive Care Review Group. Cancer 88(1):226–237
Sato I, Higuchi A, Yanagisawa T et al (2015) Parent's perceived provision of information regarding diagnosis to children with brain tumors. Open J Nurs 5:451–464
Schaefer KG, Block SD (2009) Physician communication with families in the ICU: evidence-based strategies for improvement. Curr Opin Crit Care 15(6):569–577
Sharman M, Meert KL, Sarnaik AP (2005) What influences parents' decisions to limit or withdraw life support? Pediatr Crit Care Med 6(5):513–518
Simon CM, Siminoff LA, Kodish ED, Burant C (2004) Comparison of the informed consent process for randomized clinical trials in pediatric and adult oncology. J Clin Oncol 22(13):2708–2717
Singh RK, Raj A, Paschal S, Hussain S (2015) Role of communication for pediatric cancer patients and their family. Indian J Palliat Care 21(3):338–340
Slavin LA, O'Malley JE, Koocher GP, Foster DJ (1982) Communication of the cancer diagnosis to pediatric patients: impact on long-term adjustment. Am J Psychiatry 139(2):179–183
Snaman JM, Kaye EC, Torres C et al (2016a) Helping parents live with the hole in their heart: the role of health care providers and institutions in the bereaved parents' grief journeys. Cancer 122:2757–2765
Snaman JM, Kaye EC, Torres C et al (2016b) Parental grief following the death of a child from cancer: the ongoing odyssey. Pediatr Blood Cancer 63(9):1594–1602
Snaman JM, Kaye EC, Cunningham M et al (2016) Going straight to the source: a pilot study of bereaved parent-facilitated communication training for pediatric subspecialty fellows. Pediatr Blood Cancer 64(1):156–162
Snaman JM, Kaye EC, Levine DR et al (2017) Empowering bereaved parents through the development of a comprehensive bereavement program. J Pain Symptom Manage 53(4):767–775
Snethen JA, Broome ME, Knafl K et al (2006) Family patterns of decision-making in pediatric clinical trials. Res Nurs Health 29(3):223–232
Spinetta JJ, Jankovic M, Eden T et al (1999) Guidelines for assistance to siblings of children with cancer: report of the SIOP Working Committee on Psychosocial Issues In Pediatric Oncology. Med Pediatr Oncol 33(4):395–398
Spinetta JJ, Masera G, Jankovic M et al (2003) Valid informed consent and participative decision-making in children with cancer and their parents: a report of the SIOP working committee on psychosocial issues in pediatric oncology. Med Pediatr Oncol 40(4):244–246
Spinetta JJ, Jankovic M, Masera G et al (2009) Optimal care for the child with cancer: a summary statement from the SIOP Working Committee on psychosocial issues in pediatric oncology. Pediatr Blood Cancer 52(7):904–907
Sposito AM, de Montigny F, Sparapani Vde C et al (2015) Puppets as a strategy for communication with Brazilian children with cancer. Nurs Health Sci 18(1):30–37
Standley JM, Hanser SB (1995) Music therapy research and applications in pediatric oncology treatment. J Pediatr Oncol Nurs 12(1):3–8
Stark D, Kiely M, Smith A et al (2002) Anxiety disorders in cancer patients: their nature, associations, and relation to quality of life. J Clin Oncol 20(14):3137–3148
Steele AC, Kaal J, Thompson AL et al (2013) Bereaved parents and siblings offer advice to health care providers and researchers. J Pediatr Hematol Oncol 35(4):253–259
Strauss RP, Sharp MC, Lorch SC, Kachalia B (1995) Physicians and the communication of "bad news": parent experiences of being informed of their child's cleft lip and/or palate. Pediatrics 96(1 Pt 1):82–89
Surbone A (2008) Cultural aspects of communication in cancer care. Support Care Cancer 16(3):235–240
Szmuilowicz E, Neely KJ, Sharma RK et al (2012) Improving residents' code status discussion skills: a randomized trial. J Palliat Med 15(7):768–774
The AM, Hak T, Koëter G, van Der Wal G (2000) Collusion in doctor-patient communication about

imminent death: an ethnographic study. BMJ 321(7273):1376–1381
The Conversation Project. Pediatric starter kit: having the conversation with your seriously ill child. http://theconversationproject.org/wpcontent/uploads/2016/05/TCP_PediatricSK_Forms.pdf. Accessed 28 June 2016
Thompson LA, Knapp C, Madden V, Shenkman E (2009) Pediatricians' perceptions of and preferred timing for pediatric palliative care. Pediatrics 123(5):e777–e782
Tucquet B, Leung M (2014) Music therapy services in pediatric oncology: a national clinical practice review. J Pediatr Oncol Nurs 31(6):327–338
Tulsky JA, Arnold RM, Alexander SC et al (2011) Enhancing communication between oncologists and patients with a computer-based training program: a randomized trial. Ann Intern Med 155(9):593–601
Valdez-Martinez E, Noyes J, Bedolla M (2014) When to stop? Decision-making when children's cancer treatment is no longer curative: a mixedmethod systematic review. BMC Pediatr 14:124
VitalTalk. http://www.vitaltalk.org/about-us. Accessed 28 June 2016
Vollenbroich R, Duroux A, Grasser M et al (2012) Effectiveness of a pediatric palliative home care team as experienced by parents and health care professionals. J Palliat Med 15(3):294–300
de Vries MC, Houtlosser M, Wit JM et al (2011) Ethical issues at the interface of clinical care and research practice in pediatric oncology: a narrative review of parents' and physicians' experiences. BMC Med Ethics 12:18
Wallin AE, Steineck G, Nyberg T, Kreicbergs U (2016) Insufficient communication and anxiety in cancer-bereaved siblings: a nationwide longterm follow-up. Palliat Support Care 14:488–494
Weaver MS (2014) Know guilt. J Clin Oncol 32(7):699–700
Weaver MS, Heinze KE, Kelly KP et al (2015) Palliative care as a standard of care in pediatric oncology. Pediatr Blood Cancer 62(S5):S829–S833
Weaver MS, Heinze KE, Bell CJ et al (2016) Establishing psychosocial palliative care standards for children and adolescents with cancer and their families: an integrative review. Palliat Med 30:212–223
Weeks JC, Cook EF, O'Day SJ et al (1998) Relationship between cancer patients' predictions of prognosis and their treatment preferences. JAMA 279(21):1709–1714
Weir RF, Peters C (1997) Affirming the decisions adolescents make about life and death. Hastings Cent Rep 27(6):29–40
Wheeler B (2015) Music therapy handbook. Guilford Press, New York
Widger K, Friedrichsdorf S, Wolfe J et al (2016) Protocol: evaluating the impact of a nation-wide train-the-trainer educational initiative to enhance the quality of palliative care for children with cancer. BMC Palliat Care 15:12
Wiener L, Zadeh S, Battles H et al (2012) Allowing adolescents and young adults to plan their end-of-life care. Pediatrics 130(5):897–905
Wolfe L (2004) Should parents speak with a dying child about impending death? N Engl J Med 351(12):1251–1253
Wolfe J, Klar N, Grier HE et al (2000) Understanding of prognosis among parents of children who died of cancer: impact on treatment goals and integration of palliative care. JAMA 284(19):2469–2475
Wright AA, Zhang B, Ray A et al (2008) Associations between end-of-life discussions, patient mental health, medical care near death, and caregiver bereavement adjustment. JAMA 300(14):1665–1673
Young B, Dixon-Woods M, Windridge KC, Heney D (2003) Managing communication with young people who have a potentially life threatening chronic illness: qualitative study of patients and parents. BMJ 326(7384):305
Young B, Ward J, Salmon P et al (2011) Parents' experiences of their children's presence in discussions with physicians about Leukemia. Pediatrics 127(5):e1230–e1238
Zabora J, BrintzenhofeSzoc K, Curbow B et al (2001) The prevalence of psychological distress by cancer site. Psychooncology 10(1):19–28
Zachariae R, Pedersen CG, Jensen AB et al (2003) Association of perceived physician communication style with patient satisfaction, distress, cancer-related self-efficacy, and perceived control over the disease. Br J Cancer 88(5):658–665
Zelcer S, Cataudella D, Cairney AEL, Bannister SL (2010) Palliative care of children with brain tumors: a parental perspective. Arch Pediatr Adolesc Med 164(3):225–230
Zwaanswijk M, Tates K, van Dulmen S et al (2007) Young patients', parents', and survivors' communication preferences in paediatric oncology: results of online focus groups. BMC Pediatr 7:35
Zwaanswijk M, Tates K, van Dulmen S et al (2011) Communicating with child patients in pediatric oncology consultations: a vignette study on child patients', parents', and survivors' communication preferences. Psychooncology 20(3):269–277

Considerations for Cancer-Directed Therapy in Advanced Childhood Cancer

5

Angela M. Feraco, Luca Manfredini, Momcilo Jankovic, and Joanne Wolfe

Key Points

- Cancer-directed therapy may have an important role in the care of children with advanced cancer.
- Cancer control can be viewed as a continuum.
- As the field of cancer therapeutics evolves, honest prognostic communication becomes increasingly nuanced.
- Decisions about whether and how to utilize cancer-directed therapy in the setting of advanced cancer should reflect the values of the patient, family, and healthcare system.

A.M. Feraco, M.D., M.M.Sc. (✉)
Department of Pediatric Oncology, Dana-Farber Cancer Institute and Boston Children's Hospital, 450 Brookline Avenue, Boston, MA 02215, USA
e-mail: angela_feraco@dfci.harvard.edu

L. Manfredini, M.D.
Department of Neurosciences, Paediatric Chronic Pain and Palliative Care Service, Rehabilitation and Continuity of Care, Institute G. Gaslini, Genoa, Italy

M. Jankovic, M.D.
Department of Paediatric Haemato-Oncology, Monza and Brianza Foundation for Children and Mothers, Hospital San Gerardo, Monza, Italy

J. Wolfe, M.D., M.P.H.
Department of Psychosocial Oncology and Palliative Care, Dana-Farber Cancer Institute, Boston, MA, USA

5.1 Cancer-Directed Therapy and Cancer Control

Marc is a 15-year-old adolescent male with relapsed osteosarcoma with pulmonary metastases and multiple bony lesions. Which factors may affect decision-making around whether and how to utilize cancer-directed therapy for Marc?

Cancer-directed therapy refers to any pharmacologic, surgical, or radiation therapy that is thought to have proven or potential antineoplastic activity (Orkin 2015). Combination cytotoxic chemotherapy has been the mainstay of pharmacologic cancer treatment, but a new generation of biologic and immunotherapies is rapidly altering the landscape of pharmacologic cancer-directed therapy for children with advanced cancer (Yu et al. 2010; von Stackelberg et al. 2016). Cancer control can be viewed as a continuum, ranging from little to no control (an actively growing tumor) to total control (cancer that has been completely treated and does not return). Achieving total control of childhood cancer is frequently referred to as achieving cure.

J. Wolfe et al. (eds.), *Palliative Care in Pediatric Oncology*, Pediatric Oncology,
https://doi.org/10.1007/978-3-319-61391-8_5

5.2 The Concept of "Cure" in Childhood Cancer

Prior to the 1960s, most childhood malignancies were fatal. The American Children's Cancer Study Group reported in 1969 that the 5-year survival of children with acute leukemia treated between 1957 and 1964 was 0.8%—just 15 of 1770 children (Pierce et al. 1969). Over the next 20 years, the use of multi-agent dose-dense chemotherapy, in combination with local control surgery (when applicable) or radiation, led to substantial long-term survival rates in acute leukemia, Hodgkin's lymphoma, and Wilms' tumor, among others. As the duration of expected remission lengthened, the term "cure" was increasingly used to describe the intended outcome of cancer-directed therapy (Mauer 1987). The term "cure" was used to mean "little or no expectation of return of disease," but frequently did not mean the restoration of health commensurate to that enjoyed prior to the initial cancer diagnosis (Mauer 1987).

The term "cure" is now frequently used with children and families when discussing cancer-directed therapy—in the current treatment era, a majority of children diagnosed with cancer are expected to experience lifelong disease eradication (Howlader et al. 2017). There are psychological, social, and financial benefits to using this term, and it may reflect a reality of unaltered life expectancy for some childhood cancer survivors (Pui et al. 2003). However, the term *cure* also suggests a dichotomy between cancers that can be cured and cancers that cannot—and by extension, children who can be cured and children who cannot. This dichotomy fails to take into account the frequently complex illness trajectories that children with cancer and their families experience (Feraco et al. 2017). Children with favorable-risk cancers sometimes die of infection or from unintended effects of cancer-directed therapy, while children with advanced cancer may live for many years with active disease while receiving multiple extended courses of cancer-directed therapy (Huo et al. 2016).

Frequently, the current literature distinguishes between cancer-directed therapy administered with "curative intent" and contrasts this with cancer-directed therapy administered with "palliative intent" (Weeks et al. 2012; von Stackelberg et al. 2011; Kang et al. 2013). Here, "palliative intent" is often taken to mean that the prescribing oncologist does not believe that there is an effective antineoplastic regimen that can be expected to provide effective, long-lasting cancer control (Kang et al. 2013; Bluebond-Langner et al. 2007). This nomenclature risks suggesting that palliation, the treatment of bothersome symptoms, is only a priority when we do not expect to eradicate cancer and that perhaps the goals of treating symptoms and treating cancer are mutually exclusive. It may also suggest that cancer-directed therapies are the only tools available to address symptoms. Notably, while oncologists use the term "palliative" to describe cancer-directed treatments (Kang et al. 2013), parents do not (Bluebond-Langner et al. 2007). Particularly in an era of changing paradigms in cancer-directed therapy, such as the increasing use of targeted agents and immunotherapies, which may substantially alter present prognostic estimates (Yu et al. 2010; von Stackelberg et al. 2016), this nomenclature falls short. As these treatments help us to reappraise what it means to gain control of childhood cancer, they should also encourage us to reexamine our approach to prognostic discussions.

5.3 Prognostic Discussions in the Setting of Advanced Childhood Cancer and Relationship to Use of Cancer-Directed Therapy

Discussing prognosis is an important component of family-centered childhood cancer care (Sisk et al. 2017; Mack and Joffe 2014; Mack et al. 2006). The goal is to convey honest, nuanced prognoses and make recommendations that incorporate our best understanding of patient and family preferences, cancer biology, available treatments, and the healthcare system. In adults with advanced lung cancer, there has been concern that focusing on selecting and administering cancer-directed therapy allows both oncologists and patients to sidestep honest discussions of prognosis (The et al. 2000). Likewise, research among adults with advanced cancer suggests that accurate prognostic understanding is associated with a preference for less intensive care, including less cancer-directed therapy (Weeks et al. 1998, 2012). Children and young adults with advanced cancer frequently receive cancer-directed therapy in the final days and weeks of life (Kang et al. 2013; Mack et al. 2015; Wolfe et al. 2015). Parents of children with advanced cancer may be slower to understand that cancer cannot be cured than treating oncologists (Wolfe et al. 2000a; Rosenberg et al. 2014). However, parents may value cancer-directed therapy for children with advanced cancer without expecting the outcome to be cure (Bluebond-Langner et al. 2007; Kamihara et al. 2015). Symptom reports from children with advanced cancer suggest that ongoing high-intensity cancer-directed therapy is associated with increased symptom burden, but that low-intensity cancer-directed therapy may be associated with a lessened symptom burden (Wolfe et al. 2015). However, retrospective reports by pediatric oncologists suggest that low-intensity cancer-directed therapy may fall short of expectations for symptom management and enhancement of quality of life (Kang et al. 2013). Thus, discussions of prognosis and the role of cancer-directed therapy should be individualized and nuanced. Table 5.1 provides example language that may be helpful to elicit patients' and parents' views about cancer-directed therapy. Discussions of possible treatment should address the likelihood of cure but also provide anticipatory guidance about what the child and family may expect in terms of possible life extension with cancer, symptoms attributable to treatment, and function during remaining life. Figure 5.1 summarizes the interacting factors that must be evaluated when considering cancer-directed therapy in the setting of advanced cancer. Just as time-limited trials of life-sustaining therapies may be useful for some children in the end-of-life period, time-limited trials of cancer-directed therapies with frequent reappraisal may be appropriate for some children with advanced cancer.

For Marc, there are no proven treatments that can completely control (cure) relapsed osteosarcoma, since his multifocal bony disease precludes the possibility of surgical resection. The expected illness course is death from progressive disease in months to years (Chou et al. 2005; Kempf-Bielack et al. 2005). Cancer-directed therapies may offer possibilities of cancer control that could lead to life extension but may also require substantial investment of time and produce additional burdensome symptoms or even lead to toxic death (Wolfe et al. 2000b, 2015). A discussion of the likely illness course and considerations of cancer-directed therapy should take into account Marc's and his family's preferences regarding time spent in the hospital or oncology clinic, acceptable routes of medication administration, and likelihood of side effects, as well as likelihood of short-term disease control without a realistic possibility for disease eradication.

Table 5.1 Exploring factors relevant to recommendations about cancer-directed therapy

Gauging illness and prognostic understanding	"What is your understanding of your/your child's illness?" "What is your sense of what to expect during the next few weeks/months?"
Eliciting views of cancer-directed therapy	"Given where we are with your/your child's illness, what are your hopes and worries as we consider whether more cancer treatments may be helpful?"
Reassessing the role of cancer-directed therapy	"When we began this treatment, we said we would carefully consider the degree to which it was helping or hurting. What is your sense of how the treatment is affecting you/your child and your family life now?"

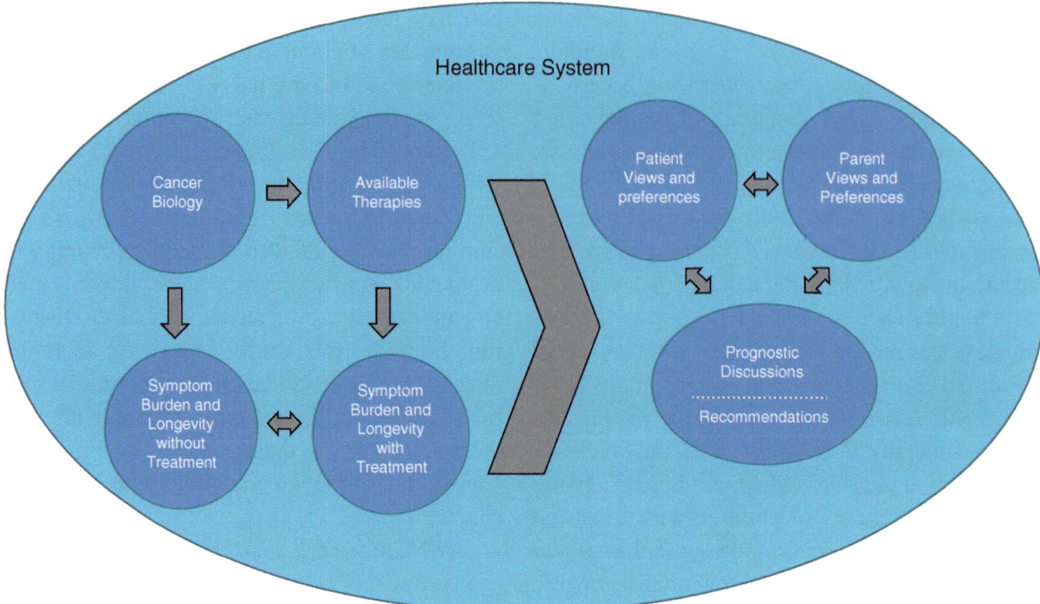

Fig. 5.1 Factors shaping recommendations regarding cancer-directed therapy in advanced childhood cancer. On the left-hand side of the figure, attributes of the cancer's biology and child's clinical status determine which available therapies may be most relevant and contribute to the oncologist's assessment of the likely illness course and symptom burden with and without cancer-directed treatments. These factors are incorporated into prognostic discussions, which elicit and incorporate patient and parent views and preferences. Finally, synthesis of these factors within the local healthcare system context leads to individualized recommendations

5.4 Parent, Patient, and Healthcare System Factors

Parents frequently seek cancer-directed therapy for children with advanced cancer, even when there is little expectation of successfully controlling cancer growth (Kang et al. 2013; Bluebond-Langner et al. 2007). Bluebond-Langner and colleagues suggest that for many parents, seeking additional options for cancer-directed therapy becomes central to the parenting role (Bluebond-Langner et al. 2007). They feel they must "leave no stone unturned" (Bluebond-Langner et al. 2007). Alternatively, parents may engage in a process of reappraising and resetting their goals and priorities in light of changes in a child's illness trajectory or evolution in the family's understanding of the illness' likely course (Hill et al. 2014). Importantly, bereaved parents may hold different views about cancer-directed therapy, believing in retrospect that children receiving cancer-directed therapy incurred suffering without benefit (Mack et al. 2008).

Although parents are legally responsible for decisions regarding the role of cancer-directed therapy, children are frequently actively engaged in decisions regarding their cancer care. Older children and adolescents are capable of participating in decision-making about the role of cancer-directed therapy during the end-of-life period (Hinds et al. 2005; Bluebond-Langner et al. 2010). For example, in a multi-institutional American study of informed consent conferences with families considering enrollment onto a phase I trial, the affected child with cancer was present for the informed consent conference 98% of the time (Hazen et al. 2015). Adolescents with advanced cancer may wish to pursue cancer-directed therapy as an expression of their regard for a loved one, such as a parent, or may derive personal benefit from a sense of acting to maintain health for as long as possible (Hinds et al. 2005). Alternatively, adolescents may acknowledge burdensome symptoms and decide that foregoing cancer-directed therapy is more consistent with living as well as possible.

Workforce factors, care environment, and healthcare payment model factors may also contribute significantly to decision-making around disease-directed therapy in the setting of advanced cancer (Miller et al. 2012). Although there is increasing emphasis on integration of palliative care and disease-directed care throughout the illness trajectory for children with cancer (Levine et al. 2017), healthcare payment models may not always allow for cancer-directed therapy in patients who would benefit from intensive home-based symptom management, such as through the use of hospice services. Thus, open communication with the patient and family that explores hopes, worries, priorities, and perspectives as well as detailed knowledge of the local healthcare system are crucial to ensure sound recommendations regarding the potential role for cancer-directed therapy.

In discussions with his primary oncologist and an interdisciplinary pediatric palliative care team, Marc and his parents were able to express their hopes, worries, and priorities. They were able to express their understanding that there were no proven treatments to achieve remission of Marc's osteosarcoma, given disseminated disease that could not be surgically removed. Marc enjoyed being outdoors and wanted to be able to take walks in the woods near his home for as long as possible. He was not interested in traveling to centers far from his home, but did not mind continuing to attend the oncology clinic at which he had received his initial treatment. He had substantial pain from his bony lesions. Ifosfamide and etoposide were administered with a goal of controlling cancer growth to assist with pain treatment and to extend life. Long-acting opiate medications and gabapentin were administered to treat bony nociceptive and neuropathic pain. Marc's pain improved substantially with these cancer-directed and symptom-directed treatments, but he disliked spending 1 week out of every 3 weeks in the hospital or clinic to receive chemotherapy. Additionally, due to effects of his chemotherapy and multiple antiemetics (including dexamethasone), he had a high symptom burden: fatigue, muscle aches, diarrhea, and hyperglycemia, as well as profound myelosuppression that required additional visits for transfusions of red blood cells and platelets.

After three cycles of ifosfamide and etoposide, Marc and his family, together with his oncology and palliative care teams, decided that the high symptom burden associated with his intensive cancer-directed therapy was too costly. However, he was interested in pursuing other potential treatments that would carry less of a symptom burden. Marc's oncology team and palliative care team collaborated and offered Marc treatment with monthly zoledronic acid, an intravenous bisphosphonate found to be tolerable in osteosarcoma (Goldsby et al. 2013) with evidence of preclinical efficacy and radiation therapy. Marc received both of these treatments as an outpatient. His bony pain lessened substantially for a period of several months, allowing him to enjoy walks in the woods during multiple seasons. Fifteen months after Marc's osteosarcoma relapse, he died of progressive disease.

5.5 Summary

In summary, cancer control may be understood as a continuum, and the potential role for cancer-directed therapy in the setting of advanced cancer is determined by considering the interplay of (1) patient and family preferences, (2) the patient's clinical status, (3) cancer biology and novel/targeted therapeutics, (4) likely symptom burden associated with giving versus withholding a particular medication/therapy, and (5) the healthcare system in which care is rendered. Marc's story illustrates potential roles for cancer-directed therapy in the advanced cancer setting and demonstrates an approach that incorporates a time-limited trial of cancer-directed therapy with active reappraisal of the associated symptom burden and subsequent selection of less-intensive cancer-directed therapy. Nuanced prognostic discussions and serial explorations of goals and symptoms should guide decision-making with regard to selecting, continuing, or discontinuing cancer-directed therapy.

References

Bluebond-Langner M, Belasco JB, Goldman A, Belasco C (2007) Understanding parents' approaches to care and treatment of children with cancer when standard therapy has failed. J Clin Oncol 25(17):2414–2419

Bluebond-Langner M, Belasco JB, DeMesquita Wander M (2010) "I want to live, until I don't want to live anymore": involving children with life-threatening and life-shortening illnesses in decision making about care and treatment. Nurs Clin North Am 45(3):329–343

Chou AJ, Merola PR, Wexler LH et al (2005) Treatment of osteosarcoma at first recurrence after contemporary therapy: the Memorial Sloan-Kettering Cancer Center experience. Cancer 104(10):2214–2221

Feraco AM, Dussel V, Orellana L et al (2017) Tumor talk and child-well being: perceptions of "good" and "bad" news among parents of children with advanced cancer. J Pain Symptom Manage 53:833–841

Goldsby RE, Fan TM, Villaluna D et al (2013) Feasibility and dose discovery analysis of zoledronic acid with concurrent chemotherapy in the treatment of newly diagnosed metastatic osteosarcoma: a report from the children's oncology group. Eur J Cancer 49(10):2384–2391

Hazen RA, Zyzanski S, Baker JN, Drotar D, Kodish E (2015) Communication about the risks and benefits of phase I pediatric oncology trials. Contemp Clin Trials 41:139–145

Hill DL, Miller V, Walter JK et al (2014) Regoaling: a conceptual model of how parents of children with serious illness change medical care goals. BMC Palliat Care 13(1):9

Hinds PS, Drew D, Oakes LL et al (2005) End-of-life care preferences of pediatric patients with cancer. J Clin Oncol 23(36):9146–9154

Howlader N, Noone AM, Krapcho M, et al (eds) (2017) SEER Cancer Statistics Review, 1975–2014. National Cancer Institute, Bethesda, MD. https://seer.cancer.gov/csr/1975_2014/, based on November 2016 SEER data submission, posted to the SEER web site

Huo JS, Symons HJ, Robey N, Borowitz MJ, Schafer ES, Chen AR (2016) Persistent multiyear control of relapsed T-cell acute lymphoblastic leukemia with successive donor lymphocyte infusions: a case report. Pediatr Blood Cancer 63:1279–1282

Kamihara J, Nyborn JA, Olcese ME, Nickerson T, Mack JW (2015) Parental hope for children with advanced cancer. Pediatrics 135(5):868–874

Kang TI, Hexem K, Localio R, Aplenc R, Feudtner C (2013) The use of palliative chemotherapy in pediatric oncology patients: a national survey of pediatric oncologists. Pediatr Blood Cancer 60(1):88–94

Kempf-Bielack B, Bielack SS, Jurgens H et al (2005) Osteosarcoma relapse after combined modality therapy: an analysis of unselected patients in the Cooperative Osteosarcoma Study Group (COSS). J Clin Oncol 23(3):559–568

Levine DR, Mandrell BN, Sykes A et al (2017) Patients' and parents' needs, attitudes, and perceptions about early palliative care integration in pediatric oncology. JAMA Oncol doi:10.1001/jamaoncol.2017.0368 (published online 9 March 2017 ahead of print)

Mack JW, Joffe S (2014) Communicating about prognosis: ethical responsibilities of pediatricians and parents. Pediatrics 133(Suppl 1):S24–S30

Mack JW, Wolfe J, Grier HE, Cleary PD, Weeks JC (2006) Communication about prognosis between parents and physicians of children with cancer: parent preferences and the impact of prognostic information. J Clin Oncol 24(33):5265–5270

Mack JW, Joffe S, Hilden JM et al (2008) Parents' views of cancer-directed therapy for children with no realistic chance for cure. J Clin Oncol 26(29):4759–4764

Mack JW, Chen K, Boscoe FP et al (2015) High intensity of end-of-life care among adolescent and young adult cancer patients in the new york state medicaid program. Med Care 53(12):1018–1026

Mauer AM (1987) The concept of cure in pediatric oncology. Altered realities. Am J Pediatr Hematol Oncol 9(1):58–61

Miller EG, Laragione G, Kang TI, Feudtner C (2012) Concurrent care for the medically complex child: lessons of implementation. J Palliat Med 15(11):1281–1283

Orkin SH (2015) Nathan and Oski's hematology and oncology of infancy and childhood, 8th edn. Elsevier Saunders, Philadelphia, PA

Pierce MI, Borges WH, Heyn R, Wolff JA, Gilbert ES (1969) Epidemiological factors and survival experience in 1770 children with acute leukemia treated by members of Children's Study Group A between 1957 and 1964. Cancer 23(6):1296–1304

Pui CH, Cheng C, Leung W et al (2003) Extended follow-up of long-term survivors of childhood acute lymphoblastic leukemia. N Engl J Med 349(7):640–649

Rosenberg AR, Orellana L, Kang TI et al (2014) Differences in parent-provider concordance regarding prognosis and goals of care among children with advanced cancer. J Clin Oncol 32(27):3005–3011

Sisk BA, Kang TI, Mack JW (2017) Prognostic disclosures over time: parental preferences and physician practices. Cancer doi:10.1002/cncr.30716 (published online 3 April 2017 ahead of print)

von Stackelberg A, Volzke E, Kuhl JS et al (2011) Outcome of children and adolescents with relapsed acute lymphoblastic leukaemia and non-response to salvage protocol therapy: a retrospective analysis of the ALL-REZ BFM study group. Eur J Cancer 47(1):90–97

von Stackelberg A, Locatelli F, Zugmaier G et al (2016) Phase I/phase II study of blinatumomab in pediatric patients with relapsed/refractory acute lymphoblastic leukemia. J Clin Oncol 34(36):4381–4389

The AM, Hak T, Koeter G, van Der Wal G (2000) Collusion in doctor-patient communication about imminent death: an ethnographic study. BMJ 321(7273):1376–1381

Weeks JC, Cook EF, O'Day SJ et al (1998) Relationship between cancer patients' predictions of prognosis and their treatment preferences. JAMA 279(21):1709–1714

Weeks JC, Catalano PJ, Cronin A et al (2012) Patients' expectations about effects of chemotherapy for advanced cancer. N Engl J Med 367(17):1616–1625
Wolfe J, Klar N, Grier HE et al (2000a) Understanding of prognosis among parents of children who died of cancer: impact on treatment goals and integration of palliative care. JAMA 284(19):2469–2475
Wolfe J, Grier HE, Klar N et al (2000b) Symptoms and suffering at the end of life in children with cancer. N Engl J Med 342(5):326–333
Wolfe J, Orellana L, Ullrich C et al (2015) Symptoms and distress in children with advanced cancer: prospective patient-reported outcomes from the PediQUEST study. J Clin Oncol 33(17):1928–1935
Yu AL, Gilman AL, Ozkaynak MF et al (2010) Anti-GD2 antibody with GM-CSF, interleukin-2, and isotretinoin for neuroblastoma. N Engl J Med 363(14):1324–1334

Palliative Care in Hematopoietic Stem Cell Transplantation

6

Monika Führer

6.1 Introduction

Over the past four decades, hematopoietic stem cell transplantation (HSCT) has become an important part of the standard therapy for a number of malignant hematological disorders and some solid tumors in children. The modern era of HSCT has begun with the new insights in the significance of histocompatibility in the 1970s. Two immunological mechanisms are relevant in HSCT—the recognition and destruction of the foreign tissue in a host-versus-graft reaction (graft rejection) by the recipient and the immunological recognition of the recipient tissue by immune-competent cells in the graft initiating a graft-versus-host (GvH) reaction.

To overcome the host-versus-graft reaction and allow the engraftment of hematopoietic stem cells (HSC), a highly immunosuppressive and cytotoxic conditioning treatment regimen is necessary prior to BMT. The collection of HSCs is an invasive procedure for the donor. HSCs are either harvested by multiple needle aspirations from the hip bones in a sterile operation room under general anesthesia or collected over several hours by peripheral blood apheresis after stimulation with granulocyte-colony stimulating factor (G-CSF). The collected HSCs are transplanted by intravenous transfusion.

The clinical course after HSCT can be complicated and patients often need intense supportive care for several weeks. The conditioning treatment typically causes severe organ toxicity and painful mucosal damage resulting in deficient barrier function. Notably, therapy-related mortality has been significantly decreased in the last two decades (Svenberg et al. 2016). Fifty to eighty percent of pediatric HSCT patients with hematologic malignancies survive and are cured of their disease. Many children also recover fully from the complications of the procedure and reach a normal quality of life (Conter et al. 2014; Pession et al. 2013; Suttorp et al. 2009).

In both autologous and allogeneic HSCT treatment, toxicity and infections due to impaired immune defense cause the main side effects in the acute posttransplant period. In autologous HSCT no immunological problems result since the patient's own cryopreserved stem cells are infused as rescue after high-dose myelotoxic chemotherapy. In the allogeneic setting, however, graft-versus-host disease (GvHD) remains a major complication.

Within some diagnoses such as acute lymphoblastic leukemia, high-dose myeloablative chemotherapy, in combination with total body irradiation, has conventionally been used as the conditioning regimen before HSCT because of

M. Führer
Dr. von Hauner Children's Hospital, University Clinics Munich, Munich, Germany
e-mail: Monika.Fuehrer@med.uni-muenchen.de

J. Wolfe et al. (eds.), *Palliative Care in Pediatric Oncology*, Pediatric Oncology,
https://doi.org/10.1007/978-3-319-61391-8_6

its profound immunosuppressive effect and its proven antitumor efficacy. Studies comparing the outcome according to donor match have shown a higher risk for relapse in identical twins (Gale et al. 1994) and a lower risk of relapse in recipients who developed GvHD (Ringden et al. 2009). Thus, an alloreactive response to recipient tumor cells called graft-versus-tumor (GVT)/graft-versus-leukemia (GvL) effect was postulated. In the 1990s donor lymphocyte infusions were for the first time used to induce remissions in patients with relapsed chronic myeloid leukemia (CML) after allo-HSCT (Kolb et al. 1990). Today there is ample evidence that the main therapeutic principle in allo-HSCT is an alloimmune effect directed against tumor cells. And this effect, like GvHD, is mediated by immunocompetent cells of the donor (Petersen 2007).

Since the late 1990s, non-myeloablative and reduced intensity conditioning (RIC) regimens have been developed (Slavin et al. 1998). These highly immunosuppressive regimens are used in pediatric HSCT to limit acute toxicity and enable the engraftment of T-cell-depleted grafts from human lymphocyte antigen (HLA)-mismatched or haploidentical donors (Bitan et al. 2014). The donors were mainly the parents who were willing and able to donate megadoses of peripheral HSCs after stimulation with G-CSF. In hematopoietic malignancies, rejection of HSCs after RIC was not a major problem; however, with non-myeloablative conditioning the curative potential relies entirely on the GvT effect (Lee et al. 2011).

The major throwback after allogeneic HSCT is the relapse of the malignancy. In order to improve the antileukemic or antitumor effect, the following main strategies are used: (i) lowering the tumor burden before the transplant, e.g., using modified T cells targeting specific antigens on the malignant clone (Maude et al. 2015); (ii) enhancing the posttransplant GvT effect, e.g., by adapting the posttransplant immunosuppressive therapy to the individual risk profile (Pochon et al. 2015); or (iii) intensifying the GvT effect through scheduled posttransplant infusions of increasing doses of donor T-lymphocytes or natural killer (NK) cells (Rettinger and Merker 2017).

The abovementioned strategies illustrate that HSCT has become a complex procedure that uses the allogeneic transplant as a platform for a sophisticated alloimmune therapy of the malignant disease. Molecular technology is applied to continuously monitor chimerism or, more specific, minimal residual disease, and alloimmune therapy is modified according to the results. Thus, this therapeutic approach may be extended over many years with the aim to control the malignant clone and to prevent overt relapse (Bader et al. 2015). This approach has changed the disease trajectories of children with hematologic malignancies completely as these diseases have become chronic conditions that may accompany a child's development for a decade or more. Living a decade or more under the sword of Damocles of a life-threatening illness that requires full parental involvement makes it extremely difficult to transition treatment goals when indicated, as this may be experienced as all the suffering and sacrifices have been in vain. Therefore, this process may be supported by the accompaniment of a specialized palliative care team (Lafond et al. 2015; Mahmood et al. 2016).

The following case vignette will exemplify the long and burdensome journey of HSCT the children and their families have to face. The story will show how palliative care can introduce aspects of quality of life into the transplant procedure and aftercare to reduce suffering and support families to cope with long-term sequelae and therapy failure.

Case Vignette: Anna

Anna developed acute myeloid leukemia with a rare high-risk genetic marker at the age of 9 months. She received chemotherapy according to the study protocol and was grafted in first remission at the age of 15 months with bone marrow from an unrelated HLA-identical donor after myeloablative conditioning with busulfan. The posttransplant course was uneventful, and no significant acute or chronic GvHD occurred. However, 18 months posttransplant, she developed a relapse in the bone marrow. Since Anna had not shown any major toxicity, her treating physician discussed with her parents the possibility of a second HSCT from the same donor after reduced intensity conditioning using peripheral stem cells. Anna's parents agreed. Because of the high relapse risk, the GvHD prophylaxis with cyclosporine A was tapered early and stopped at day + 60 to foster the graft-versus-leukemia effect. In the acute posttransplant period, Anna suffered from grade III gut toxicity and two episodes with bacterial infections. Her early acute GvHD grade II–III was successfully treated with a short course of steroid therapy. At 6 months after her transplant, she showed signs of chronic GvHD (cGvHD) with involvement of the skin, mucous membranes, gut, and liver. In the following months, she suffered from severe itching, alopecia, dry eyes, and progressing joint stiffness. She did not thrive and often was too weak to go to school. The immunosuppressive therapy was restarted and intensified but was not able to sufficiently control her progressing cGvHD. Despite her medical condition, she had her first day at school at age 6. After a few weeks at school, she was admitted to the ICU because of severe breathlessness. The X-ray and CT scan of her lungs confirmed the diagnosis of idiopathic pneumonia syndrome. Her condition deteriorated despite all therapeutic efforts, and she was placed on mechanical ventilation. Anna decided for herself to undergo a tracheostomy and mechanical ventilation. Her kidney and gut function worsened due to progressive cGvHD and the side effects of immunosuppressive therapy and she was started on hemofiltration. Six months after her admission, she was still in the intensive care unit (ICU) with chronic progressive multi-organ failure. After an unsuccessful attempt to discharge her for Christmas, Anna asked her mother: "Will I never see the sun again?" At that time the specialized pediatric palliative care team was called to prepare and coordinate her discharge. It took an enormous effort to finally bring her home on mechanical ventilation with a 24/7 on call specialized pediatric home palliative care service and a home nursing team. She remained on mechanical ventilation and received opioids and benzodiazepines through a patient-controlled analgesia (PCA) device. Six weeks later Anna died peacefully at home with her family around. Her brother still remembers that he was not allowed to visit his sister in the ICU. Her parents still struggle with the enormous burden the 7 months in the ICU caused to them.

6.2 Decision Making in HSCT

HSCT offers a potentially and in many cases the only possible curative treatment in advanced hematologic and some non-hematologic malignancies. Since the risk for severe toxicity, treatment-related death, or significant long-term sequelae still substantially exceeds the risks of conventional cancer therapy, HSCT is only considered after relapse or in high-risk cases.

Children and adolescents undergoing HSCT are exposed to severe physical symptoms and existential distress. An interdisciplinary approach with a focus on symptom management and quality of life is implemented by many SCT teams. Early integration of palliative care specialists to support the young patient and family is still uncommon in pediatric HSCT. Experience suggests that parents experience stressful uncertainty and worry about transplant difficulties, and many avoid focusing on thoughts about the mortality risk for their child while undergoing HSCT. Parents often prefer to concentrate on hope and immediate challenges that foster a sense of control. Thus, a mutual tacit understanding between parents and healthcare professionals leads to exclusion of this particular patient group from palliative care consultation, resulting in low rates of hospice enrollment and mainly hospital deaths (Ullrich et al. 2016a; Wolfe et al. 2000; Mack et al. 2006).

Pediatric HSCT patients and their families often face a high burden of symptoms and suffering throughout the immediate course of the transplant and sometimes for years after the transplant. Specialized pediatric palliative care (SPPC) services could provide much needed additional support during the inpatient phase of the transplant, bridge the gap to the home care setting, assist in care coordination, and take care of the physical, emotional, and spiritual suffering of the patient and the family (Roeland et al. 2010a; b; Groh et al. 2013). Furthermore, SPPC teams may be helpful in facilitating goals-of-care discussions and advance care planning before HSCT and during the posttransplant phase (Loggers et al. 2014; Ullrich et al. 2016b; Lotz et al. 2017).

Like in Anna's case, decision making is perceived as especially difficult by parents when the child is very young and unable to express his/her own wishes. While facing a life-threatening disease, parents are often concerned about exposing an infant or young child to toxic therapies with severe side effects that might impair the child's development and future well-being. This burden is even greater if the child experiences a relapse. Parents are already informed about what it means to go through HSCT, and they are aware that with every relapse, cure becomes less likely.

Therefore, palliative care counseling should be integrated in the decision-making process to address the hopes and anxieties of the patient and the parents and to honestly discuss the prognosis and the burden HSCT will cause (Mack et al. 2007). Palliative care counseling can help to create space for new perspectives where the child's and the family's quality of life (QoL) and the psychosocial and spiritual needs are considered important (Mack et al. 2009).

6.3 Acute and Chronic Toxicity

Most children are admitted to HSCT after their malignant disease has relapsed, but some are already grafted in first remission mainly because of high-risk chromosomal aberrations in the malignant clone. They enter the conditioning phase after they have undergone intensive chemotherapy and in solid tumors also surgery and radiation therapy. The toxicity of myeloablative conditioning regimen is considerable. Its cytotoxic effects especially affect all tissues with a high cell turnover like the mucous membranes, causing severe painful mucositis and enterocolitis.

There is some evidence from adult studies that integration of palliative care improves symptom control and reduces suffering during the conditioning treatment and the early posttransplantation phase (El-Jawahri et al. 2016). During the conditioning treatment, nausea and vomiting are major physical complaints. Mucositis and enterocolitis cause significant pain and often necessitate continuous i.v. opioid treatment, which should ideally be provided as patient (or parent)-controlled analgesia (PCA) (Collins et al. 1996). Furthermore, anxiety, isolation, and feelings of being powerless and completely dependent are highly prevalent and of high impact on the patients QoL. These psychosocial and existential issues warrant specific attention.

Veno-occlusive disease (VOD)/sinusoidal obstruction syndrome (SOS) is an acute and potentially life-threatening complication of HSCT that causes severe symptoms and suffering. The condition usually develops during the first 30 days after HSCT. Toxic endothelial cell lesions caused by the conditioning therapy may lead to a wide range of endothelial syndromes including VOD/SOS, capillary leak syndrome, transplant-associated microangiopathy, or diffuse alveolar hemorrhage (Mohty et al. 2015). Risk factors for VOD/SOS like young age (< 2 years), myeloablative and busulfan-based conditioning treatment, unrelated and mismatched donors, and second HSCTs are often present in children. Abdominal discomfort, pain, and significant weight gain are early symptoms; the full clinical picture of severe VOD/SOS includes all signs of multi-organ failure with impaired pulmonary and renal function and in some cases CNS involvement. Early diagnosis and treatment with defibrotide is crucial to prevent a lethal course (Richardson et al. 2016). The symptomatic management of abdominal pain, dyspnea, and edema necessitates interdisciplinary cooperation. The SPPC team can help to reduce the patient's physical suffering by optimizing symptom control and address the patients and the parents' fears by providing psychosocial support.

Subacute and chronic organ toxicity is not only caused by the conditioning treatment but also, e.g., by immunosuppressants, antibiotics, or drugs to treat fungal or viral infections. Renal toxicity is prevalent in SCT recipients who receive calcineurin inhibitors for a long time or are exposed to antiviral drugs like cidofovir (Didsbury et al. 2015). In children with long and complex transplant courses, chronic impairment of organ function is common and must be considered when, e.g., opioids or adjuvants are used for symptom management.

6.4 Infectious Complications

Mucositis together with agranulocytosis and long-lasting immunosuppression are the main causes for severe bacterial, fungal, and viral infections. Antibiotic prophylaxis and therapy is successful in most cases; however, severe pneumonia and septicemia can be life-threatening and may result in ICU referral (Fernández-García et al. 2015). Antifungal therapy is still less effective, and cure of fungal infections mainly depends on engraftment and granulocyte recovery. Even worse are the options to treat complications that are caused by viral infections that might occur especially after mismatched or unrelated transplantation. Antiviral therapy is often toxic (Caruso Brown et al. 2015), and effective control of viral infections depends on the reconstitution of T-cell immunity.

"Reduced intensity conditioning" (RIC) regimen was introduced to decrease acute toxicity and mucosal damage. This also reduced the risk of acute bacterial infections and allowed to expand HSCT to vulnerable populations and to perform second or even third HSCTs in relapsed patients. However, RIC transplants are profoundly immunosuppressive and may therefore result in delayed immune reconstitution and more viral infections especially in HLA-mismatched and HLA-haploidentical transplants (Federmann et al. 2011).

Most pediatric patients are kept in isolation in a room with laminar airflow to avoid infections. Complete isolation is ceased as soon as the child's granulocyte count rises above 500/μL. Isolation per se is frightening to most children. They are not allowed to leave their room, and depending on the unit, visitors may be required to wear face masks, sterile clothes, and even gloves. Parents may not be allowed to stay overnight and to sleep in the same room with their child. Close skin-to-skin contact is restricted, and especially younger children suffer when their parents are not able to comfort them in their familiar way. Several strategies can be used to ease the impact of isolation in an age-appropriate way. Many children enjoy the company of their familiar toys, and they love to listen to familiar music or audiotapes and to receive letters with photographs of their loved ones or small gifts sent by their classmates. Keeping in touch with friends and family using digital communication or social media and continuing favorite activities can help to avoid feelings of isolation and abandonment. In addition, a teacher or child care worker can offer lessons and activities that help to maintain a sense of normality and to structure the days.

During acute infection patients experience a variety of symptoms like fever, pain, weakness, and dyspnea. Since parents are aware of the patient being defenseless during the posttransplant phase, systemic infection and associated symptoms can cause a significant decline in parental emotional functioning (Terrin et al. 2013). In addition to the anti-infective treatment, the symptoms should be assessed, and symptom-directed treatment should be adjusted to the current needs of the child. Experience suggests that only when physical distress is adequately controlled, patient and parents are able to make use of additional psychosocial and spiritual support.

6.5 Acute and Chronic GvHD

After successful engraftment, acute GvHD can be a major problem during the first 100 days. GvHD is almost absent in identical twins (syngenic HSCT) and less prevalent in HLA-identical sibling donors when compared to matched unrelated or mismatched donors. Despite careful selection of unrelated donors according to HLA types and GvHD prophylaxis with immunosuppressive agents in recipients, acute GvHD can occur within days after engraftment and can cause mild to severe organ damage. The main target organs of aGvHD are the skin, liver, and intestine. Today lethal aGvHD is very rare.

There is growing evidence that inflammation due to tissue damage caused by the conditioning treatment is an important trigger for aGvHD (van der Zouwen et al. 2012). Since many children lack sibling donors, transplants from an alternative donor, e.g., matched unrelated donor or haploidentical parent, have become increasingly important. As noted previously, especially in haploidentical transplants, RIC is used in combination with T-cell-depleted grafts to avoid inflammation and aGvHD.

Chronic graft-versus-host disease (cGvHD) is defined as an immunoregulatory disorder that occurs after allogeneic HSCT and shares features of autoimmunity and immunodeficiency (Lee 2017). cGvHD plays a major role for QoL and long-term survival after childhood HSCT. It can evolve from aGvHD or arise independently. cGVHD and its treatment and complications are the major cause of late non-relapse mortality and morbidity (Wilhelmsson et al. 2015). In many cases limited cGvHD can be successfully controlled with corticosteroids and immune-suppressive therapy; however, in a small proportion of children, cGvHD evolves into a chronic, progressive, and life-limiting condition that causes severe losses in QoL. Multiple attempts have been made to define and classify cGvHD and to develop new treatment options that avoid the side effects of long-term steroid treatment. Photophoresis has been applied successfully in adult patients and increasingly also in pediatric cGvHD patients (Weitz et al. 2015). Beyond that, third-party mesenchymal stem cells have recently been successfully used to control cGvHD, so far without any major adverse events. Children with extensive cGvHD and their families may benefit from SPPC to optimize symptom control (see Table 6.1), offer psychosocial support, and thereby as much as possible allow for home-based care.

Table 6.1 Symptoms, assessment, and supportive/palliative treatment of chronic GvHD (Lawitschka et al. 2014; Wiener et al. 2014; Hildebrandt et al. 2011; Meier et al. 2011; Dietrich-Ntoukas et al. 2012; Marks et al. 2011; Packman et al. 2010; Fiuza-Luces et al. 2015)

Organ	Symptom	Assessment	Treatment
Skin, nails, and hair	Itching Skin discoloration, rash, bladders, sores Skin tightness, thick skin, edema Skin pain Hair loss, nail peeling	Timing (e.g., day and/or night); dependence on, e.g., temperature, drugs; association with handling and care procedures Risk factors for sores Vigilance for skin infection; taking cultures Evaluation of alopecia: scarring or non-scarring scalp alopecia?	*Avoiding triggers*: strict UV protection (clothing, sun blocks) *Basic skin care*: lukewarm shower, avoid rubbing, regular lubrication, ointments and creams with urea (3–10%), glycerol or dexpanthenol, cold black tea compresses *Topical treatment* with steroids and calcineurin inhibitors (e.g., tacrolimus), intralesional steroids *Pruritus*: polidocanol-based emollients; wet wrap treatment; high-dose antihistamine, gabapentin *Extracorporeal photopheresis (ECP)*, PUVA therapy *Psychosocial support*: camouflage for post-inflammatory hypo- and hyperpigmentation; finding a funny cap/hat/wig; distraction and relaxation exercises
Mouth	Mouth dry, pain, bothersome Problems eating, pain while eating Erythema, edema, inflammation, ulcers	Association with specific foods or textures (salty, spicy, hot, dry?) Sjörgren-like syndrome, xerostomia, dental caries, gingival recession, dental loss	*Diet* according to preferences Pilocarpin, artificial saliva, salivary gland stimulation with sugar-free gum, dental healthcare *Topical* steroids and/or tacrolimus Local anesthetics (lidocaine), CO_2 laser

Table 6.1 (continued)

Organ	Symptom	Assessment	Treatment
Eyes	Eyes bothersome, dry, hurting, foreign body sensation, itchiness No clear sight	Ophthalmological examination (Schirmer's test and microbial swabs)	*Lubricants*, preservative-free eye drops/synthetic tears, ointment *Topical* treatment with corticosteroids/cyclosporine Prophylactic/therapeutic topical antibiotics *Glasses* and/or sunglasses, occlusive eye wear
Gastrointestinal tract	Poor appetite, certain foods cannot be eaten Difficulty swallowing Belly pain, diarrhea, constipation	Eating preferences, preferred textures, and temperature Local/mucosal infections (Candida, C. diff.) Medication causing pain, diarrhea, constipation	Adaptation of meals according to preferences, careful substitution of vitamins and micronutrients (e.g., iron substitution causing pain/constipation) Consequent prophylaxis and treatment of constipation (polyethylene glycol, bisacodyl, naltrexone) Mild exercise program (physiotherapy) Adaptation of physician prescription of necessary intake (amount of calories and fluids)
Lung	Breathing problems Shortness of breath: walking, running Coughing Need of oxygen	Sensations that are associated with breathing problems (pain, headache, palpitation, sweating, anxiety) Occasions of dyspnea (while exercising, daily activities, resting) Cough (productive, nonproductive, hurting) Pulmonary function test, chest X-ray, high-resolution CT Exclusion/detection of infection (bronchoalveolar lavage)	Early topical treatment with inhaled steroids (e.g., budesonide, fluticasone) and beta-agonists (e.g., salbutamol) Systemic treatment with steroids (pulse therapy) Treatment of chronic bacterial colonization of the airways and sino-bronchial syndrome with tobramycin inhalation Continuous azithromycin therapy Antifibrotic therapy with imatinib; anti-inflammatory treatment with montelukast Morphine for treatment of dyspnea Noninvasive/invasive ventilation and tracheostomy
Muscle, joints/fascia	Muscles/joints bothersome, pain Muscles weak, cramping Tight joints, difficulty moving, unable to run	Fasciitis, (poly)myositis, myalgia, and arthralgia	Physiotherapy, especially thermal modalities, stretching, joint mobilization, and lymphatic drainage to avoid contractures Systemic therapy with steroids (myositis) or extracorporeal photopheresis (ECP) (fasciitis)
Genital	Vaginal burn, pain Phimosis	Regular examination: fibrosis, scarring, adhesions? Sex hormone levels?	Hormone substitution Topical hormones (estrogen), steroids, tacrolimus
Emotion	Depression Anxiety Sleeping disturbance	Health-related quality of life Testing for neurocognitive function Situations, procedures, thoughts, and memories that trigger anxiety	Behavioral therapy: guided imagery, distraction, progressive muscle relaxation Support groups and creative therapy programs (art, music, dance) Parent support interventions, family interventions Pharmacological interventions: antidepressants, melatonin
General condition	Loss of weight Loss of energy, need to sleep a lot Osteopenia	Health-related QoL Hormone analysis (growth hormone, thyroid hormone)	Physical exercise, rehabilitative medicine Hormone substitution, infection prophylaxis, bisphosphonate therapy

6.6 Secondary Malignant Neoplasms After SCT

Secondary malignant neoplasms (SNMs) are one of the most serious late complications in childhood cancer survivors. HSCT survivors represent a high-risk group for secondary cancer, especially those who have undergone very intensive treatment with high doses of chemotherapy or radiotherapy or those who have experienced prolonged immune deficiency due to delayed T-cell recovery. The cumulative incidence for secondary malignant neoplasms (SMNs) comes up to 10–15% by 15-year posttransplant and continues to rise for several decades after completion of treatment, so far with no evidence of a plateau (Choi et al. 2014). Most secondary malignancies occur due to previous treatment, but some may be related to genetic or other environmental factors.

Posttransplant lymphoproliferative disorders (PTLDs), which usually manifest as EBV-related B-cell non-Hodgkin lymphoma (NHL), occur in most cases very early, i.e., within months post-HSCT. Three to five years after chemotherapy with alkylating agents or topoisomerase II inhibitors, secondary acute myeloid leukemia or myelodysplastic syndrome may rarely develop, while solid tumors appear later, i.e., after 10–15 years mainly after radiotherapy (Nelson et al. 2015). Age at total body irradiation (TBI) was significant for the occurrence of SMN with children <10 years old at the time of TBI having a 55-fold higher risk of developing a solid SMN and remained elevated in children 10 to 19 years old with a fourfold increased risk (Lee et al. 2015). Some patients who are grafted suffer from an underlying condition similar to Fanconi anemia, which significantly increases the probability of SMN because of an extensive susceptibility to ionizing radiation (Deeg et al. 1996). Today the trend in pediatric HSCT is to avoid radiation-based conditioning regimens especially in small children below the age of 3 or in patients with a cancer predisposition.

A SMN often causes deep despair in the patient and the parents, especially when a cancer-predisposing condition is diagnosed. Sensitive counseling is important in these cases where families must not only cope with the life-limiting disease of their child but also have to face the possibility that additional family members might be affected in the future.

The therapeutic choices and the prognosis of SMNs are different and depend on the type of the SMN and whether an underlying condition is present. Early detection and treatment may positively affect the prognosis of solid tumors, which underlines the importance of prevention (e.g., UV protection) and surveillance after HSCT. The prognosis of secondary myelodysplastic syndrome (MDS) or secondary AML is unfavorable (Danner-Koptik et al. 2013). In most cases treatment of secondary AML/MDS requires another allogeneic HSCT, which often results in severe acute and chronic side effects and significant mortality in many of these heavily pretreated patients.

The majority of PTLDs are associated with Epstein-Barr virus infection (EBV). Compared to children who received a solid organ transplant, the risk of PTLD is relatively low after allogeneic HSCT (1–2% of recipients) but may be significantly higher in patients with delayed immune reconstitution. Specific risk factors were identified, e.g., T-cell depletion of the graft (up to 24%), use of antithymocyte globulin (ATG) for GVHD prophylaxis, unrelated or HLA-mismatched grafts, and chronic GVHD (Bomken and Skinner 2015). Reduced intensity conditioning (RIC) regimen might be associated with an increased risk of PTLD (Cohen et al. 2007). During the relatively short period of highest PTLD risk, intensive monitoring of EB virus load offers the possibility to effectively control PTLD by lowering thc immunosuppressive therapy or treating the B-cell expansion with the anti-CD20 monoclonal antibody rituximab (Llaurador et al. 2016). In some cases cytotoxic chemotherapy is necessary and prognosis is still less favorable in patients with CNS involvement (Styczynski et al. 2016).

Since many pediatric cancer patients are surviving after their HSCT into adulthood, these patients should be educated about their risk for SMN and the necessity of surveillance. When a SMN occurs after HSCT, SPPC should be considered to help reduce the overwhelming burden the families have to carry in view of a secondary cancer. The SPPC team can help to clarify therapeutic goals and to develop strategies that reduce the burden of repeated hospitalizations, diagnostic procedures, and treatment. The SPPC team can also address that sufficient symptom control may receive less attention, especially in cases with PTLD, where symptoms can be unspecific and diffuse.

6.7 Quality of Life and Long-Term Sequelae After HSCT

Survival after HSCT has been improved significantly during the last two decades. However, survivors are at risk of developing long-term physical, emotional, and social problems (Ness et al. 2005). Most long-term survivors of pediatric HSCT have impaired fertility and carry a high risk for morbidity, including endocrine dysfunction, musculoskeletal disorders, and cardiopulmonary abnormalities (Chow et al. 2016). In 2011 Armenian et al. reported the long-term health-related outcomes in survivors of childhood cancer treated with conventional chemotherapy, autologous SCT, and allogeneic HSCT. Fifty-nine percent of HSCT survivors reported ≥2 chronic health conditions and 25.5% severe/life-threatening conditions. Compared with survivors after conventional chemotherapy, HSCT survivors show significantly elevated risks for severe/life-threatening conditions, functional impairment, and activity limitation. Long-term sequelae like cardiac dysfunction, growth retardation, gonadal failure, neurocognitive impairment, and organ dysfunctions may result from the combined effects of pre-HSCT chemo- and radiotherapy, HSCT-related conditioning, and post-HSCT complications such as chronic GvHD and immune deficiency (Armenian et al. 2011). Increased risks were also found for motor impairments, hearing loss, vision loss, and persistent pain. Cataracts were a frequent adverse effect. Adverse effects on cognitive abilities are more likely in younger children and in patients who have received cranial irradiation and/or TBI (Gurney et al. 2006; Willard et al. 2014).

Longitudinal studies assessing the health-related quality of life (HQoL) in children and adolescents post-HSCT found that pre-HSCT psychosocial functioning is predictive of post-HSCT distress and functioning. A certain trajectory can be described with the lowest level of HQoL about 10 days posttransplant and a steady increase until 6 months posttransplant. In about 20% of patients, HQoL remains low with a strong association between psychosocial and physical functioning. Compromised emotional functioning, worry, and reduced communication during the acute phase of the HSCT predicted reduced physical functioning and worry 1 year post-HSCT (Packman et al. 2010). These data underline the need of additional support in the field of emotional functioning and communication.

6.8 End-of-Life Care in SCT

HSCT remains a high-risk procedure, and a significant number of HSCT recipients still die of relapse, acute treatment-related complications, or progressing chronic conditions. Organ toxicity, severe infections, and extensive cGvHD have a significant impact on the symptoms and suffering of pediatric HSCT patients at the end of life. Little is known about the specific needs of children at the end of life following HSCT. Bradshaw et al. reported that children who died after HSCT were more likely to experience pulmonary or cardiovascular complications. They had a do-not-resuscitate (DNR) order in place for a shorter period of time before death and were less likely to die at home, when compared to children who died after conventional chemotherapy (Bradshaw et al. 2005). Children who died after HSCT spent more days in the hospital in their last month of life; they were more likely to be intubated in the last 24 h of their life and they more often died in the intensive care unit (ICU). The location of death was less often planned and hospice was less often involved, hence HSCT parents were more likely to have preferred an alternative location for their child when compared to non-HSCT parents. In the HSCT group, death occurred more often after life-sustaining treatment was withdrawn. Discussions to forgo resuscitation were held with equal frequency in both groups; however, in the HSCT group, these discussions occurred later and resulted in fewer DNR orders. Children in the HSCT group were more likely to suffer highly from their last cancer-directed therapy. On average, children in the HSCT group suffered more from physical and psychologic symptoms than children in the non-HSCT group (Ullrich et al. 2010).This intense suffering warrants early integration of SPPC in the care of pediatric HSCT patients. Ullrich et al. found that although pediatric HSCT patients were mainly dying in a medicalized setting, integration of pediatric palliative care reduced interventions such as intubation or cardiopulmonary resuscitation close to the end of life (EOL), and facilitated EOL communication and ACP. Pediatric HSCT patients may benefit from early integration of SPPC since Ullrich et al. also found that patients who received palliative care for at least 1 month were more likely to receive hospice care (Ullrich et al. 2016b).

6.9 Psychosocial and Spiritual Aspects

HSCT presents many psychological challenges for the pediatric patient and the family. In most families, distress in HSCT begins with the consent process. Since HSCT is only considered if the child's disease is not likely to be cured by conventional chemotherapy, parents are at that point faced with the possibility of treatment failure and death from cancer. On the one hand, HSCT is the only chance for cure, but on the other hand, this complex procedure is connected with multiple risks for serious acute complications and long-term sequelae that are difficult to predict for a given child. Parent outlook on their child's survival and future health might have an important impact on decision making and coping; however, only little is known about parental hopes and fears. Ullrich et al. found that most parents frequently think about the immediate difficulties the transplantation might cause but avoid concerning themselves with thoughts about the risk of future worsening health or possible death of their child (Ullrich et al. 2016a).

Almost all pediatric patients experience significant anxiety before HSCT (Vrijmoet-Wiersma et al. 2009). Many patients already show high levels of emotional distress when they are hospitalized for the conditioning phase, and the distress continues to escalate during the first weeks after the transplant (Meyers et al. 1994). There is some evidence that up to 80% of pediatric HSCT patients show symptoms of post-traumatic stress 3 months after HSCT and that these symptoms persist in a significant number of children at 12 months after the transplantation (Stuber et al. 1991). Children and adolescents particularly suffer from social isolation that might persist beyond the actual HSCT procedure due to frequent hospital admissions and chronic health conditions (Packman et al. 2010).

The HSCT process has also been shown to be difficult for siblings, both donors and non-donors. However, the impact on siblings' acute and long-term emotional and social well-being is still being widely neglected. Packman et al. found that siblings are at risk of developing emotional reactions such as post-traumatic stress disorder, anxiety, and overall low self-esteem. A qualitative study by Wilkins and Woodgate in siblings found that "interruption" of the normal family life was a main theme. Siblings felt a sense of isolation from their families (Wilkins and Woodgate 2007a). The same authors report seven themes siblings identified as helpful during the HSCT process:

(1) Include me in the definition of "family."
(2) Be caring.
(3) Share information with me.
(4) Give me choices.
(5) Help me share feelings.
(6) Provide opportunities for me to meet my peers.
(7) Create a healthy hospital environment (Wilkins and Woodgate 2007b).

New behavior problems, anxiety, and low self-esteem were reported more frequently among siblings who were donating bone marrow

(Pillay et al. 2012). MacLeod et al. studied whether the success of the HSCT has an impact on sibling donor distress. They found that sibling donors often feel responsible for the survival of their sibling. But both the donors of successful and unsuccessful HSCTs stated that there was "no choice" for them to refuse in the consent process and that the psychological distress by far outweighed the physical aspects of the donation (MacLeod et al. 2003).

Parental distress during the consent process and in the immediate transplant phase is particularly high if a sibling is the donor. Parents are concerned with the health of both the child patient as well as the sibling donor (Hutt et al. 2015). They worry about putting the healthy donor child at risk through the general anesthesia and the bone marrow harvest, especially if the donating child is much smaller and younger than the patient.

In one study, at the time of admission for HSCT, 66% of mothers scored above the clinical cutoff on a depression inventory, and during the week before HSCT, 8% of mothers experienced clinically significant depression and 50% met the clinical cutoff for anxiety disorder (Manne et al. 2004). According to Jobe-Shields et al., parents are at risk of developing a depressive symptomatology. These parents may become less responsive to their children's needs and are thereby putting their children at risk for additional psychological and social problems (Jobe-Shields et al. 2009). Parental mental health is an important factor for a child's adjustment to its medical illness. As a means of coping, Forrinder et al. recommends that families empower themselves by participating actively and asking questions pertaining to their child's illness and the procedures involved (Forinder and Norberg 2014). A more supportive family environment may reduce distress during the HSCT process. Phipps and Mulhern found that the results of pre-HSCT assessment of family conflict and family cohesiveness and expressiveness were predictive of a child's adjustment 6–12 months after HSCT (Phipps and Mulhern 1995).

Providing psychological support to strengthen parents with their coping would be beneficial not only to the parents but would also foster the psychological well-being of the sick child and the siblings. Strengthening the family cohesion throughout the HSCT process is important; moreover, open and honest communication in the family can support the emotional well-being of the sick child and the siblings (Kazak et al. 2007).

Importantly, studies suggest for the pediatric patient the use of both cognitive-behavioral techniques and pharmacological interventions to prevent suffering due to severe symptoms and painful medical interventions which result in both short-term reduction of distress and long-term improvement in coping strategies (Kazak et al. 2005).

6.10 Care Structures and Team Aspects

While prognosis and potential for life-threatening complications are often explicitly discussed by SCT clinicians, advanced care planning is often deferred until later in the course when complications arise. However, there is some evidence from adult HSCT that advance care planning is perceived as helpful und does not undermine the patients' and the families' trust in the medical staff nor does it decrease their willingness to fully engage in the HSCT (Loggers et al. 2014).

Children and families may especially benefit from SPPC when they are faced with advanced and progressing life-shortening conditions like uncontrolled cGvHD, SMN, or relapse regardless of the ongoing attempts to treat the condition. Internationally different organizational models for SPPC exist. Some are hospital based (Feudtner et al. 2013), others are part of a free-standing children's hospice (Siden et al. 2014), some provide inpatient counseling only, and some have an outpatient clinic or provide specialized pediatric home palliative care with a 24/7 on call visiting service (Groh et al. 2013). Essential for the acceptance by the families and the quality of care in this very vulnerable patient group is the close cooperation with the HSCT specialist team and the composition of the SPPC team, which should at least offer medical and nursing care by specialized pediatric palliative care physicians and nurses and psychosocial support by a social worker or child care specialist, a psychologist or psychotherapist (or family therapist), and a chaplain.

References

Armenian SH, Sun C-L, Kawashima T et al (2011) Long-term health-related outcomes in survivors of childhood cancer treated with HSCT versus conventional therapy: a report from the Bone Marrow Transplant Survivor Study (BMTSS) and Childhood Cancer Survivor Study (CCSS). Blood 118(5):1413–1420. https://doi.org/10.1182/blood-2011-01-331835

Bader P, Kreyenberg H, von Stackelberg A et al (2015) Monitoring of minimal residual disease after allogeneic stem-cell transplantation in relapsed childhood acute lymphoblastic leukemia allows for the identification of impending relapse: results of the ALL-BFM-SCT 2003 trial. J Clin Oncol 33(11):1275–1284. https://doi.org/10.1200/JCO.2014.58.4631

Bitan M, He W, Zhang MJ et al (2014) Transplantation for children with acute myeloid leukemia: a comparison of outcomes with reduced intensity and myeloablative regimens. Blood 123(10):1615–1620. https://doi.org/10.1182/blood-2013-10-535716

Bomken S, Skinner R (2015) Secondary malignant neoplasms following haematopoietic stem cell transplantation in childhood. Children 2:146–173. https://doi.org/10.3390/children2020146

Bradshaw G, Hinds PS, Lensing S, Gattuso JS, Razzouk BI (2005) Cancer-related deaths in children and adolescents. J Palliat Med 8(1):86–95. https://doi.org/10.1089/jpm.2005.8.86

Caruso Brown AE, Cohen MN, Tong S et al (2015) Pharmacokinetics and safety of intravenous cidofovir for life-threatening viral infections in pediatric hematopoietic stem cell transplant recipients. Antimicrob Agents Chemother 59(7):3718–3725. https://doi.org/10.1128/AAC.04348-14

Choi DK, Helenowski I, Hijiya N (2014) Secondary malignancies in pediatric cancer survivors: perspectives and review of the literature. Int J Cancer 135(8):1764–1773

Chow EJ, Anderson L, Baker KS et al (2016) Late effects surveillance recommendations among survivors of childhood hematopoietic cell transplantation: a children's oncology group report. Blood Marrow Transplant 22(5):7827–7895. https://doi.org/10.1016/j.bbmt.2016.01.023

Cohen J, Cooper N, Chakrabarti S et al (2007) EBV-related disease following haematopoietic stem cell transplantation with reduced intensity conditioning. Leuk Lymphoma 48:256–269. https://doi.org/10.1080/10428190601059837

Collins JJ, Geake J, Grier HE (1996) Patient-controlled analgesia for mucositis pain in children: a three-period crossover study comparing morphine and hydromorphone. J Pediatr 129(5):722–728

Conter V, Valsecchi MG, Parasole R et al (2014) Childhood high-risk acute lymphoblastic leukemia in first remission: results after chemotherapy or transplant from the AIEOP ALL 2000 study. Blood 123(10):1470–1478. https://doi.org/10.1182/blood-2013-10-532598

Danner-Koptik KE, Majhail NS, Brazauskas R et al (2013) Second malignancies after autologous hematopoietic cell transplantation in children. Bone Marrow Transplant 48(3):363–368. https://doi.org/10.1038/bmt.2012.166

Deeg HJ, Socié G, Schoch G et al (1996) Malignancies after marrow transplantation for aplastic anemia and Fanconi anemia: a joint Seattle and Paris analysis of results in 700 patients. Blood 87(1):386–392

Didsbury MS, Mackie FE, Kennedy SE (2015) A systematic review of acute kidney injury in pediatric allogeneic hematopoietic stem cell recipients. Pediatr Transplant 19(5):460–470. https://doi.org/10.1111/petr.12483

Dietrich-Ntoukas T, Cursiefen C, Westekemper H et al (2012) Diagnosis and treatment of ocular chronic graft-versus-host disease: report from the Germn-Austrian-Swiss consensus conference on clinical practice in chronic GVHD. Cornea 31(3):299–310

El-Jawahri A, LeBlanc T, Van Dusen H et al (2016) Effect of inpatient palliative care on quality of life 2 weeks after hematopoietic stem cell transplantation: a randomized clinical trial. JAMA 316(20):2094–2103. https://doi.org/10.1001/jama.2016.16786

Federmann B, Hägele M, Pfeiffer M et al (2011) Immune reconstitution after haploidentical hematopoietic cell transplantation: impact of reduced intensity conditioning and CD3/CD19 depleted grafts. Leukemia 25(1):121–129. https://doi.org/10.1038/leu.2010.235

Fernández-García M, Gonzalez-Vicent M, Mastro-Martinez I et al (2015) Intensive care unit admissions among children after hematopoietic stem cell transplantation: incidence, outcome, and prognostic factors. J Pediatr Hematol Oncol 37(7):529–535. https://doi.org/10.1097/MPH.0000000000000401

Feudtner C, Womer J, Augustin R et al (2013) Pediatric palliative care programs in children's hospitals: a cross-sectional national survey. Pediatrics 132(6):1063–1070. https://doi.org/10.1542/peds.2013-1286

Fiuza Luces C, Garatachea N, Simpson RJ et al (2015) Understanding graft-versus-host disease. Preliminary findings regarding the effects of exercise in affected patients. Exerc Immunol Rev 21:80–112

Forinder U, Norberg AL (2014) Posttraumatic growth and support among parents whose children have survived stem cell transplantation. J Child Health Care 18(4):326–335. https://doi.org/10.1177/1367493513496666

Gale RP, Horowitz MM, Ash RC et al (1994) Identical twin bone marrow transplants for leukemia. Ann Intern Med 120:646–652

Groh G, Borasio GD, Nickolay C et al (2013) Specialized pediatric palliative home care: a prospective evaluation. J Palliat Med 16(12):1588–1594. https://doi.org/10.1089/jpm.2013.0129

Gurney JG, Ness KK, Rosenthal J et al (2006) Visual, auditory, sensory, and motor impairments in long-term survivors of hematopoietic stem cell transplantation performed in childhood: results from the bone marrow transplant survivor study. Cancer 106(6):1402–1408

Hildebrandt GC, Fazekas T, Lawitschka A et al (2011) Diagnosis and treatment of pulmonary chronic GVHD: report from the consensus conference on clinical practice in chronic GVHD. Bone Marrow Transplant 46:1283–1295

Hutt D, Nehari M, Munitz-Shenkar D et al (2015) Hematopoietic stem cell donation: psychological perspectives of pediatric sibling donors and their parents. Bone Marrow Transplant 50:1337–1342

Jobe-Shields L, Alderfer MA, Barrera M et al (2009) Parental depression and family environment predict distress in children before stem cell transplantation. J Dev Behav Pediatr 30(2):140–146. https://doi.org/10.1097/DBP.0b013e3181976a59

Kazak AE, Simms S, Alderfer MA et al (2005) Feasibility and preliminary outcomes from a pilot study of a brief psychological intervention for families of children newly diagnosed with cancer. J Pediatr Psychol 30:644–655

Kazak AE, Rourke MT, Alderfer MA et al (2007) Evidenced-based assessment, intervention, and psychosocial care in pediatric oncology: a blueprint for comprehensive services across treatment. J Pediatr Psychol 32:1099–1110

Kolb HJ, Mittermüller J, Clemm C et al (1990) Donor leukocyte transfusions for treatment of recurrent chronic myelogenous leukemia in marrow transplant patients. Blood 76:2462–2465

Lafond DA, Kelly KP, Hinds PS, Sill A, Michael M (2015) Establishing feasibility of early palliative care consultation in pediatric hematopoietic stem cell transplantation. J Pediatr Oncol Nurs 32(5):265–277. https://doi.org/10.1177/1043454214563411

Lawitschka A, Güclü ED, Varni JW et al (2014) Health-related quality of life in pediatric patients after allogeneic SCT: development of the PedsQL stem cell transplant module and results of a pilot study. Bone Marrow Transplant 49:1093–1097

Lee SJ (2017) Classification systems for chronic graft-versus-host disease. Blood 129(1):30–37

Lee KH, Lee JH, Lee JH et al (2011) Reduced-intensity conditioning therapy with busulfan, fludarabine, and antithymocyte globulin for HLA-haploidentical hematopoietic cell transplantation in acute leukemia and myelodysplastic syndrome. Blood 118(9):2609–2617. https://doi.org/10.1182/blood-2011-02-339838

Lee SJ, Wolff D, Kitko C (2015) Measuring therapeutic response in chronic graft-versus-host disease. National Institutes of Health Consensus Development Project on criteria for clinical trials in chronic graft-versus-host disease: IV. The 2014 Response Criteria Working Group Report. Biol Blood Marrow Transplant 21:984–999

Llaurador G, McLaughlin L, Wistinghausen B (2016) Management of post-transplant lymphoproliferative disorders. Curr Opin Pediatr 29(1):34–40

Loggers ET, Lee S, Chilson K et al (2014) Advance care planning among hematopoietic cell transplant patients and bereaved caregivers. Bone Marrow Transplant 49(10):1317–1322. https://doi.org/10.1038/bmt.2014.152

Lotz JD, Daxer M, Jox RJ, Borasio GD, Führer M (2017) “Hope for the best, prepare for the worst”: A qualitative interview study on parents’ needs and fears in pediatric advance care planning. Palliat Med 31(8):764–771

Mack JW, Wolfe J, Grier HE, Cleary PD, Weeks JC (2006) Communication about prognosis between parents and physicians of children with cancer: parent preferences and the impact of prognostic information. J Clin Oncol 24(33):5265–5270

Mack JW, Cook EF, Wolfe J et al (2007) Understanding of prognosis among parents of children with cancer: parental optimism and the parent-physician interaction. J Clin Oncol 25(11):1357–1362

Mack JW, Wolfe J, Cook EF et al (2009) Peace of mind and sense of purpose as core existential issues among parents of children with cancer. Arch Pediatr Adolesc Med 163(6):519–524. https://doi.org/10.1001/archpediatrics

MacLeod KD, Whitsett SF, Mash EJ et al (2003) Pediatric sibling donors of successful and unsuccessful hematopoietic stem cell transplants (HSCT): a qualitative study of their psychosocial experience. J Pediatr Psychol 28(4):223–231

Mahmood LA, Casey D, Dolan JG, Dozier AM, Korones DN (2016) Feasibility of early palliative care consultation for children with high-risk malignancies. Pediatr Blood Cancer 63(8):1419–1422. https://doi.org/10.1002/pbc.26024

Manne S, DuHamel K, Ostroff J et al (2004) Anxiety, depressive, and posttraumatic stress disorders among mothers of pediatric survivors of hematopoietic stem cell transplantation. Pediatrics 113:1700–1708

Marks C, Stadler M, Häusermann P et al (2011) German–Austrian–Swiss Consensus Conference on clinical practice in chronic graft-versus-host disease (GVHD): guidance for supportive therapy of chronic cutaneous and musculoskeletal GVHD. Br J Dermatol 165(1):18–29

Maude SL, Teachey DT, Porter DL, Grupp SA (2015) CD19-targeted chimeric antigen receptor T-cell therapy for acute lymphoblastic leukemia. Blood 125(26):4017–4023. https://doi.org/10.1182/blood-2014-12-580068

Meier JK-HH, Wolff D, Pavletic S et al (2011) Oral chronic graft-versus-host disease: report from the International Consensus Conference on clinical practice in cGVHD. Clin Oral Invest 15:127–139

Meyers CA, Weitzner M, Byrne K, Valentine A et al (1994) Evaluation of the neurobehavioral functioning of patients before, during, and after bone marrow transplantation. J Clin Oncol 12:820–826

Mohty M, Malard F, Abecassis M et al (2015) Sinusoidal obstruction syndrome/veno-occlusive disease: current situation and perspectives-a position statement from the European Society for Blood and Marrow Transplantation (EBMT). Bone Marrow Transplant 50(6):781–789. https://doi.org/10.1038/bmt.2015.52

Nelson AS, Ashton LJ, Vajdic CM (2015) Second cancers and late mortality in Australian children treated by allogeneic HSCT for haematological malignancy. Leukemia 29(2):441–447. https://doi.org/10.1038/leu.2014.203

Ness KK, Bhatia S, Baker KS et al (2005) Performance limitations and participation restrictions among childhood cancer survivors treated with hematopoietic stem cell transplantation: the bone marrow transplant survivor study. Arch Pediatr Adolesc Med 159(8):706–713

Packman W, Weber S, Wallace J, Bugescu N (2010) Psychological effects of hematopoietic SCT on pediatric patients, siblings and parents: a review. Bone Marrow Transplant 45:1134–1146

Pession A, Masetti R, Rizzari C et al (2013) Results of the AIEOP AML 2002/01 multicenter prospective trial for the treatment of children with acute myeloid leukemia. Blood 122(2):170–178. https://doi.org/10.1182/blood-2013-03-491621

Petersen SL (2007) Alloreactivity as therapeutic principle in the treatment of hematologic malignancies. Studies of clinical and immunologic aspects of allogeneic hematopoietic cell transplantation with nonmyeloablative conditioning. Dan Med Bull 54(2):112–139

Phipps S, Mulhern R (1995) Family cohesion and expressiveness promote resilience to the stress of pediatric bone marrow transplant: a preliminary report. J Dev Behav Pediatr 16:257–263

Pillay B, Lee SJ, Katona L et al (2012) The psychosocial impact of haematopoietic SCT on sibling donors. Bone Marrow Transplant 47:1361–1365

Pochon C, Oger E, Michel G et al (2015) Follow-up of post-transplant minimal residual disease and chimerism in childhood lymphoblastic leukaemia: 90 d to react. Br J Haematol 169(2):249–261. https://doi.org/10.1111/bjh.13272

Rettinger E, Merker M, Salzmann-Manrique E et al (2017) Pre-emptive immunotherapy for clearance of molecular disease in childhood acute lymphoblastic leukemia after transplantation. Biol Blood Marrow Transplant 23(1):87–95. https://doi.org/10.1016/j.bbmt.2016.10.006. Epub 2016 Oct 11

Richardson PG, Riches ML, Kernan NA et al (2016) Phase 3 trial of defibrotide for the treatment of severe veno-occlusive disease and multi organ failure. Blood 127(13):1656–1665. https://doi.org/10.1182/blood-2015-10-676924

Ringden O, Pavletic SZ, Anasetti C et al (2009) The graft-versus-leukemia effect using matched unrelated donors is not superior to HLA-identical siblings for hematopoietic stem cell transplantation. Blood 113(13):3110–3118

Roeland E, Mitchell W, Elia G et al (2010a) Symptom control in stem cell transplantation: a multidisciplinary palliative care team approach. Part 1: physical symptoms. J Support Oncol 8(3):100–116. Review

Roeland E, Mitchell W, Elia G et al (2010b) Symptom control in stem cell transplantation: a multidisciplinary palliative care team approach. Part 2: psychosocial concerns. J Support Oncol 8(4):179–183. Review

Siden H, Chavoshi N, Harvey B et al (2014) Characteristics of a pediatric hospice palliative are program over 15 years. Pediatrics 134(3):e765–e772. https://doi.org/10.1542/peds.2014-0381

Slavin S, Nagler A, Naparstek E (1998) Nonmyeloablative stem cell transplantation and cell therapy as an alternative to conventional bone marrow transplantation with lethal cytoreduction for the treatment of malignant and nonmalignant hematologic diseases. Blood 91(3):756–763

Stuber M, Nader K, Yasuda P (1991) Stress responses after pediatric bone marrow transplantation: preliminary results of a prospective longitudinal study. J Am Acad Child Adoles Psychiatr 30:952–957

Styczynski J, van der Velden W, Fox CP et al (2016) Management of Epstein-Barr Virus infections and post-transplant lymphoproliferative disorders in patients after allogeneic hematopoietic stem cell transplantation: Sixth European Conference on Infections in Leukemia (ECIL-6) guidelines. Sixth European Conference on Infections in Leukemia, a joint venture of the Infectious Diseases Working Party of the European Society of Blood and Marrow Transplantation (EBMT-IDWP), the Infectious Diseases Group of the European Organization for Research and Treatment of Cancer (EORTC-IDG), the International Immunocompromised Host Society (ICHS) and the European Leukemia Net (ELN) Haematologica 101(7):803-811. doi: https://doi.org/10.3324/haematol.2016.144428. Review

Suttorp M, Claviez A, Bader P et al (2009) Allogeneic stem cell transplantation for pediatric and adolescent patients with CML: results from the prospective trial CML-paed I. Klin Padiatr 221(6):351–357. https://doi.org/10.1055/s-0029-123952

Svenberg P, Remberger M, Uzunel M et al (2016) Improved overall survival for pediatric patients undergoing allogeneic hematopoietic stem cell transplantation—a comparison of the last two decades. Pediatr Transplant 20(5):667–674. https://doi.org/10.1111/petr.12723

Terrin N, Rodday AM, Tighiouart H et al (2013) Parental emotional functioning declines with occurrence of clinical complications in pediatric hematopoietic stem cell transplant. Support Care Cancer 21(3):687–695

Ullrich CK, Dussel V, Hilden JM et al (2010) End-of-life experience of children undergoing stem cell transplantation for malignancy: parent and provider perspectives and patterns of care. Blood 115(19):3879–3885

Ullrich CK, Rodday AM, Bingen K et al (2016a) Parent outlook: how parents view the road ahead as they embark on hematopoietic stem cell transplantation for their child. Biol Blood Marrow Transplant 22(1):104–111. https://doi.org/10.1016/j.bbmt.2015.08.040

Ullrich CK, Lehmann L, London WB et al (2016b) End-of-life care patterns associated with pediatric palliative care among children who underwent hematopoietic stem cell transplant. Biol Blood Marrow Transplant 22(6):1049–1055. https://doi.org/10.1016/j.bbmt.2016.02.012

Vrijmoet-Wiersma CMJ, Egeler RM, Koopman HM et al (2009) Parental stress before, during, and after pediatric stem cell transplantation: a review article. Support Care Cancer 17:1435–1443. https://doi.org/10.1007/s00520-009-0685-4

Weitz M, Strahm B, Meerpohl JJ (2015) Extracorporeal photopheresis versus alternative treatment for chronic graft-versus-host disease after haematopoietic stem cell transplantation in paediatric patients. Cochrane Database Syst Rev 12:CD009898. https://doi.org/10.1002/14651858.CD009898.pub3

Wiener L, Baird K, Crum C et al (2014) Child and parent perspectives of the chronic graft-versus-host disease (cGVHD) symptom experience: a concept elicitation study. Support Care Cancer 22(2):295–305

Wilhelmsson M, Vatanen A, Borgström B et al (2015) Adverse health events and late mortality after pediatric allogeneic hematopoietic SCT-two decades of longitudinal follow-up. Bone Marrow Transplant 50(6):850–857. https://doi.org/10.1038/bmt.2015.43

Wilkins KL, Woodgate RL (2007a) An interruption in family life: siblings' lived experience as they transition through the pediatric bone marrow transplant trajectory. Oncol Nurs Forum 34:E28–E35

Wilkins KL, Woodgate RL (2007b) Supporting siblings through the pediatric bone marrow transplant trajectory: perspectives of siblings of bone marrow transplant recipients. Cancer Nurs 30(5):E29–E34. https://doi.org/10.1097/01.NCC.0000290811.06948.2c

Willard VW, Leung W, Huang Q et al (2014) Cognitive outcome after pediatric stem-cell transplantation: impact of age and Total-body irradiation. J Clin Oncol 32(35):3982–3989

Wolfe J, Klar N, Grier HE et al (2000) Understanding of prognosis among parents of children who died of cancer: impact on treatment goals and integration of palliative care. JAMA 284(19):2469–2475

van der Zouwen B, Kruisselbrink AB, Jordanova ES et al (2012) Alloreactive effector T cells require the local formation of a proinflammatory environment to allow crosstalk and high avidity interaction with nonhematopoietic tissues to induce GVHD reactivity. Biol Blood Marrow Transplant 18(9):1353–1367. https://doi.org/10.1016/j.bbmt.2012.06.017

Easing of Physical Distress in Pediatric Cancer

7

Sergey Postovsky, Amit Lehavi, Ori Attias, and Eli Hershman

Key Points

- Physical suffering is a main contributor to global suffering of the ill child and his family.
- Alleviating physical distress may significantly attenuate the psychological distress and vice versa.
- Palliative care should be implemented throughout the whole time span of the disease, from the moment of initial diagnosis until cure or death.
- Fatigue and pain are the most frequent physical symptoms.
- Pain management includes integrative treatment with multimodal pharmacological approach and non-pharmacologic interventions.
- Regional analgesia techniques can improve pain control and reduce systemic analgesia requirements.
- Respiratory symptoms, air hunger (dyspnea) as one of the most prevalent, distressing, and frightening symptoms during the last weeks of life, should be addressed with treatment of reversible causes, medications, and ventilatory support.
- Nausea and vomiting management can be challenging due to its multifactorial nature. Causes unrelated to the gastrointestinal systems should be addressed, combined with antiemetic medications.
- Constipation is usually multifactorial. Opioids and other drugs represent its most common and frequently treatable cause:
  - Cachexia is a complex and debilitating clinicobiochemical syndrome frequently encountered in pediatric oncology, especially in advanced stages of disease. Anorexia may contribute to development of cachexia. Treatment is frequently difficult and directed primarily at the underlying cancer.
  - Involvement of central nervous system in pediatric cancer patients is

S. Postovsky, M.D. (✉)
Division of Pediatric Oncology/Hematology, Ruth Rappaport Children's Hospital,
Rambam Health Care Campus, Haifa, Israel
e-mail: s_postovsky@rambam.health.gov.il

A. Lehavi, M.D.
Pediatric Anesthesiology Unit, Ruth Rappaport Children's Hospital, Rambam Health Care Campus,
Haifa, Israel

O. Attias, M.D. • E. Hershman, M.D.
Department of Pediatric Intensive Care, Ruth Rappaport Children's Hospital,
Rambam Health Care Campus, Haifa, Israel

J. Wolfe et al. (eds.), *Palliative Care in Pediatric Oncology*, Pediatric Oncology,
https://doi.org/10.1007/978-3-319-61391-8_7

> quite a common phenomenon. Since in many instances this involvement has treatable causes, their timely recognition and treatment may be of utmost importance for the preservation of quality of life in palliative setting.

7.1 Introduction

Easing physical distress is one of the central and most important considerations in proper delivering of palliative care to a child suffering from cancer throughout the whole time span of his disease from the moment of initial diagnosis till cure or death.

Physical distress makes the child and his family seek medical assistance before the diagnosis and remains one of the main objectives for care during the illness and frequently after the cure of cancer is achieved.

It is especially pertinent to the situations when the cure of a child suffering from cancer is impossible. Traumatic recollections of parents about the last weeks, days, and hours spent by their child and accompanying by physical suffering may have profound impact on their own lives. Research has shown that such impact may be long-acting (Wolfe et al. 2000; Pritchard et al. 2008; Heath et al. 2010; Theunissen et al. 2007; Kreicbergs et al. 2005; von Lützau et al. 2012; Jalmsell et al. 2006; Mack et al. 2005). All available efforts should be exercised in order to achieve efficient control of physical suffering. Despite that in many contemporary medical settings such as pediatric oncology departments of modern tertiary hospitals in Western Europe and North America there are actively functioning comprehensive pediatric palliative programs, their efficacy in achieving satisfactory control of physical suffering of pediatric cancer patients is not always optimal (Wolfe et al. 2008; Postovsky and Ben Arush 2004; Schmidt et al. 2013).

There is significant gap in perception of efficacy of control of physical symptoms between medical staff and parents of dying child. In general, medical staff believe that easing of physical suffering of a child during the last phase of life is more efficacious than do the child's parents (Mack et al. 2005).

It is important to remember that it is parents who continue to live with the trauma of constant recollections about how their child spent their last days and hours. That's why it is parents who are ultimate judges of the efficacy of provided palliative care to their children.

Children with cancer suffer from wide specter of physical symptoms with fatigue and pain being the most frequent (Wolfe et al. 2000; Pritchard et al. 2008; Heath et al. 2010; Theunissen et al. 2007; Kreicbergs et al. 2005; von Lützau et al. 2012; Jalmsell et al. 2006; Mack et al. 2005).

Physical suffering is multifactorial and stems from many causes, particularly due to the disease itself, side effects of anticancer treatment and its consequences, as well as various painful procedures the child undergoes during cancer treatment.

Physical distress may reflect injury to practically every organ and system in a pediatric cancer patient, and therefore symptoms of physical distress may vary in form, intensity, location, and its ability to interfere with a child's everyday activity and life.

Physical suffering is a main part of global suffering which besets the ill child, his parents, and other members of his family and also other persons involved. Proper and timely delivered pediatric palliative care directed at the easing of physical distress also greatly facilitates easing of both psychological and existential distress and preserving the dignity of the child and surrounding family members. To successfully deal with physical distress as a part of global suffering, there is a need for an interprofessional approach involving various specialists working as an interdisciplinary team (Wolfe et al. 2008; Postovsky and Ben Arush 2004; Schmidt et al. 2013).

Suffering is not only physical among people irrespective of their age (Cassel 1982). Every suffering bears certain meanings, and, therefore, proper assessment of physical distress should always take into account its emotional, psychological, and existential impact on an ill child.

Recognizing suffering in children is sometimes a difficult task. Children's ability to express their distress may differ depending on age; developmental level; medical, cognitive, and psychological status; as well as cultural background. There are a number of validated tools to assess physical distress in suffering child with cancer in a timely and objective manner (Collins et al. 2000; Wolfe et al. 2015). Despite these tools, it is the physician with his tender heart, caring soul, and inquisitive mind who is responsible for delivering palliative care for the child with cancer and his family. Meticulous attention to symptoms and signs of physical distress and its timely recognition and assessment facilitate the achievement of gratifying results both for the suffering child and medical providers (Postovsky and Ben Arush 2004).

7.2 Fatigue

Fatigue is reported by pediatric oncology patients and by parents to be one of the most common symptoms causing physical distress (Wolfe et al. 2000; Zhukovsky et al. 2015). Fatigue may interfere with each and every aspect of child's life thus exerting a global negative effect. Fatigue may negatively influence both physical and psychological well-being of a child with advanced cancer.

Cancer-related fatigue is defined as a distressing, persistent, subjective sense of physical, emotional, and/or cognitive tiredness or exhaustion related to cancer or cancer treatment that is not proportional to recent activity and that significantly interferes with usual functioning (Bower et al. 2014). This definition of fatigue is primarily used for adult oncology patients who have completed anticancer treatment. The definition of fatigue in pediatric oncology may differ from that of adult oncology since it does not include developmental characteristics specific for children at different phases of their motor, cognitive, and social development. Diagnosis of fatigue in children with cancer who are very young may be especially difficult due to their inability to verbally convey their feelings.

Cancer-induced fatigue is multifactorial phenomenon with many factors contributing to its initiation and progression (Ryan et al. 2007). Causes of fatigue may be divided into the following groups:

- Cancer related
- Treatment related
- Psychological

Anemia One of the relatively frequent causes of fatigue in oncology is underlying anemia that may result from either the disease itself or as a side effect of anticancer treatment (Ullrich and Mayer 2007; Ullrich et al. 2010). Symptomatic anemia should be recognized in a timely manner and treated. Children with symptomatic anemia usually receive packed cells transfusions. The use of erythropoietin for correction of anemia in pediatric patients with advanced cancer is uncommon and should be considered in terms of goals of care and life expectancy (Ullrich et al. 2010).

Hypothyroidism is another possible cause of fatigue; therefore, any child with unexplained fatigue should have the TSH and free T4 levels tested. It is especially true in cases of children who were previously treated with radiotherapy directed at neck region.

Unremitting symptoms and side effects of medications used to treat them can both contribute to fatigue. For example, pain and/or opioids, especially when initiated, and/or other adjuvants for pain treatment medications with sedative effects (e.g., antidepressants, benzodiazepines, some antiepileptics), may contribute and worsen fatigue in pediatric oncology patients.

Carnitine deficiency One mechanism contributing to fatigue in cancer patients involves abnormalities in adenosine triphosphate synthesis caused by carnitine deficiency (Hockenberry et al. 2009). This deficiency may result from chemotherapy. Several trials in adults with cancer with low-level plasma carnitine identified that levocarnitine supplementation may be effective in alleviating chemotherapy-induced fatigue

(Graziano et al. 2002; Cruciani et al. 2012). Studies in children with cancer have yielded inconsistent results. In one pediatric study of 67 children with cancer, a majority of evaluated patients were found to have decreased carnitine plasma levels after at least 1 week of chemotherapy including cisplatin, ifosfamide, or doxorubicin (Hockenberry et al. 2009). However, the same group of authors more recently published results of another study of 58 patients and concluded that plasma levels of carnitine were not associated with administration of the same chemotherapy agents (Hooke et al. 2015). Clearly, more research should be done in order to further clarify the role of carnitine in development of cancer-induced fatigue, especially among pediatric oncology patients.

Chemotherapy and other forms of anticancer drug therapy may contribute to fatigue. The expanding use of biologically active small molecules in treatment of various cancers both in adults and children has led to more deep understanding of side effects of these drugs. In pediatric oncology, the use of biologic therapy is especially frequent in patients with recurrent or progressive disease. Fatigue as a side effect of such drugs as imatinib, sunitinib, and sorafenib has been reported in 30–50% of cases (Brown 2011; Torino et al. 2009). Potentially, many other drugs used as "targeted therapy" may cause fatigue as well.

Deconditioning Many children with cancer, especially with advanced disease, spend a lot of time in hospital or at home, and their physical activity is significantly limited. As a result of prolonged periods of limited physical activity, many children with cancer become physically deconditioned, and this may worsen their fatigue. Many pediatric oncology patients experience *sleep disturbances* (Olson 2014; Crabtree et al. 2015; Orsey et al. 2013), and increase in physical activity may lead to qualitative and quantitative improvement of sleep in these children (Braam et al. 2013). Methods aimed at increasing physical activity even in severely debilitated children with advanced cancer may, therefore, decrease severity of fatigue caused by sleep disturbances.

Treatment of fatigue Given the high prevalence of fatigue in children with advanced cancer, it is obvious that successful management of this symptom is very challenging. Importantly, all treatable causes of fatigue should be recognized and addressed in a manner consistent with goals of care. Frequently, packed cell transfusion and adjustment of medications with sedative effects (when feasible) may be helpful. Correction of dehydration and maintenance of normal electrolyte balance may also be useful.

Pharmacologic treatment of fatigue in children with advanced cancer has not been properly evaluated, and evidence for use of drugs as methylphenidate in this population of pediatric patients is limited. Based on results driven from adult oncology studies and extrapolating data obtained from use of methylphenidate in children with attention deficit disorders, as well as anecdotal experience, methylphenidate may be considered in children with advanced cancer (Reineke-Bracke et al. 2006; Sharp et al. 2013). Typical starting doses are as low as 2.5 mg, one to three times a day as needed in older children. Further titration depends on the individual response.

Children with advanced cancer experience significant psychological, social, and existential distress. Depression and other psychological disturbances may contribute to fatigue (Hwang et al. 2003). Providing psychological and spiritual support is therefore of paramount importance, as well as consultation by pediatric psychiatrist in selected cases.

Since fatigue in pediatric advanced cancer is a multifactorial phenomenon, its treatment should be ideally guided by an interdisciplinary team.

7.3 Pain

7.3.1 Case Presentation

Sam is a 16-year-old boy with osteogenic sarcoma of the left proximal humerus extending to the distal part of his left arm. On chest CT performed at the time of initial metastatic work-up, multiple bilateral lung metastases were detected.

Despite initial chemotherapy, his tumor continued to progress locally causing severe pain especially in the proximal portion of his left arm. Repeated chest CT showed further progression of his lung metastases. Sam and his family declined further second-line chemotherapy and preferred to proceed to alternative methods of treatment with nonconventional approaches. Because of very extensive tumor involvement of the entire humerus and surrounding soft tissues and widespread metastatic pulmonary disease, radical resection of the primary tumor (left upper extremity amputation) was not recommended. Instead, a conservative surgical approach was performed with gross resection of tumor mass and insertion of a prosthesis with subsequent local radiation therapy. Surgery resulted in satisfactory control left upper arm pain for several weeks; however, with renewed local recurrence, he began to experience increasing pain despite continuation of use of oral opioids. Since his pain at that time originated only from one location and was rendered as both somatic and neuropathic in nature, a brachial plexus blockade was performed, using an interscalene approach, providing analgesia to the shoulder, upper arm, and elbow. This approach allowed him to gradually discontinue systemic opioids and resolution of side effects including constipation, slowed mental processing, and pruritis. Unfortunately, after period of several weeks of comfort, Sam began experiencing very severe pain along his entire left arm and hand and within left part of his upper back. He was reluctant to be treated with oral analgesics, and instead, intravenous patient-controlled analgesia (PCA) was initiated. Sam was able to control his pain and regulate the intensity acceptable to him. Opioid side effects were managed. At the end of his life, as his disease progressed further and signs of respiratory distress appeared and worsened, Sam was treated with continuous infusion of morphine and midazolam carefully titrated in order to control both pain and respiratory distress.

Pain management is a cornerstone in the treatment of children with cancer. Pain, particularly combined with anxiety and fatigue, is very common and has a significant influence on the child's overall well-being. In children with advanced cancer, pain is highly prevalent. A recently published study found that among other common distressing symptoms, pain was reported 48% of the time among children with advanced cancer. Furthermore, in the last 12 weeks of life, pain prevalence was even higher, at 62% (Wolfe et al. 2015).

7.3.2 Teamwork, the Multimodal Pharmacological Approach, and Integrative Treatment

Pediatric pain management in general, and in advance cancer in particular, requires teamwork and may include palliative care, pediatric pain and sedation services, anesthesia, psychosocial care, child life, physical therapy, spiritual support, and many other services. In developed countries, such services are built-in parts of the palliative care team. In contrast, such services are often inaccessible to children with cancer in many places worldwide.

Non-pharmacologic interventions are inherent and essential parts of the integrative treatment and are discussed in detail elsewhere in the textbook and should always be considered in conjunction with medication.

The World Health Organization (WHO) 2012 guidelines

The WHO guidelines on the pharmacologic treatment of persistent pain in children with medical illnesses, including cancer, were updated in 2012. The guidelines outline a few key general concepts for pain management:

- A two-step strategy should be employed: step one for mild pain and step two for moderate to severe pain.
- Dosing at regular intervals (or continuously) should be offered instead of "as needed" treatment.
- Appropriate routes of administration should be used.
- Treatments should be adapted to the necessities of individual children.

Following WHO guidelines has been shown to provide pain control to a majority of children for a significant period over the course of their illness (Zernikow et al. 2006).

7.3.3 Pain Categories and Causes

Pain characteristics can identify the underling pathophysiology and direct the approach to treatment. Characteristics to consider include the time frame in which it appears and for how long it persists, the anatomical location, and the way it is described. Nevertheless, pain subtypes are often related entities. One can find, for example, pain syndromes in which acute and chronic phases are a continuous process rather than distinct subtypes. Commonly, in the most advanced stages of pediatric cancer, pain is persistent, multifaceted, and accompanied by frequent exacerbations:

- Acute pain is defined as a new-onset event. This type of pain is related to tissue damage, is often short-lived, and resolves after healing, though not in the most advanced states of disease. Acute pain is common, usually procedure related, and can be incidental or breakthrough pain:
  - Incidental acute pain is pain that is associated with changes in body position, such as in a patient with a pathological fracture.
  - Breakthrough pain is an acute event of pain flare-up in a child with otherwise controlled pain. This type of pain is relatively prevalent, and younger children may experience breakthrough pain more than teenagers (Friedrichsdorf et al. 2007).
- Chronic pain is defined as pain that lasts more than 12 weeks. In advanced cancer, the pain arises from persistent etiology such as tumor growth, metastatic invasion, and pathological fractures. Such pain can also be related to anticancer treatments, such as chemotherapy, radiotherapy, or late effects of surgery, among other treatments. Chronic pain with no clear organic cause, a well-known illness in pain clinics, is rarely relevant in advanced cancer.

Pain is further classified as nociceptive (somatic or visceral) or neuropathic pain:

- Nociceptive pain arises from damage to a non-neural tissue and is due to activation of nociceptors, sensory receptors of the peripheral somatosensory nervous system (International Association for the Study of Pain (IASP)):
  - Somatic pain is usually well localized and may be described as sharp if superficial or dull and throbbing if it arises from deep tissue. Typical examples of deep somatic pain in children with cancer include pain experienced with bone metastasis of neuroblastoma or sarcoma.
  - Visceral pain arises from internal organs, such as the intestine, kidneys, liver, and peritoneum. This type of pain is poorly localized and dull and may be described as a deep pressure or spasm. It is usually observed in cases with retroperitoneally located tumors or abdominal lymph node involvement in lymphoma.
- Neuropathic pain is defined as pain caused by a lesion or disease of the somatosensory nervous system. This type of pain is more difficult to describe or to localize and is occasionally accompanied by paresthesia (an abnormal sensation) or dysesthesia (an abnormal sensation that is considered to be unpleasant) (International Association for the Study of Pain (IASP)).

Young children may find neuropathic pain difficult to describe. The onset of the pain with a recent related nerve injury may contribute to the correct diagnosis. Direct neuronal damage due to tumor or metastatic invasion to the brain, spinal cord, and nerve roots or surgical injury induces neuropathic pain. Chemotherapy, especially with vincristine, is a known cause of neuropathic pain. Neuropathic pain may be less frequently diagnosed than non-neuropathic pain in children with cancer. However, neuropathic pain was described in 17% of the referrals to a multidisciplinary pediatric cancer pain service (Anghelescu et al. 2014):

- Mixed pain has no formal definition; however, a pain in which the aforementioned mechanisms coexist is common in palliative care and

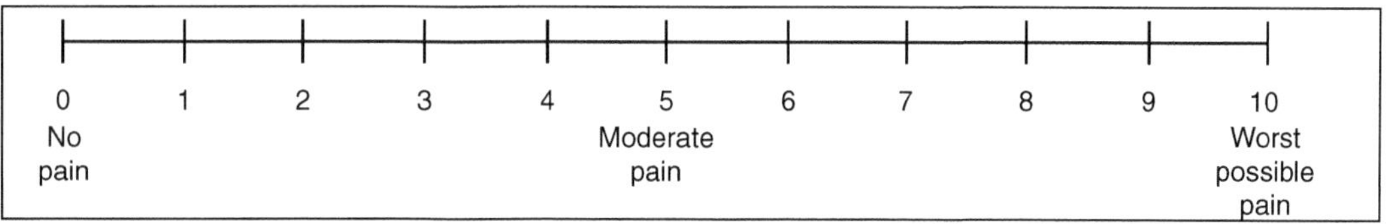

Fig. 7.1 Numeric Rating Scale

Table 7.1 Pain measurement tools

Tool	Face pain scale	Visual analog scale	Oucher	Numerical rating scale
Age	4–17 years	Above 8 years	3–12 years	Above 8 years

should be addressed accordingly with multimodal drug therapy and integrative multidisciplinary treatment.

- Procedure-related pain deserves special consideration. During the child's illness, procedural pain is one of the most common sources of pain, and it has a substantial impact on the general pain experience. Children can reach physical and psychological state in which there are no "minor" or "brief" procedures they are able to tolerate. Among children at end of life, thorough consideration should be given to every single procedure, and decisions should be made that are consistent with family goals of care. Effective procedural sedation or analgesia should always be considered when available.

7.3.4 Pain Assessment

Pain, like any other vital sign, should be assessed on a regular basis.

Pain experience is a complex product of many factors. Because of the lack of pain scales for pediatric palliative care, other tools that have been developed for pain assessment are commonly used. These tools are unidimensional, scoring pain intensity only. Multidimensional tools score more than one factor, with pain intensity being one of those factors.

It is well accepted that a child's self-report is the best way to assess and measure pain when possible. Several measuring tools have been validated for children. These tools are age adjusted and depend on the child's ability to point at the appropriate level of pain as expressed through pain symbols. The FLACC (faces, legs, activity, cry, and consolability) scale is an observational tool for children aged 3 years or younger. It was developed for acute pain assessment and functions by measuring changes in scores in response to analgesics. The FLACC scale can be used for all ages, including mentally challenged children (Voepel-Lewis et al. 2002). For children aged 8 years or above, the visual analog scale or the *numeric rating scale* (Fig. 7.1) is simple validated 0–10 scales. The child quantifies his pain status by pointing to the pain level, ranged from no pain to the worst pain ever (von Baeyer et al. 2009). The *face pain scale-revised* (Face Pain Scale; Hicks et al. 2001), the *color analog scale*, and the "Oucher" scale (The Oucher Photographic Scale; Beyer et al. 1992) are also used routinely in acute pain management (Table 7.1).

For younger children with cancer, a behavioral scale, the Hetero Evaluation Douleur Enfant (HEDEN) scale, was published for the assessment of prolonged cancer or postsurgical pain in children aged 2–6 years. In this five-category pain scale, each category is scored 0–2, for a maximal total score of 10. The pain signs are categorized as voluntary pain expression, direct expression of pain, and psychomotor inactivity. As this scale is a new tool, the translation of the numerical score into clinical implications of mild, moderate, or severe pain deserves more study (Marec-Berard et al. 2015).

7.4 Treatment

7.4.1 Basic Approach

The abovementioned two-step strategy recommends that for the first step of pain management, mild pain should be treated with ibuprofen and acetaminophen. Because children with advanced cancer mostly experience moderate to severe pain, step one drugs typically serve as adjuncts and opioid-sparing drugs. For the second step, when the pain is moderate to severe, an opioid is usually needed. Morphine remains the most common first drug of choice. However, a variety of opioids can be used based on availability, the child's response, and the side effect profile. Switching between drugs, known as opioid rotation, is one method to overcome tolerance or side effects.

The "by the clock" phrase highlights the need for regular intervals or continuous administration of analgesia as opposed to intermittent dosing "as needed."

The route of administration should be the one most convenient for the child. Oral, transdermal, trans-buccal, intravenous, and subcutaneous routes are all acceptable. Intramuscular injections and rectal application in children should be avoided.

The most important point is "adapting treatment to the individual child" including regular reassessment, dose titration, drug combination changes, breakthrough pain treatment, and side effect management.

7.4.2 Acetaminophen, Ibuprofen, and Ketorolac

Acetaminophen is an effective step one drug for mild pain (de Martino and Chiarugi 2015). The intravenous formulation can be used when children cannot tolerate oral intake. Furthermore, acetaminophen has a significant analgesic effect and is widely used for acute pain. In a study in neonates and infants after major surgery, intravenous acetaminophen reduced the morphine requirements significantly by more than 30% (Ceelie et al. 2013). There are no data on the safety of prolonged use, but repeated doses less than 75 mg per kg a day seem to be well tolerated (Heard et al. 2014). Importantly, in children continuing to receive antineoplastic therapy, acetaminophen excretion may be highly variable. Repeated doses may induce an increase in metabolism via the hepatotoxic formation of the highly reactive intermediate *N*-acetyl-p-benzoquinone imine (NAPQI) (Koling et al. 2007).

Ibuprofen and other nonsteroidal anti-inflammatory drugs (NSAIDs) also have opioid-sparing effects. The combination of acetaminophen and ibuprofen treatment can be very effective. Ketorolac, an intravenous NSAID, can be used for acute events for up to 5 days. A systematic review of perioperative pain management in children showed its opioid-sparing effect and supported the addition of NSAIDs and/or acetaminophen to systemic opioid treatment (Wong et al. 2013). In pediatric advanced cancer, the effect of NSAIDs on platelet function needs to be considered. Where available, celecoxib can be used. Compared to nonselective NSAIDs, cyclooxygenase-2 selective inhibitor such as celecoxib will not interfere with normal mechanisms of platelet aggregation and hemostasis (Leese et al. 2000). Less tolerability-related gastrointestinal adverse events such as abdominal pain, dyspepsia, nausea, diarrhea, and flatulence may offer additional advantage. NSAIDs should be avoided in children with intravascular volume depletion or preexisting renal dysfunction.

7.4.3 Tramadol

Tramadol is considered an opioid analgesic with intermediate potency; however, there is no available evidence for its effectiveness or safety in children (World Health Organization 2012). Tramadol for postoperative pain treatment in children compared to placebo has an analgesic effect; nevertheless, its efficacy and side effect profile are uncertain compared to other opioids (Schnabel et al. 2015).

7.4.4 Opioids

Opioids are the keystone of cancer pain management (Zernikow et al. 2009). Morphine remains the medicine of choice, although other opioids should be used when opioid rotation is required (Zernikow et al. 2006). High-dose opioids may be needed, especially during end-of-life pain management (Siden and Naiewajek 2003; Rasmussen et al. 2015). Care should be taken when opioids are administered to patients with impaired renal function, which is not rare among children with advanced cancer.

Children differ in their responses to specific opioids. The causes for this variability may involve genetic variants and different metabolism (Nielsen et al. 2015). A trial of more than one opioid may be needed to provide adequate analgesia with acceptable tolerability.

The oral route is preferable whenever possible. Immediate-release drugs are used for the titration phase and for breakthrough pain. Once the child's pain is controlled, a slow-release product can be started (Table 7.2).

Intravenous administration is the appropriate route for rapid titration in cases of severe pain (Table 7.3). However, the need for alternate routes is common. Subcutaneous (low-volume) infusion of concentrated morphine or a hydromorphone solution may be an effective alternative (Morlion et al. 2015).

Starting dosages are for the treatment of opioid-naïve patients. Significantly higher doses are needed to control severe pain. In principle, there is no upper limit for an opioid dose. Rather, the upper dose is dictated by the child's response and side effect profile.

Table 7.2 Oral opioids (for age >1 year)

Drug	Starting oral dose (for age >1 year)
Morphine	0.3 mg/kg every 4 h
Oxycodone	0.2 mg/kg every 4–6 h
Hydromorphone	0.04–0.06 mg/kg every 4 h

7.4.5 Opioid Rotation and Combination

When the child's response to an opioid is unsatisfactory or the adverse effect intensity limits the dose needed for satisfactory analgesia, switching to another opioid is indicated.

In a retrospective study to determine the therapeutic value of opioid rotation, this action had a positive impact on managing opioid therapy during cancer pain treatment in children (Kestenbaum et al. 2014). In an adult study, for patients with chronic uncontrolled cancer pain despite dose titration, both opioid rotation and opioid combination provided significant pain relief (Drake et al. 2004).

When a child develops tolerance to an opioid, she/he may exhibit some degree of tolerance to the new one. However, it is assumed that tolerance is incomplete, and generally speaking, following conversion, dose reductions of 25–50% are recommended.

Cross-tolerance may be incomplete, symmetrical (changing from A to B will produce an equal cross-tolerance in the opposite direction), or asymmetrical and may be unidirectional. Practically, converting opioids should be undertaken with caution, as it is not simply a matter of using an opioid equipotency calculation. A review with practical information on performing opioid rotation in (adult) clinical practice was recently published (Kim et al. 2015).

Opioid common side effects (Table 7.4)—general key points:

Table 7.3 Continuous intravenous opioid doses (for age >1 year)

Drug	Loading dose	Starting infusion dose
Morphine	0.05 mg/kg	0.02–0.04 mg/kg/h
Fentanyl	1 μg/kg	0.5–1 μg/kg/h
Hydromorphone	10 μg/kg	1–2 μg/kg/h

Table 7.4 Selected adverse effects of opioid use

Adverse effect	Management	Example	Remarks
Constipation (discussed in details bellow; see page)	Stool softeners *and* stimulants	Bisacodyl Polyethylene glycol Lactulose	Should be prescribed when opioids are commenced
Nausea	Serotonin antagonist	Ondansetron	
Pruritus	Anti-histamine Serotonin antagonist Opioid rotation Low dose naloxone	Hydroxyzine Ondansetron	Limited efficacy

- Look for other contributing factors. Some of the adverse effects are not unique to opioids and could be partially due to other causes such as chemotherapy-induced nausea, multidrug therapy drowsiness, etc.
- Adjunct nonopioid analgesia may enable opioid dose reduction.
- Opioid rotation and alternative route may reduce side effects.
- Alternative analgesia if appropriate such as regional or neuroaxial block (epidural, intrathecal) may temporarily eliminate the need for opioids altogether.

7.4.6 Patient-, Parent-, and Nurse-Controlled Analgesia (PCA) (Table 7.5)

PCA is a method based on a programmable pump that delivers continuous analgesia as background infusion and an option to deliver rescue boluses activated by the patient. This method has a number of advantages: it can serve as a continuous drug delivery system, and boluses are given with out delay when needed. Therefore, the child has some control over the pain relief. Children as young as 6 years can use a PCA device, which has several safety features. The child's control button is pneumatic, meaning that a drowsy child cannot push hard enough to activate the system. It has a lockout time interval in which the number of demand requests is documented, but the drug is not delivered. Counting the number of self-activations, both within and outside of the safety lockout time, enables the child's daily dose needs to be more easily adjusted. See Table 7.5 for dosing considerations.

Table 7.5 PCA dose (for age >1 year)

Drug	PCA dose (μg/kg)	Continuous dose (μg/kg/h)
Morphine	10–30	5–10
Fentanyl	0.5–1	0.2–0.5
Hydromorphone	2–5	1–2

The lockout time interval is usually 4–6 min. A maximal dose every 4 h can be programmed.

Continuous infusion is recommended to achieve more stable analgesia, especially during sleep. An adequate analgesia should result in approximately one to two button activations per hour; otherwise, the continuous infusion rate or rescue demand dose should be adjusted. PCA is an effective tool for acute pain management, breakthrough pain, and titration phase before commencing the use of long-acting opioids for chronic pain.

PCA analgesia by proxy, nurse, or parent may be operated when a child is unable to activate the system himself. With appropriate institutional standards, guidelines, and caregiver education, PCA has been safely used in pediatric oncology (Smith and Peppin 2014) and in children (including those younger than 6 years old) following major surgery (Anghelescu et al. 2012). Nurse-controlled analgesia may be needed at the last phase of the child's life, when it may become psychologically difficult for parents to deliver parent-controlled analgesia. PCA has been successfully used in end-of-life care (Howard et al. 2010).

Fentanyl transdermal is an option for nonopioid-naïve patients when an alternative route is not satisfactory. A patch is applied to an intact skin area for 72 h. In some cases, patch replacement is needed after 48 h because the analgesic effect seemed to fade earlier than expected. The time to reach a steady state seems to be longer, the drug's clearance rate is higher, and the elimination half-life is shorter in children than in adults. The conversion ratio is 12.5 μg/h fentanyl for every oral daily dose equivalent of morphine (45 mg) (Anghelescu et al. 2015); however, dose adjustments should be performed according to the clinical situation. Dose adjustments should only be made every 3–6 days, as it may take this long to reach equilibrium with each change.

Ketamine is an *N*-methyl-D-aspartate (NMDA) receptor antagonist. It blocks the NMDA receptors in the spinal dorsal horn, which are involved in central pain sensitization. Ketamine is being used extensively for anesthesia and procedural sedation-analgesia. Additionally, sub-anesthetic low-dose ketamine may be used for analgesia to potentiate the effect of opioids and mitigation of tolerance. Ketamine can be delivered intermittently or as a continuous intravenous and subcutaneous infusion. The initial dose for continuous infusion is 0.1–0.2 mg/kg/h. In a small case series, ketamine improved pain control and had an opioid-sparing effect. Ketamine (20 or 40 μg/kg/mL) has been added to morphine PCA for mucositis pain and improved analgesia without increased side effects (Zernikow et al. 2007).

Methadone is a unique opioid that can offer effective analgesia in cases where significantly high doses of other opioids are insufficient. Furthermore, in addition to its opioid receptor activity, methadone is an antagonist at the NMDA receptor, which may benefit children with neuropathic and mixed pain (James et al. 2010). One approach to starting oral methadone is as follows: start at 0.1 mg/kg every 4 h for the first three doses, and then change to every 12 h, given its long half-life. No dose adjustments should be made for 72 h given its long half-life. Methadone has complex pharmacokinetics-pharmacodynamics and multiple drug interactions. Individual dose adjustments and close follow-up are essential for effective and safe treatment. Methadone usage is less common than other opioids (Anghelescu 2011), and consultation with a pain or palliative care expert may be helpful.

Table 7.6 Tricyclic antidepressant and gabapentin doses

Drug	Initial dose	Maintenance dose[a]
Amitriptyline Nortriptyline (age >6 years)	0.1 mg/kg (max. 5 mg) once, at night	0.5 mg/kg (25 mg) once, at night
Gabapentin (age >3 years)	2 mg once, at night	5–10 mg/kg three times a day[b]

[a]Gradually increasing as required over 1 week
[b]Higher doses can be used if required and tolerated

7.4.7 Additional Treatment for Neuropathic Pain

Opioids are also among first-line treatments for neuropathic pain. Opioids are commonly combined with non-pharmacological therapy and adjunct drugs. Adjunct drugs, such as nonsteroidal anti-inflammatory drugs, tricyclic antidepressants (nortriptyline), gabapentinoids (gabapentin) (Table 7.6), and NMDA blocker (ketamine) combinations, are usually commenced; however, this practice is not evidence based. An expert opinion on the management of neuropathic pain in children with cancer was recently published (Friedrichsdorf and Nugent 2013).

7.4.8 Dexamethasone

Dexamethasone may be considered as an adjunct drug in cases with pain due to cerebral edema, spinal cord compression, or bone metastasis. In some adult studies, significant pain reduction was noted; however, the evidence of its efficacy for pain control is weak (Haywood et al. 2015).

7.4.9 Additional Strategies for Management of Refractory Pain

Anxiolytics can be helpful in the management of refractory pain and when using high-dose opioids resulting in myoclonus. The level of sedation can be adjusted to the desired level; occasionally, a relatively small dose of benzodiazepine or another anxiolytic agent is satisfactory.

7.4.10 Palliative Sedation

Palliative sedation is accepted as a method of easing suffering at end of life for children with refractory pain that does not respond to multimodal therapy. Palliative sedation can be safely used even at home (Korzeniewska-Eksterowicz et al. 2014). Typical agents used to achieve sedation include infusions of midazolam or pentobarbital.

7.4.11 Regional Pain Relief Techniques in Pediatric Palliative Care

Judicious integration of regional anesthesia into a multimodal analgesia plan can potentially improve pain control and reduce systemic analgesia requirements and side effects and typically does not interfere with a patient dying in their preferred location (Anghelescu et al. 2010). As regional anesthesia requires significant skills and experience, early involvement of pediatric pain services or pediatric anesthesia service may yield an optimal palliative pain control plan (Anghelescu et al. 2010).

As opposed to systemic analgesia aiming at modulation of pain in either cerebral or spinal level, regional techniques aim at disrupting the neuronal transmission of the pain: the nociceptive stimuli transmitted from the sensory end plate to the peripheral nerves, through the dorsal root ganglia and spinal roots, up the spinal cord to the brain. Local anesthetics, opioids, and various other substances can be administered along those pathways, minimizing or preventing nociceptive signals from reaching the brain. The nociceptive transmission can be blocked at multiple levels (Fig. 7.2):

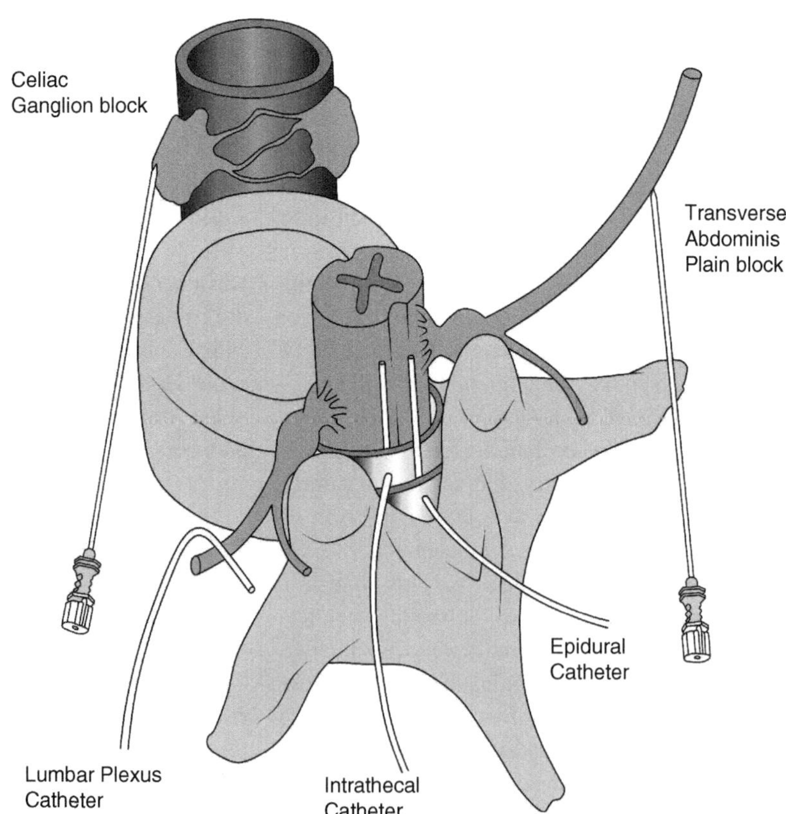

Fig. 7.2 Schematic illustration of various regional anesthesia needle and catheter techniques

- The receptor level using topical and local anesthetics
- The peripheral nerve using peripheral nerve blocks
- The ventral ramus using truncal plain blocks such as transverse abdominis plain (TAP) block or intercostal block
- At the dorsal root ganglion using paravertebral infiltration
- The root level using epidural techniques
- The spinal cord level, using intrathecal administration of medications

Disrupting the transmission can be achieved in a number of different ways, depending on the clinical settings, life expectancy, and available skills and resources (Fig. 7.3):

- *Single injections of* local anesthetics, commonly mixed with steroids and other adjuvants, will provide transient analgesia, usually lasting hours to few days, are easy to perform, minimize the risk of infection, and do not require connection to external devices.
- *Catheter techniques* are based on insertion of small-bore plastic catheters, commonly under ultrasound or X-ray guidance, to the subarachnoid or epidural space, in proximity to nerve plexuses or peripheral nerves. Medications can then be administered either continuously or intermittently, providing analgesia for days to weeks. Continuous infusion using electric infusers or, more commonly, mechanical elastomer or spring-loaded infuser is commonly used for long-term analgesia in outpatient settings.
- *Nerve ablation* using either surgical interventions, intraneural injections of chemical agents such as phenol or ethyl alcohols, cryoablation, and radiofrequency ablations may provide long-term or permanent regional pain relief.

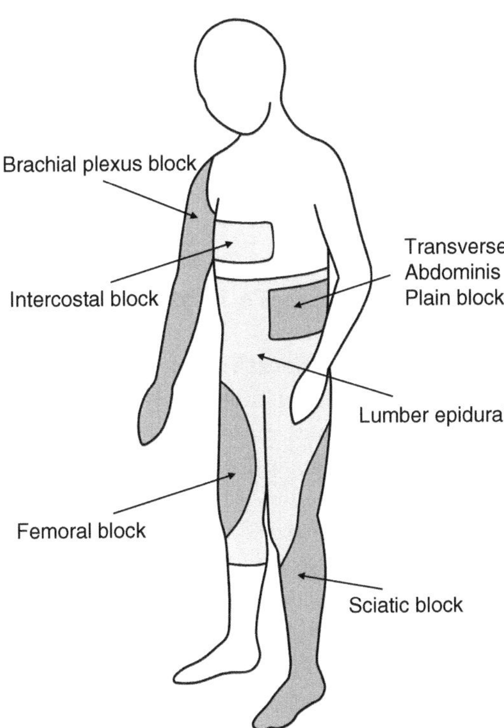

Fig. 7.3 Sensory distribution of various regional anesthesia techniques

7.4.12 Topical Anesthesia

Direct administration of local anesthetics, as well as morphine to skin ulcers, wounds, pressure sores, and mucosal surfaces, is simple, safe, and highly effective. Topical anesthetics at moderate concentrations such as lidocaine 2–4% and EMLA® cream (5% lidocaine/prilocaine mixture) are commonly used, while morphine sulfate 2% mouthwash has shown good results in severe cases of oral mucositis.

7.4.13 Peripheral Nerve Blocks

Catheter techniques are commonly used in perioperative settings, with excellent results and minimal serious complications (Walker et al. 2015). Catheter continuous brachial plexus block (Cooper et al. 1994) and femoral block (Pacenta et al. 2010) have been used in adults and children with advanced cancer and intractable pain. In selected patients, when limb mobility is not required and life expectancy is short, ultrasound-guided phenol ablation of selected peripheral nerves has been used for analgesia (Fu et al. 2013).

7.4.14 Brachial Plexus Blocks

The brachial plexus, originating from C5-T1 spinal roots, provides motor, sensory, and sympathetic innervation to the upper extremity. Blocks can be performed at the root level using an intrascalene approach which provides analgesia to the shoulder, upper arm, and elbow, at the division level using a supraclavicular approach or at the cord level using an infraclavicular approach to provide analgesia to the arm, elbow, and hand below the shoulder.

7.4.15 Lumbar Plexus Blocks

The lumbar plexus, originating from T12-L5 spinal roots, provides sensory and sympathetic innervation to the lower extremity. Blocks can be performed at the root or division level, using paravertebral techniques, or, more commonly, either at the femoral nerve—to provide analgesia to the anterior aspect of the thigh and knee—or at the sciatic nerve, providing analgesia to the posterior thigh, lower leg, and foot. Single-injection techniques; long-term, catheter techniques; and nerve destruction have been described with good results as part of palliative care pain relief (Pacenta et al. 2010; Chambers 2008)

7.4.16 Truncal Blocks

7.4.16.1 Transverse Abdominal Plain (TAP) Block

The low thoracic and high lumber ventral rami provide sensory innervation to the abdominal wall, which can be effectively blocked either bilaterally or unilaterally using either a single injection of local anesthetic or a continuous catheter technique. Nerve ablation based on TAP block using 33–70% alcohol was reported as an analgesic modality for intractable abdominal wall cancer pain with good long-term results, lasting from 17 days to 6 months (Sakamoto et al. 2012; Hung et al. 2014).

7.4.16.2 Intercostal Block

The intercostal nerves provide somatic innervation to the chest wall. Intercostal nerve blocks using local anesthetics and steroids (Gulati et al. 2015) can provide short-lasting analgesia. Both cryoablation (Sepsas et al. 2013) and radiofrequency ablation (Gulati et al. 2015) have been used with good results for pain relief at end of life.

7.4.16.3 Paravertebral Block

Administration of local anesthetic into the paravertebral space at high and low thoracic and lumbar levels can provide unilateral analgesia and may reduce the sympathetic block commonly involved in epidural and intrathecal techniques.

7.4.17 Sympathetic Ganglion Blocks

7.4.17.1 Celiac Block and Ablation

The celiac ganglia, located adjacent to the aorta at the level of the celiac artery, are part of the sympathetic prevertebral chain and provide a significant part of the somatic innervation of the intra-abdominal organs. In selected cases, blocking the celiac plexus may provide complete pain relief until death (Mercadante and Nicosia 1998). Celiac nerve block can be performed either percutaneously, endoscopically, or directly during abdominal surgery.

7.4.18 Neuroaxial Techniques

7.4.18.1 Intrathecal Techniques

Long-term intrathecal administration of opioids and local anesthetics can provide excellent pain control. Due to the tight dose-dependent nature of the somatic distribution of the analgesic effect of intrathecal local anesthetic, intrathecal catheters can provide near-absolute analgesia. Long-term use of percutaneous intrathecal catheters carries the risk of meningitis and encephalitis; thus, the use of an implanted pump with medication reservoir may be a better option for children with intractable pain who have a life expectancy greater than a few weeks (Galloway et al. 2000; Aram et al. 2001; de Pinto and Naidu 2015). Cord destruction with intrathecal phenol has been reported in case reports (Shimazaki et al. 2003).

7.5 Respiratory Symptoms

7.5.1 Case Presentation

Paul, a 12-year-old boy with metastatic osteosarcoma involving the lungs, was admitted to the oncology ward because of a runny nose and a cough accompanied by shortness of breath and desaturation that suddenly appeared. A do-not-resuscitate order was in place. On admission to ward, he was treated with oxygen enrichment which resolved his desaturation, but did not relieve his shortness of breath. Accordingly, morphine treatment was started at a dose of 25 mcg per kg with gradual and partial improvement in his dyspnea. In consultation with the palliative team given impression of parents and nursing staff that there was a significant component of anxiety, midazolam was cautiously added to his treatment regimen. However, no benefit was shown, and midazolam treatment was discontinued accordingly. Thereafter, he was begun on high-flow nasal cannula (HFNC) with significant clinical benefit. After 3 days of treatment, there was again a sudden worsening in his respiratory distress. Auscultation revealed decreased air sounds bilaterally together with percussion dullness over the lung bases. A chest X-ray demonstrated bilateral pleural effusions. The palliative team was involved again, and decision to perform bilateral pleural taps was made. Under ultrasound guidance with local anesthesia, 18 gauge intravenous cannulas were temporally advanced into the pleural spaces with considerable removal of bilateral transudate fluid which resulted in great improvement in the boy respiratory distress.

7.6 Introduction

Respiratory symptoms occur in 30–80% of children with advanced cancer (Wolfe et al. 2000; Jalmsell et al. 2006). These symptoms are distressing and have long-term impact especially for the parents (van der Geest et al. 2014). Overall, there are insufficient data to advance our understanding of symptoms and their characteristics during end of life for children (Liben et al. 2014). In this chapter, we will describe the management of the most common and distressing respiratory symptoms encountered in pediatrics: dyspnea, cough, hemoptysis, and retained secretions. Much of the evidence is extrapolated from adult studies.

As previously noted, the management of any symptom should include a holistic approach that takes into consideration the interaction of physical, psychological, social, and spiritual factors (Liben et al. 2014). The clinical teams should set goals for the treatment such as reduction in symptom burden and address it clearly with the parents so that if these objectives are not achieved, treatment can rapidly be withdrawn especially when treatment itself adds to patient's burdens.

7.7 Dyspnea

Dyspnea is the term for the sensation of breathlessness (air hunger). Since this is a subjective experience, only the patient can judge its severity—a challenge in a population in which many are nonverbal or have not acquired descriptive language. Although pediatric dyspnea scale can aid assessment, it may still be unreliable or difficult to perform in some patient groups (Pianosi et al. 2006). As a result, many studies rely on the parents or staff perspectives.

Dyspnea is one of the most distressing and frightening symptoms experienced by children and witnessed by parents (Craig et al. 2015) with increasing prevalence and intensity during the last weeks of life (Heyse-Moore et al. 1991). Wolfe et al. found that in the last month of life, 80% of the children with cancer suffer from dyspnea, according to their parents. In approximately 48% of children, the dyspnea is associated with "a lot" or "a great deal" of suffering (Wolfe et al. 2000). Drake et al. found that the overall prevalence of dyspnea in the dying children during the last week of life is 46.7% (Drake et al. 2003). Blume et al. found that parents of children with advanced heart disease report difficulty breathing in the last month of life to be associated with "a lot" or "a great deal" of suffering in 77% of children under 2 years and 62% of those over 2 years (Blume et al. 2014).

Dyspnea is a complex multisystem disorder with evidence of neurohormonal abnormalities, peripheral and respiratory muscle dysfunction, and a whole host of other changes outside the cardiorespiratory system (Ban Banzett et al. 2000; Booth et al. 1996; Evans et al. 2002; Frost et al. 1985; Gaytan and Pasaron 1998). Dyspnea can occur as a continuous symptom; it can occur slowly or show acute exacerbation. Amplitudes are mostly of short duration but occur spontaneously or triggered by certain events and may result in anxiety that itself may exacerbate dyspnea resulting in a vicious cycle (Clemens and Klaschik 2011; Thomas and von Gunten 2002).

7.8 Treatment of Dyspnea

7.8.1 Air and Oxygen

Oxygen is often the first treatment to be thought of by both patients and staff when faced with dyspnea, and it is by far the most frequently prescribed therapy for cancer patients with dyspnea in the hospital setting (Escalante et al. 1996). However, there is an ongoing debate about its role in the management of dyspnea (Philip et al. 2006). Two studies by Bruera et al. (1992, 1993) involved significantly hypoxemic patients ($n = 1$ and $n = 14$) and revealed benefit from supplemental oxygen. Booth et al. (1996) ($n = 33$) also found relief of dyspnea with oxygen. On the other hand, two studies by Clemens et al. (Clemens and Klaschik 2011; Clemens et al. 2009) that involved palliative care patients ($n = 46$ and $n = 26$) failed to show significant decrease in intensity of dyspnea including hypoxic and non-hypoxic patients. Interestingly, there is one large multicenter study that showed no benefit of oxygen over room air (administered through a similar route), suggesting that the benefit of oxygen administration may only be through providing cool airflow, rather than the oxygen itself (Abernethy et al. 2010). However, this study showed that patients with higher baseline dyspnea derived more benefit from oxygen with most benefit occurring in the first 48 h.

Given the controversial evidence from these studies together with the knowledge that oxygen is a pharmacological agent and, like any other drug, it can have adverse effects such as drying of airways and absorption atelectasis (Spathis et al. 2006), it seems rational to offer a trial of airflow prior to considering oxygen (using something as simple as a handheld fan). If this proves unsuccessful, oxygen could be offered but discontinued if there is no apparent symptomatic benefit within the first 48 h. When treating children with chronic CO_2 retention with oxygen, care should be taken to avoid suppression of their hypoxic drive (Craig et al. 2015).

7.8.2 Opioids

Experimental models in humans found that moderate morphine doses produced substantial relief of laboratory dyspnea, with reduction in the ventilatory response to decreasing O_2 and rising CO_2 (Banzett et al. 2011). Recently published studies on symptomatic treatment of dyspnea with opioids showed a statistically significant benefit of opioid use in these patients (Al et al. 2002; Clemens and Klaschik 2007; Clemens and Klaschik 2008; Pauwels et al. 2001). Nevertheless, significant respiratory depression is a much feared adverse effect of the therapeutic use of opioids (Barbour et al. 2004; Thorns and Sykes 2000; Clemens et al. 2008), especially in hypoxic and opioid-naïve patients and in patients pretreated with strong opioids (Clemens et al. 2008). For this reason, Clemens et al. (2008) conducted a prospective study that included 46 patients with mild to severe dyspnea. Their study found that intermittent application of strong opioids significantly reduced the intensity of dyspnea both in hypoxic and in non-hypoxic patients, without significantly increasing carbon dioxide partial pressure or decreasing oxygen saturation even in opioid-naïve patients. Even though different opioids are in use, morphine remains the most common drug for symptomatic treatment of dyspnea.

Based on Craig et al. (2015), the following approach should be used to treat dyspnea in children with advanced cancer:

1. *Opioid-naïve children*: start with one quarter of a standard pain management dose (e.g., morphine 0.1 mg/kg/dose).
2. *Children established on opioids for pain management*: increase the breakthrough dose by 25%.
3. *Children with chronic dyspnea*: consider long-acting opioids (Currow et al. 2011) (divide the daily dose of oral morphine by six and give as sustained-release oral morphine, may increase to half daily dose of oral morphine).
4. May consider the use of intranasal opioids.
5. Do not use fentanyl or nebulized opioids.

The role of nebulized morphine or other opioids in alleviation of dyspnea in pediatric palliative care has not been evaluated, and today its use in this setting is controversial. The highest concentration of μu receptors is found in alveoli (Zebraski et al. 2000). Alveolar system is primarily responsible for gas exchange in lungs, whereas delivery of oxygen to alveoli and evacuation of CO_2 from them is mediated through more proximal part of respiratory system, namely, trachea and bronchial tree. This system is frequently unable to deliver effective concentration of nebulized opioids and other drugs to alveoli due to multiple causes including the presence of secretions within upper airways and hypoventilation secondary to weakness of respiratory musculature. Frequent occurrence of atelectasis and compression of pulmonary parenchyma by accumulated fluid in pleural cavity further hamper proper delivery of morphine and other opioids to alveoli. Moreover, a significant portion of the opioids potentially may become bounded to μu receptors that are located in high concentration on epithelial linings of oral and nasal cavities. Thus, summarily, the probability of therapeutic effect of nebulized morphine given in such form for alleviation of dyspnea is very low. As stated earlier, there are no published data from prospective randomized studies showing efficacy of nebulized morphine for alleviating respiratory distress in pediatric cancer patients. Scarce data originating from adult oncology practice are inconclusive as well (Charles et al. 2008; Ben-Aharon et al. 2008). Thus to better understand the role of nebulized opioids, prospective and randomized studies are needed to clarify whether nebulized opioids are absorbed via the lungs and if they have a local effect in reducing the sensation of breathlessness (Penson et al. 2002).

7.8.3 Anxiolytics

The relationship between anxiety and dyspnea is not clear. However, many patients report anxiety concurrent with their feeling of air hunger. Dyspnea can lead to anxiety, and anxiety can exacerbate dyspnea (Clemens and Klaschik 2011). Opioids can break this cycle by decreasing dyspnea, as previously mention. Anxiolytics (such as benzodiazepines) are commonly prescribed for the acute phase of anxiety. Yet, their efficacy and safety given along with opioids for the treatment of dyspnea are still in question. With regard to efficacy, Mitchell-Heggs et al. conducted a placebo-controlled single-blind study of patients with COPD and showed that moderate doses of diazepam improved dyspnea (Mitchell-Heggs et al. 1980). In contrast, subsequent double-blind studies of diazepam or alprazolam in patients with COPD found no benefit over placebo (Stark et al. 1981; Woodcock et al. 1981; Man et al. 1986). Regarding safety, clinical (Gililand et al. 1996; NaviganteA 2003) studies have not shown an impact on ventilation when opioids and benzodiazepines were used in combination. Clemens et al. (Clemens and Klaschik 2011) showed in a prospective nonrandomized study with 26 patients who suffered from moderate to severe dyspnea that neither an increase in $paCO_2$ nor a decrease in SaO_2 was found in both hypoxic and non-hypoxic patients after application of the opioid in combination with lorazepam. Dyspnea and anxiety intensity were significantly reduced, and none of the patients showed undesirable side effects of this combination therapy. Craig et al. (2015) in their conclusion on the use of anxiolytics for the treatment of dyspnea summarized the data as not sufficiently robust to recommend the widespread use of anxiolytics for the management of dyspnea in children. However, anxiolytics may be considered on an individual patient basis, together with opioids, especially if anxiety is a significant factor.

7.9 High-Flow Nasal Cannula (HFNC) and Noninvasive Ventilation (NIV)

HFNC and NIV are two modalities that have been gaining attention as alternative respiratory support strategies for patients who are spontaneously breathing but have an increased work of breathing due to variety of conditions such as asthma and COPD exacerbation, respiratory infections, and congestive heart failure. Benefit in children with advanced cancer is unknown.

HFNC delivers up to 40 L/min of humidified heated oxygen through a nasal cannula. In addition to high-flow oxygenation, it also provides nasopharyngeal washout and positive distending pressure and decreases airway resistance and the metabolic cost of breathing, all of which may alleviate dyspnea (Dysart et al. 2009).

NIV provides ventilatory support without using an invasive artificial airway. Positive-pressure ventilation delivered through a variety of interfaces (mouth piece or nasal, face or helmet mask) has become the main method providing noninvasive ventilatory support. This support can be achieved through using a variety of ventilatory modes (e.g., volume ventilation, pressure support, bi-level positive airway pressure (BiPAP), etc.).

Nava et al. (2013) assessed the acceptability and effectiveness of NIV versus oxygen therapy in decreasing dyspnea and the amount of opioids needed in patients with solid tumors, acute respiratory failure, and life expectancy less than 6 months. In a multicenter, stratified, randomized feasibility study, 200 patients were randomly allocated to NIV or oxygen treatment, while morphine was used in both groups. Their findings showed that dyspnea decreased more in the NIV group than the oxygen group, as did patients' need for morphine. Improvements in dyspnea and the reduced need for morphine occurred predominantly in the hypercapnic patients ($PaCO_2 > 45$ mm Hg).

Hui et al. (2013) conducted a randomized trial of HFNC versus NIV with BiPAP for 2 h in advanced cancer patients with persistent dyspnea. The goals of this study were to examine the changes in dyspnea, physiologic parameters, and adverse effects with these modalities. They found that dyspnea improved with both modalities in a before-and-after comparison. However, no significant differences in dyspnea relief were detected between the two modalities. Respiratory rate reduction was not statistically significant with both treatments. BiPAP was associated with a decrease in heart rate. HFNC also was associated with a significant decrease in systolic blood pressure and improvement in oxygen saturation. The authors did not identify any significant adverse effects with BiPAP and HFNC, but patients reported less trouble sleeping while on HFNC compared with BiPAP.

Considering the above data, it seems reasonable to consider HFNC or NIV for the child with advanced cancer, if tolerated, especially if reversible causes, such as infection, can be addressed. Furthermore, in addition to reducing dyspnea, NIV may allow more effective use of morphine or other sedative analgesia without causing excessive sleepiness or progressive CO2 retention. Nevertheless, clinical team should set clear goals and discuss the expectations clearly with the parents or other family members. Although NIV is referred as "noninvasive," in reality NIV can be a very invasive procedure for an individual child and family. This procedure can be poorly tolerated and can be associated with complications that contribute to distress, including mask discomfort, nasal congestion and dryness, agitation, claustrophobia, and aspiration (Gay 2009). Initiation of NIV therefore should be considered when consistent with child and family goals of care.

7.9.1 Management of Underlying Causes

When possible, treatment should be directed at reversible causes, without neglecting concurrent symptomatic treatment. Cancer-related causes of dyspnea include primary lung tumors (uncommon in children), lung metastases, pleural and pericardial effusions, pneumothorax, and superior vena cava syndrome. Tumor mass can be treated with resection, chemotherapy, or radiotherapy. Pleural or pericardial effusions can be drained by ultrasound-guided thoracocentesis or pericardiocentesis, respectively. In the case of intractable pleural effusion, pleurodesis with doxycycline may be attempted (Hoffer et al. 2007). Antibiotics may be appropriate for infections. Anticoagulants can prevent and treat thrombotic pulmonary emboli. Bronchodilators such as salbutamol can treat reversible bronchospasm.

7.9.2 Cough and Retained Secretions

Cough in the pediatric palliative care setting is usually due to acute or chronic infection, recurrent aspiration, gastroesophageal reflux, or malignant disease. To be able to cough effectively, the patient must have the ability to create an adequate airstream velocity, and the secretions must be loose enough to be cleared. Ineffective cough can lead to persistent and distressing coughing which can further increase pain and dyspnea.

7.9.3 Treatment of Cough and Secretions

As with dyspnea, cough and secretions treatment can be divided into symptomatic managements and underlining cause managements. However, symptomatic management must be addressed alongside any disease-directed interventions.

7.9.4 Opioids

The most effective antitussive agents are opioids. The antitussive action is different from the analgesic effect and thought to act both on central brainstem opioid receptors and on receptors located peripherally in airway sensory nerve endings (MacRedmond and O'Connell 1999). Adult studies have not shown any one opioid to be superior to another (Morice et al. 2007; Wee et al. 2012; Yancy et al. 2013). Dose information for pediatric patients is lacking, and Craig et al. (2015) suggest 25–50% of the starting pain dose. For children already receiving opioids for pain, there are no data to support or to oppose the addition of a separate opioid or for increasing opioid dose above the dose needed for pain management (Craig et al. 2015).

7.9.5 Nonopioids

The antitussive benefit of nonopioids drugs even in adult patients is inconclusive (Yancy et al. 2013; Molassiotis et al. 2010). In children, antitussives, antihistamines, antihistamine-decongestants, and antitussive/bronchodilator combinations have shown no benefit over placebo in the treatment of acute cough (Smith et al. 2014). Although sodium cromoglycate was shown to be more effective than placebo for cough in adults with advanced lung cancer (Moroni et al. 1996), there is no evidence for its effectiveness for the management of prolonged, nonspecific cough in children.

Local anesthetics such as lidocaine 2% or bupivacaine 0.25% can be delivered locally to the airways by inhalation. Their use has shown some benefit in adults by attenuation of capsaicin-induced cough (Choudry et al. 1990). However, the evidence is insufficient to support their use in pediatric patients. Furthermore, their effect is transient, and the antitussive effect is accompanied by bronchospasm and oropharyngeal anesthesia leading to an increased risk of aspiration of airway secretions and food.

Gabapentin or pregabalin, probably by acting via central mechanism, can also be used for the treatment of chronic cough (Ryan 2015; Gibson and Vertigan 2015). Although gabapentin is recommended for unexplained chronic cough in updated American College of Chest Physicians (ACCP) guidelines (Gibson et al. 2016), its use for chronic cough is not approved. Additionally, there are no data on its use for this purpose in children.

7.9.6 Management of Underlying Causes

A common reversible cause of cough is gastroesophageal reflux. Reducing feed volumes and/or commencing continuous feeding can be an effective intervention, alongside or in place of antacids and prokinetics. Recurrent aspiration, especially in children with impaired swallow, may be reduced by changing from oral to feeding tube or gastrostomy feeding. Oropharyngeal accumulation of secretions may be managed with postural drainage, suctioning, and physiotherapy, in addition to anticholinergic medication.

Bronchospasm and infections should be managed appropriately especially in children with underlying respiratory diseases like cystic fibrosis or asthma. Cough induced by airway inflammation can be reduced by inhaled corticosteroids combined with long-acting beta-agonists (Nannini et al. 2013). Cough induced by airway compression due to tumor mass should be treated with tumor mass reduction techniques.

7.9.7 Airway Clearance

7.9.7.1 Loosening Secretions

If the sputum is thick, expectorants (e.g., glyceryl guaiacolate) or mucolytics (e.g., acetylcysteine) may be used in order to reduce the viscosity of secretions and make each cough more productive. However, the data on their effectiveness in reducing cough intensity is not significant. Moreover, their use should be cautioned in patient with neuromuscular diseases due to their inability to cough out the liquified mucus. Nebulized 0.9% saline and hypertonic saline are both effective in loosening secretions. Hypertonic saline is superior to lower concentrations but may be less well tolerated in the pediatric population (Kellett and Robert 2011). For better tolerance and to prevent bronchospasm, they should be combined with bronchodilators.

7.9.7.2 Improving Cough Strength

Intensive chest physiotherapy is very important for children with increased secretions viscosity or with inability to effectively clear their airways. Patients can be assisted by the use of a mechanical insufflation/exsufflation, which increases peak cough flow and improves secretion clearance (Chatwin et al. 2003; Chatwin and Simonds 2009; Moran et al. 2013).

7.9.8 Gastrointestinal Tract Problems

7.9.8.1 Case Presentation

Tom is a 15-year-old boy who was diagnosed with intra-abdominal desmoplastic small cell tumor. His primary originated from left retroperitoneal space, and he had widespread metastatic disease with involving intra- and retroperitoneal lymph nodes and massive hepatic spread. His presenting symptoms were prominent nausea and vomiting. He received chemotherapy consisting of alternating courses of VDC (vincristine, doxorubicin, and Cytoxan) and IE (ifosfamide and etoposide). This chemotherapy was regarded as moderately emetogenic, and his treatment during chemotherapy courses consisted of combination of 5-HT3 receptor inhibitor ondansetron and dexamethasone. This antiemetic therapy was only partially effective, and neurokinin-1 antagonist, aprepitant (Emend), was added to subsequent courses of chemotherapy with satisfactory effect. Unfortunately, improvement in clinical status was short-lived, and after several weeks of therapy, the child presented with recurrent severe nausea and vomiting along with signs of complete bowel obstruction. A nasogastral tube was inserted, and treatment with ondansetron and dexamethasone was continued. In order to decrease intestinal secretions, subcutaneous octreotide 15 mcg/kg/day BID was started. Because of inability to use the GI tract for enteral nutrition, total parenteral nutrition was administered via central line. Given limited life expectancy and the fact that most of his abdominal cavity was involved with progressive, refractory cancer, surgical intervention was not recommended. Tom remained relatively comfortable on these therapies and died approximately 6 weeks after bowel obstruction was diagnosed. He did not developed intestinal perforation during this period.

7.9.8.2 Nausea and Vomiting

In children with cancer, especially with advanced disease, there are usually several concurrent causes of nausea and vomiting (N&V), many not restricted to the GI tract. The vomiting center is located within the medulla oblongata in humans, and signals coming to this center may originate from at least one of three sources: brain cortex, area postrema, and GI tract. The receptors located within the cortex respond to increased intracranial pressure frequently encountered in children with involvement of CNS by progressive primary tumors or by metastatic spread from a distant source. Modifying effect on nausea and vomiting resulting from stimulation of cortical receptors exerts such factors as anxiety, panic, fear, and other conditions of emotional stress and instability. A well-known phenomenon is anticipatory N&V in children, especially in adolescents and young adults which occurs even before chemotherapy is started.

Receptors located in area postrema are susceptible to various chemical substances, including chemotherapy and other drugs. It is not uncommon for children with advanced cancer to receive opioids, sometimes in high doses. Such prolonged opioid therapy frequently becomes the main cause of drug-associated N&V in this population of pediatric patients (Smith et al. 2012). Opioids contribute to development of N&V in many ways: first, by direct stimulation of chemoreceptor trigger zone in CNS. Second, opioids can cause N&V by decreasing gut motility with resultant gastrointestinal paresis and constipation. Constipation is the only side effect of opioid therapy which is not resolved spontaneously with time; therefore, it is not prudent to wait for the alleviation of nausea in cases when these symptoms are mainly secondary to GI distention. In such situations, opioid rotation may or may not be efficacious, and the best therapeutic approach is prevention of constipation.

Distention of intestines caused by intrinsic (constipation) or extrinsic factors (enlarged lymph nodes, intestinal adhesive disease) is the third reason why children experience N&V. Previous or current radiotherapy, vincristine and other alkaloids, and other drugs leading to decreased intestinal motility (paclitaxel) frequently play a detrimental role in development and worsening of N&V.

N&V exert their detrimental effect both on physical and psychological well-being since children experiencing these symptoms frequently limit their physical activity and are unable to go to school and interact with peers. This, in turn, leads in decreased self-esteem.

While evaluating the child with advanced cancer experiencing N&V, the treating clinician should take into account that the etiology is frequently multifactorial, especially in children whose disease is progressing and unresponsive to anticancer therapy. For example, consider a child with recurrent medulloblastoma with leptomeningeal spread experiencing severe pain and receiving concurrently second-line chemotherapy and opioids. In this child, contributing causes of N&V may be increased intracranial pressure (ICP), direct involvement of the cortex by disseminated disease, use of emetogenic chemotherapy, use of opioids which cause N&V both by stimulating chemoreceptors in the medulla oblongata and by worsening constipation, and, therefore, intestinal distention.

The severity of N&V may be assessed by using various tools developed and validated in pediatric population including pediatric cancer patients in last years (Baxter et al. 2011; Dupuis et al. 2006). As in cases of assessing a child with other symptoms, the clinician should take into account that any such symptom is end product of interaction of objective and subjective experiences of an ill child. It is not uncommon to encounter child who objectively had only one or two vomiting episodes but reports severe distress from these symptom.

Treatment of N&V begins with identification of all causes of these symptoms and should be provided as soon as the problem and its causes are recognized. Management of nausea and vomiting in pediatric patients sometimes can be challenging due to its multifactorial nature and resistance to interventions. Since the vomiting center localized in the medulla oblongata mediates its activity through such neurotransmitters as acetylcholine and histamine and chemoreceptor trigger zones of the cortex, area postrema, and intestines through dopamine and serotonin, these molecular substances represent the main targets for antiemetic therapy (Roila et al. 1998; Roila et al. 2005). The 5-hydroxytryptamine3 (5-HT3) receptor antagonists occupy the central role in treatment of chemotherapy-induced nausea and vomiting (CINV) (Patel et al. 2016; Jordan et al. 2011). Efficacy of these drugs in children with advanced cancer has not been systematically evaluated despite their common use in this setting.

Combinations of a 5-HT3 antagonist and dexamethasone show increased efficacy with respect to 5-HT3 antagonists alone (Kris et al. 2011). Among several 5-HT3 antagonists, ondansetron (Zofran) and granisetron (Kytril) are used especially widely. Both medicines are available in oral and intravenous forms. Although these two drugs have been shown to have similar clinical activity in various studies (Vrabel 2007), in clinical practice one drug may be found more effective than the other at individual level; therefore, rotation of 5-HT3 antagonists may be justified in selected cases when previously administered 5-HT3 antagonist has been noneffective.

The use of such neurokinin-1 (NK1) antagonist such as aprepitant in children with advanced cancer has been reported recently and was shown to be effective in this population (Bodge et al. 2014; Kang et al. 2015). Some of commonly drugs used for treatment of N&V are shown in Table 7.7.

Along with specific antiemetic therapy, other measures should be undertaken directed at other causes of N&V. Thus, if there is evidence for increased ICP, use of such agents as mannitol, furosemide, and steroids may be indicated. In selected cases, there are indications for surgical relief of increased ICP (insertion of VP shunt or ventriculostomy) even in advanced cancer when consistent with family goals. Radiotherapy in children whose ICP is the result of recurrent primary CNS tumor or metastatic spread to CNS may be an option as well.

In situations when the main cause of N&V is use of chemotherapy, thorough consideration should be given to whether or not this therapy should be continued. Thoughtful discussion with the child and family should reevaluate goals of care and continuation of cancer-directed therapy.

In cases of severe N&V caused by gastroparesis, sometimes the only therapeutic intervention that can bring alleviation is nasogastric tube insertion which can relieve suffering practically immediately. This may be especially helpful in cases of severe N&V in children with altered level of consciousness due to CNS involvement by malignant process.

In cases when intestinal obstruction due to mechanical causes is the primary cause of severe N&V, consideration should be given to surgical intervention such as placing a venting gastrostomy or intestinal stoma. If such procedures are not indicated as in cases of severe general debilitation, very high operative risk, and very short life expectancy, more conservative approach may be appropriate. In certain instances, administration of octreotide intravenously or subcutaneously may lead to sufficient decrease of intestinal secretion, thus facilitating alleviation of symptoms of intestinal obstruction and, therefore, N&V (Currow et al. 2015; Watanabe et al. 2007; Davies et al. 2012; Mercadante and Porzio 2012).

Irrespective of any medical or surgical interventions directed at alleviation of N&V, nonpharmacological measures should be applied as well, and they should include consultation with a psychologist when appropriate, education of patients and parents about eating small portions

Table 7.7 Commonly used medications for treatment of N&V

Medication	Dose	Remarks
Prokinetic/dopamine antagonist Metoclopramide	Prokinetic dose, 0.1 mg/kg/dose IV or orally every 6 h; dopamine antagonist (antiemetic) dose, 0.5–1 mg/kg/dose IV or orally every 6 h	Use with diphenhydramine to prevent extrapyramidal symptoms
Serotonin receptor antagonists Ondansetron	0.15 mg/kg/dose; up to three doses a day	
Granisetron	0.04 mg/kg PO or IV	
Anticholinergics Scopolamine	For children ≥40 kg: 1.5 mg patch behind the ear every 72 h	Not FDA approved in pediatric patients
Antivertigo agents (piperazine) Meclizine	For children >12 years of age: 25–75 mg/day orally in up to three divided doses	
Corticosteroids Dexamethasone	When used as antiemetic, 10 mg/m^2 IV or orally daily; maximum dose 20 mg daily. For increased intracranial pressure, increase dosing frequency to two to four times daily, with a maximum dose of 40 mg/day	
Somatostatin analogs Octreotide	5–10 mcg/kg/day, either as continuous 24-h IV infusion or divided twice daily and administered subcutaneously	
Atypical antipsychotic Olanzapine	2.5–5 mg/day orally, may be increased to maximum 20 mg/day. Dosing in children not established but has been used in some adolescents	Safety and effectiveness of olanzapine monotherapy not established in pediatric patients younger than 13 years
Haloperidol	0.05–0.075 mg/kg/day orally, divided and given two or three times daily	Use caution if treating patients with QT-prolonging conditions, concomitant QT-prolonging drugs, underlying cardiac abnormalities, hypothyroidism, and familial long QT syndrome
Cannabinoid Dronabinol	For children ages 6 years and older; 2.5–5 mg/m^2/dose every 4–6 h	Not recommended for children who have clinical depression
Cyproheptadine	0.25 mg/kg/24 h (8 mg/m^2/24 h) divided every 6–8 h PO	Increased appetite and weight gain

given at regular intervals, and exclusion of any food products that possess strong smells or are unpleasant for the ill child. Some patients also may benefit from acupuncture (Garcia et al. 2013), hypnosis (Richardson et al. 2007), or other forms of distraction therapy. Maintenance of good general hygiene and avoidance of any strong smelling deodorants and soaps also decrease susceptibility of vomiting trigger zone in such children.

7.9.9 Constipation

Constipation is one of the most common problems encountering among pediatric cancer patients throughout the entire course of their disease (Santucci and Mack 2007; Phillips and Gibson 2008; Constipation Guideline Committee of the North American Society for Pediatric Gastroenterology, Hepatology and Nutrition 2006). It may influence quality of life of children with cancer both through its physical impact (pain, abdominal distention, decrease in appetite, respiratory problems, etc.) and by exerting its deleterious psychological effect resulting in embarrassment, depression, and social avoidance in the ill child or adolescent. Combination of these somatic and psychological effects of constipation may result in increasing of level and intensity of global suffering of a child with cancer.

Constipation is usually multifactorial and may be caused by many factors which operate at the same time in a given child.

Causes of constipation:

1. Malignant disease itself:
   (a) Obstruction of the GI tract by tumor external to bowels such as compression by enlarged intra-abdominal lymph nodes such as in patients with lymphoma or metastatic lymph nodes of sarcoma, intra-abdominal or pelvic tumors such as teratoma, rhabdomyosarcoma, or Ewing sarcoma
   (b) Obstruction of the GI tract by tumors growing within intestinal lumen—rare cases of colonic carcinoma in childhood or intratumoral growth of primary intestinal lymphoma
2. Complications of anticancer treatment:
   (a) Drugs causing decreased intestinal motility such as vincristine and other vinca alkaloids and taxanes (Pashankar et al. 2011; Rowinsky and Donehower 1991)
   (b) Radiation
   (c) Postsurgery adhesive disease
3. Other drugs such as use of opioids, antidepressants, antihistamines, and others

Additional factors contributing to constipation include prolonged periods of decreased physical activity, dehydration, anal painful fissures, and, rarely, background dysfunction of parasympathetic nervous system such as Hirschsprung disease or such endocrine disorders as hypothyroidism along with various forms of electrolyte imbalance. Severe neurologic complication of cancer such as spinal cord compression may also result in severe constipation due to a neurogenic rectum.

The definition of constipation is varied with the age of a child since normal pattern of defecation is age related (Constipation Guideline Committee of the North American Society for Pediatric Gastroenterology, Hepatology and Nutrition 2006; Fontana et al. 1989) and depends largely on a child's diet. Healthy children older than 3 years usually have one bowel movement per day (Fontana et al. 1989). Constipation was defined by using the North American Society of Pediatric Gastroenterology, Hepatology, and Nutrition (NASPGHAN) criteria. The NASPGHAN criteria define constipation as a delay or difficulty in defecation for 2 or more weeks and sufficient to cause significant distress to the patient (Author 2006). It is common practice in pediatric oncology to define constipation for practical reasons as absence of bowel movement during at least 48 h.

The first and one of the most important steps in evaluation of a child with cancer and constipation is properly collected anamnesis. Since questions are related to one of the most intimate bodily functions, patients usually are reluctant to deliberate on this issue unless physical distress becomes almost unbearable. This is true especially for adolescents of both sexes. Hence, taking a medical history should be performed in quiet, relaxing atmosphere, preferably without participating of other family members present at this phase of patient's evaluation. If it is possible, questioning should be performed by the member of medical team of the same sex as of the patient. Education of both child and parents about the importance of early recognition of constipation for its successful prevention and treatment may significantly facilitate establishing trustful contact between treating medical staff (both physician and nurse) and an ill child and helps avoid unnecessary embarrassment for a patient. Information gathered should include not only detailed description of bowel habits such as frequency and character of bowel movements, accompanying discomfort, and pain. Questioning should also be directed at possible finding of contributing factors such as dietary habits, fluid intake, and character of regular physical activity. Children may also present with diarrhea resulting from obstipation with overflow. Physician should be aware of this possibility while taking history, especially in patients who have a history of constipation or are at high risk for constipation (Santucci and Mack 2007; Fallon and ONeill 1997).

Although constipation stems from many causes in the same patient, use of opioids and other drugs in advanced illness represents its most common and frequently treatable cause. Opioids are widely recognized as one of the main causes of constipation. Actually, constipation is the only side effect of long-use morphine and other opioids that does not abate over time (Abrahm 2000). Acute constipation was diagnosed in 57% of children receiving chemotherapy for cancer. Combined use of vincristine and opioids was associated with the development of constipation and was found as the only risk factor for its development among 35 pediatric cancer patients reported in one study (Pashankar et al. 2011). In this study, 15 children/parents (43%) perceived constipation as a significant or major problem during chemotherapy, whereas 8 children (23%) perceived constipation having a significant or major impact on lifestyle during chemotherapy.

Special attention should be given to vincristine and other vinca alkaloids. These drugs exert their therapeutic effect by the inhibition of formation and disruption of the mitotic spindle microtubule (Rowinsky and Donehower 1991). Attempts have been made by several investigators to prevent or alleviate vincristine-induced constipation by using glutamic acid as an oral agent. The exact mechanism by which glutamic acid may modify vincristine-induced neurotoxicity is not fully appreciated (Bradfield et al. 2015; Mokhtar et al. 2010). The most recently published randomized, placebo-controlled, double-blind trial of oral glutamic acid as a preventive agent in pediatric patients with cancer receiving vincristine therapy for at least 9 consecutive weeks showed no proven efficacy of this drug in children younger than 13 years (Bradfield et al. 2015). Today, routine use of glutamic acid as a drug for prevention of vincristine-induced neuropathy, including constipation, cannot be recommended.

The best and most effective method of treating constipation is its prevention. Meticulous attention should be given to all those factors that may contribute and worsen constipation. Early mobilization of patients after surgical interventions, adequate analgesia in post-op period allowing this mobilization, and proper oral and intravenous hydration greatly facilitate normal activity of the GI tract, establishing regular bowel movements. For those patients who are not able to move without assistance, such as children with spinal cord compression and debilitated children at end of life, frequent changing of body position and sufficient hydration are of paramount importance. Timely recognition and treatment of such causes of constipation as anal fissures and hemorrhoids are also very important.

There are three main interdependent mechanisms playing roles in initiation and maintenance of constipation treatment:

1. Formation of hard intestinal content
2. Absence or very weakened intestinal peristalsis
3. Difficulties in normal evacuation of rectal content

Treatment of constipation should be directed at all three components of its pathogenesis. It is common knowledge that any child who starts receiving opioids as a part of pain treatment should be given concurrently both a stool softening and stimulant for the prevention of constipation. In certain cases, when constipation is especially disturbing and more "conservative" approaches were proven to be noneffective, rectal enema can be given safely to any child with cancer who has a normal complete blood count. In the setting of neutropenia or thrombocytopenia, enemas are contraindicated since in such circumstances there is increased risk of sepsis and rectal bleeding, respectively. Evacuation of rectal content is frequently accompanied by immediate relief of abdominal pain and distention and enables the child to be more cooperative for further treatment of constipation. Several stool softeners, the main among them is docusate and osmotic agents (lactulose or magnesium sulfate), are used in advanced pediatric cancer. Based on recently published data, docusate appears to be no more effective than placebo for increasing stool frequency or softening stools and did not lessen symptoms associated with constipation (Treatments for Constipation: A Review of Systematic Reviews 2014). Stool softeners such as polyethylene glycol (PEG) may be especially helpful in children with constipation. A recently published Cochrane review of 18 studies with a total of 1643 pediatric patients concluded that polyethylene glycol preparations may increase the frequency of bowel movements in constipated children. Polyethylene glycol was generally safe, with lower rates of minor side effects compared to other agents (Gordon et al. 2013). The only stimulant with proven use in pediatric advanced illness is senna (Santucci and Mack 2007; Feudtner et al. 2014). Stimulants such as 5-HT4 agonists including prucalopride in adults with chronic constipation resulted in increased stool frequency and improved constipation-related symptoms compared with placebo (Leppert 2015). The efficacy and safety of this group of stimulants in children have not been evaluated.

Another approach that has been used with increased frequency in patients receiving opioids is concurrent use of selective inhibitor of mu receptors located in the GI tract, methylnaltrexone.

The adult methylnaltrexone dose recommended by the manufacturer is 0.15 mg/kg/dose for those weighing less than 33 kg. For those whose weight is more than 33 kg, the dose of this drug is calculated according to the weight of a patient (Compendium of Pharmaceuticals and Specialities 2011). In one retrospective study describing pediatric patients (Rodrigues et al. 2013), a mean dose 0.15 ± 0.002 mg/kg of meth ylnaltrexone was given to 15 children with median age of 14 years subcutaneously. After 14 of 19 doses administered, patients had a bowel movement within 4 h. Three patients had documented mild gastrointestinal upset following methylnaltrexone administration. None reported a reduction of pain control or opioid withdrawal symptoms. In contrast to nonselective opioid antagonist naloxone, it appears that methylnaltrexone does not cause rebound of pain or opioid withdrawal syndrome after its administration. These data were confirmed in another small retrospective study published recently (Flerlage and Baker 2015). Contraindications for administration of methylnaltrexone include mechanical gastrointestinal obstruction and acute surgical abdomen (Compendium of Pharmaceuticals and Specialities 2011). Nevertheless, the use of naloxone for prevention of opioid-induced constipation is still widely used when this drug is given as a combination in one tablet with prolonged-release (PR) oxycodone. A combination of PR oxycodone with PR naloxone (Targin®, Targiniq®, Targinact®) in one tablet with a fixed 2:1 ratio is available for the treatment of patients with severe pain (Burness and Keating 2014; Leppert 2014). Although use of this combination is not approved yet by FDA in children, clinical data accumulated from its use in adult oncology and limited experience of its use in older children with cancer suggest its clinical efficacy and relative safety in pediatric population as well.

Rotation of opioids with hydrophilic properties to those with lipophilic ones may lead to less constipation since GI tract predominantly has opioid receptors which are more avid to hydrophilic substances than lipophilic (Mercadante et al. 2001). If this is the case, switching from morphine, oxycodone, or hydromorphone to fentanyl or methadone may be beneficial for children with opioid-induced constipation. Unfortunately, in clinical practice such opioid rotation is not universally efficacious (Wirz et al. 2009). Nevertheless, a trial of opioid rotation in such situation should be considered.

Another cause of constipation sometimes encountered in practice of pediatric oncology, especially in patients with advanced intra-abdominal cancer, is mechanical intestinal obstruction. In such situation, a trial of treatment with octreotide may be conducted. Published data suggest that such treatment may be efficacious and may mitigate the need for colostomy or other surgical interventions. In the setting of end-of-life care, administration of octreotide may lessen intraintestinal secretion and, thus, lead to decrease of intraintestinal pressure above the level of obstruction, in turn reducing abdominal pain (Currow et al. 2015; Watanabe et al. 2007; Davies et al. 2012; Mercadante and Porzio 2012).

7.10 Anorexia and Cachexia

Cachexia, is a complex and debilitating clinico-biochemical syndrome frequently encountered in pediatric oncology, especially in advanced stages of disease. The role of cachexia is difficult to overestimate. Its presence negatively affects physical well-being, decreases resistance to infections, shortens survival, and leads to decreased self-esteem and ultimately to profound psychological distress (Loeffen et al. 2015; Sala et al. 2004; Morley et al. 2006). The causes of cachexia in pediatric oncology patients are numerous and often multifactorial. Cachexia occurs more frequently in children with advanced cancer who were treated with multiple lines of therapy and who have recurrent disseminated disease. The prevalence of malnutrition at diagnosis averages 50% in children with cancer in developing countries, whereas, in industrialized countries, it is related to the type of tumor and the extent of the disease, ranging from <10% in patients with standard-risk acute lymphoblastic leukemia to 50% in patients with advanced neuroblastoma (Sala et al. 2004). At end of life, the prevalence of cachexia among pediatric oncology population is nearly 100% (Wolfe et al. 2000; Jalmsell et al. 2006).

Although cachexia is a frequently diagnosed medical condition, there is no universally accepted definition. One of the proposed definitions of cachexia is that it is a complex metabolic syndrome associated with the underlying illness and is characterized by the loss of muscle with or without loss of fat mass (Aoyagi et al. 2015). The hallmark of cachexia, weight loss in cancer patients, is due to depletion of both adipose tissue and skeletal muscle mass, while the nonmuscle proteins are relatively preserved, thus distinguishing cachexia from simple starvation (KCH 1992).

Initiation and development of cachexia in cancer patients is mediated by secretion of various proinflammatory factors including interleukins (IL) 1 and 6, tumor necrosis factor (TNF), interferons, and signal transducers and activators of transcription 3 (STAT3) which are recognized as the most important (Santucci and Mack 2007; Morley et al. 2006; Aoyagi et al. 2015; KCH 1992; Tisdale 2009; Tisdale 2008; Brinksma et al. 2012). Increased secretion of these molecules leads to a metabolically abnormal condition sometimes referred to as a "cytokine storm." These cytokines profoundly alter the metabolic status of an ill child shifting the metabolic balance toward catabolic state. Complex changes observed in this condition ultimately result in profound skeletal and fat tissue wasting (Fig. 7.4).

Anorexia is defined as a disorder characterized by a loss of appetite, and its severity may vary and be graded according to the Common

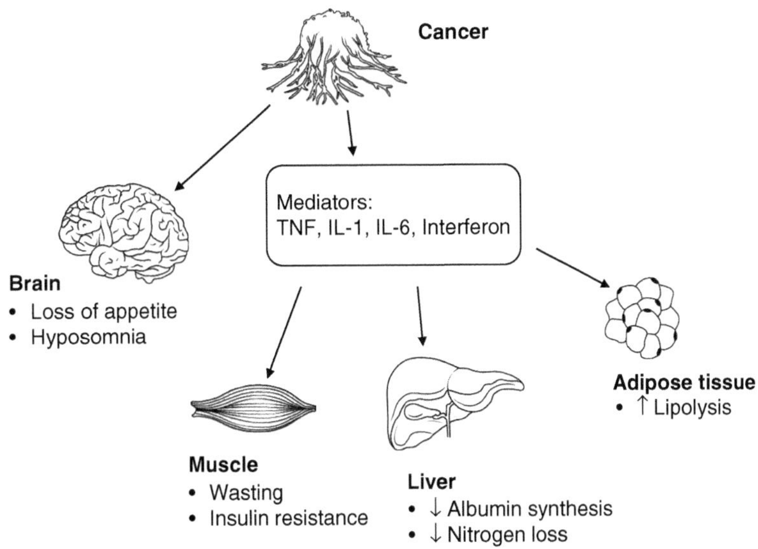

Fig. 7.4 Pathogenic mechanisms in developing cancer cachexia

Terminology Criteria for Adverse Events (CTCAE) (2009). Although anorexia and cachexia frequently occur concurrently, each has their distinct causes and pathogenetic mechanisms. Anorexia frequently accompanies cachexia, but cachexia may be diagnosed without anorexia. In cases when both entities are present, anorexia may exacerbate cachexia. Anorexia leads to decreased protein and caloric intake, which in turn may result in weight loss in children with cancer, but this process does not necessarily cause increased secretion of proinflammatory cytokines characteristic for cachexia.

The most common causes of anorexia are anticancer treatment itself, especially moderately and highly emetogenic chemotherapy and radiotherapy, particularly when directed at CNS or abdomen. In addition, typical complications of chemo- and radiotherapy such as severe and poorly controlled mucositis also contribute to anorexia. Functional or anatomical causes leading to intestinal distention and constipation should also be considered as important factors in the development of decreased oral intake.

The therapeutic approach to cachexia is complex and not always successful. While considering strategies to treat cachexia, the goals of such treatment should be clarified. Sometimes there is a discrepancy between the treating physician and child and parents in understanding the goals of cachexia treatment, especially at end of life. Parents tend to see a causative relationship between anorexia and cachexia and consider decreased food intake to be the primary cause of cachexia. Therefore, education of parents and explanation of pathogenetic mechanisms leading to cachexia may be helpful.

The best management strategy of cancer cachexia in children with cancer is to treat the underlying cancer. Unfortunately, this is often not possible in children with more advanced stages of disease which accounts for the majority of children with cachexia.

Consultation of pediatric dietician can be very helpful in the management of anorexia in children with cancer. They can provide suggestions about high-calorie foods which may be more palatable for the child. Supplementary nutrition, although an important treatment modality for some patients, is rarely fully effective in completely reversing the wasting associated with cachexia and can be experienced as highly burdensome. Furthermore, nutritional support can be a highly emotion-laden experience for families and clinicians, especially at end of life. Many believe that forgoing nutrition and fluids in a terminally ill child contradicts the very essence of compassionate care. This point of view is frequently supported by parents and other lay persons who tend to think that withholding fluids and food may accelerate the child's demise. Given the fact that most pediatric cancer patients have a central line in place during their last phase of life, it may also seem tempting to use it as a vehicle for providing nutrition to the child with cachexia. Thus it is important to provide education about the potential drawbacks of total parenteral nutrition (TPN), which may occur with even higher frequency in debilitated cancer patients. Given the risks and logistics of providing parenteral nutrition, in the absence of an obstruction, tube feedings may provide some comfort for children and the families, although these too can be experienced as burdensome. Decisions about supplemental nutrition and its mode of delivery are thus highly complex and should be carefully considered in light of mutual goals of families and providers.

It should be kept in mind that nutrition via a feeding tube or IV has little effect on increasing skeletal muscle mass and most weight gain can be attributed to an increase in adipose tissue. In these instances, addressing psychological, spiritual, and existential concerns, especially in adolescent and young adults using specialized help of interdisciplinary team members, may facilitate better management of anorexia and cachexia (Santucci and Mack 2007).

Medications that have been used in patients with cachexia are based on knowledge of pathogenesis of this syndrome. However, the use of various drugs in cachectic pediatric patients stems mainly from the data accumulated in adult oncology (Tisdale 2006) (Table 7.8).

Table 7.8 Selected medications for increasing of appetite

Name/brand name	Recommended dose	Side effects	Comments
Cyproheptadine Periactin (antihistamine)	Pediatrics >13 years: 2 mg four times per day May gradually increase over 3 weeks to 8 mg four times per day Maximum dose: 32 mg/day	Constipation, diarrhea, edema, nausea, polyuria, vomiting, xerostomia, ataxia, drowsiness, dizziness, euphoria, hallucinations, headache, hepatic dysfunction, hypotension, irritability, photosensitivity, poluyuria	Non-FDA-labeled indications for loss of appetite
Dexamethasone Decadron (corticosteroid)	0.05–0.5 mg/kg/day	Bruising, Cushingoid appearance, delayed healing, headache, immune suppression, insomnia, muscle weakness, adrenal suppression, bone thinning, cataracts, insulin resistance, protein breakdown, water retention	Optimal dose not known, no increase in lean body mass
Dronabinol, Marinol (cannabinoid)	Individual dosing	Somnolence, dizziness	Lack of consistent evidence on effectiveness in pediatric population

As in all other situations of advanced illness, thorough consideration to of potential benefits and harms should be discussed when considering medication therapy for cachexia. All medication used for this condition possess potential severe adverse effects. Importantly, any plan of care should take into account cultural and religious preferences in such delicate and sensitive situations.

7.11 Neurological Problems

7.11.1 Case Presentation

Sandra is a 16-year-old girl with alveolar soft-part sarcoma (ASPS) of the right thigh. She underwent complete macroscopic resection of her tumor and received 54 Gy of radiation therapy directed at involved field. She had been in complete clinical and radiological remission for 3 years when she began experiencing tingling pain in her left leg. Physical examination revealed increased sensitivity during percussion above L1–2. MRI of lumbar spine showed a lytic lesion located within left part of L1 vertebral body with soft tissue component extending into left intervertebral space and compressing adjacent nerve roots. The diagnosis of impending spinal cord compression was made. Sandra underwent urgent needle biopsy from soft tissue part of tumor, and diagnosis of recurrent metastatic ASPS was established. Immediately after biopsy, she received IV dexamethasone in a dose of 1 mg/kg with subsequent doses 0.2 mg/kg every 6 h. This therapy resulted in significant reduction of her leg pain. Neurological status remained practically normal. Sandra also received radiotherapy in total dose 45 Gy directed at the involved field. No other metastatic foci were detected, and Sandra and her parents decided to not pursue any kind of further therapy at this stage of her disease. Six months later, she began experiencing headaches, frequent episodes of morning vomiting, and nausea. Her gait gradually became unsteady. On physical examination, bilateral papilledema was noted. MRI of brain revealed a space-occupying lesion in posterior fossa with evidence for secondary obstructive hydrocephalus. Sandra received therapy with IV mannitol 20% in a dose of 0.3 g/kg four times a day with IV dexamethasone in the same manner as she received at the time of her SCC. She underwent VP shunt insertion as a first step and surgical removal of ASPS metastasis. Approximately 2 months later, Sandra was brought to ER unconscious with status epilepticus. She was treated with continuous IV drip of midazolam and underwent urgent brain MRI that showed multiple foci of brain metastases. At that stage of disease, clinicians and parents decided together not to pursue further interventions. Sandra was continued on midazolam IV with ever-increasing doses to keep her seizures under control, and she died soon after without regaining her consciousness.

Involvement of central nervous system in pediatric cancer patients is quite a common phenomenon and may occur as a result of many causes. The most common cause of CNS disease in children is a cancer itself. Both benign and malignant tumors of CNS may lead to severe disability and, ultimately, death. Death of children with CNS tumors usually ensues as result of local effects of tumors. Such malignant tumors of CNS as medulloblastoma, supratentorial PNET, and ATRT have a propensity for dissemination, usually within CNS itself and, at times, especially for medulloblastoma, outside the CNS. For some brain tumors such as diffuse intrinsic pontine glioma (DIPG), combining radiation therapy with an intensive focus on quality of life is the best approach (Veldhuijzen van Zanten et al. 2016). Management of children with DIPG is challenging. Involvement of such critical part of brainstem as pons may cause multiple neurological deficits, including swallowing problems with resultant aspiration leading to recurrent pulmonary infections and development of increased airway reactivity. Radiation therapy has been proven to prolong survival for several months in such patients, but as disease progresses further, new neurologic symptoms and signs may appear. If the tumor grows in caudal direction, hemiparesis may develop. In relatively rare cases of upward progression of DIPG, obstructive hydrocephalus may develop, which may lead to increased intracranial pressure. In such situations, the child with DIPG may demonstrate not only focal neurological deficits but present with headache, nausea, and vomiting. Since the majority of DIPG are high-grade gliomas, some patient may also develop leptomeningeal spread (Postovsky et al. 2008; Sethi et al. 2011). In addition to suffering caused by disease itself, children with DIPG and other tumors of CNS develop physical distress as a result of antitumor therapy. Multifaceted and sometimes debilitating morbidity may develop as a result of neurosurgeries, radiation treatment, and drug therapy. For example, prolonged use of steroid therapy in children with DIPG and other high-grade gliomas inevitably results in the development of many of its side effects which contribute to significant physical distress of the child.

Symptoms and signs that are encountered in advanced CNS tumors often profoundly interfere with quality of life and have a tendency for worsening over the course of the disease. In such situation, symptom management may become extremely complex and demanding. Involvement of many specialists (neurologist, physiotherapist, and others) may facilitate better providing intensive symptom management to these patients. Unfortunately, there are no well-developed protocols describing the management of a child with CNS tumors at end of life, and care is often provided on a case-based level. Development of such specialized protocols may improve care in this very difficult to manage group of patients (Vallero et al. 2014). Notwithstanding these problems, even in this group of patients, successful home-based care is possible (Kuhlen et al. 2016). When suffering of a child with a CNS malignant tumor at end of life becomes unbearable and nonresponsive to all other therapeutic approaches, palliative sedation may be indicated (Postovsky et al. 2007).

During past several decades, we have witnessed an increase in incidence of metastatic spread to CNS of various solid tumors in children. This increased occurrence of CNS involvement may be explained by at least two factors: first, children with cancer, even if considered incurable and will ultimately die from their cancer, generally live longer owing to modern methods of treatment allowing treating physicians to prolong the lives of such patients. That, in turn, provides enough time for distant metastases to develop in previously rarely seen locations such as the brain and spinal cord. Second, widespread use of MRI which has become a routine method of evaluation of practically any pediatric cancer patient with symptoms and signs suggestive of CNS involvement allows detection of CNS disease with relative ease and confidence (Sethi et al. 2011).

Various solid tumors have been reported as a source for metastatic spread to CNS in childhood cancer, among them various types of sarcomas and Wilms tumor being the most common (Postovsky et al. 2003; Kebudi et al. 2005; Paulino et al. 2003; Suki et al. 2014). Many patients with advanced hematological malignancies, especially with acute lymphoblastic leukemia, develop leptomeningeal disease toward the end of life (Morris et al. 2003).

Many interventions used in pediatric oncology and other treatment modalities such as radiotherapy and previous neurosurgeries may themselves affect CNS functions and cause physical distress. Such antitumor drugs as vincristine, ifosfamide, and high-dose methotrexate (HD-MTX) may cause seizures. Today, when many children with advanced cancer continue chemotherapy, these side effects may occur and should be considered in differential diagnosis of pediatric oncologic patient with new onset of seizures. Such seizures tend to be generalized in contrast to focal seizures, which occur more frequently in patients with primary brain tumors or with metastatic spread secondary to solid tumors outside of CNS (Wusthoff et al. 2007). Management of seizures in children with advanced cancer does not principally differ from such in other groups of children.

Along with CNS involvement, chemotherapy and other drugs may affect peripheral nervous system such as vincristine-induced peripheral neuropathy. This neuropathy has been described in patients receiving ifosfamide and cisplatin as well (Boyette-Davis et al. 2015). Although taxanes are not frequently used in practice of pediatric oncology, they may also cause peripheral neuropathy (Hurwitz et al. 1993).

Symptoms of peripheral neuropathy may be masked by other factors which may hamper the timely recognition of this potentially reversible complication of chemotherapy. The children at end of life are frequently debilitated and bedridden. They frequently receive steroids for prolong periods of time which may lead to myopathy, thus exacerbating signs of neuropathy and delaying its correct diagnosis.

Electrolyte imbalance such as hypokalemia, hypocalcemia, and hypomagnesemia often occurs in children with advanced cancer and may further lead to muscular weakness.

One of the most important and debilitating complications of advanced cancer is development of spinal cord compression (SCC) (Pollono et al. 2003). This complication unrecognized and left untreated causes permanent neurological damage and results in profound physical and psychological disability. In contrast to the time of initial diagnosis when the main cause of SCC is typically the primary tumor (Ewing sarcoma, neuroblastoma, non-Hodgkin's lymphoma, Langerhans cell histiocytosis), the most common cause of SCC in children with advanced cancer is metastatic spread. Any part of the spinal cord may be affected, with lumbar spine being the most common. Cauda equine syndrome is a clinical equivalent of SCC when there is compression below the level of spinal cord (Duong et al. 2012; Fraser et al. 2009).

Clinicians should be alert to the possibility of development of SCC in any child with advanced cancer who presents with back and/or leg pain with or without concurrent symptoms of urine retention or new onset of constipation. Any child with a suspicion of SCC should be immediately examined and should undergo pertinent imaging studies (CT and/or MRI). The opportunity for successful treatment of SCC and for preservation of patient's ambulation is reversely related to the duration of time from development of first symptoms to the start of treatment. The longer the period of immobility before starting of treatment, the less the chances are for regaining his motor function.

The treatment of SCC is complex combining use of drugs and radiotherapy and/or surgery. Dexamethasone is the drug of choice directed at the lessening of peritumoral edema. The dose is usually high (a dose of 1 to 2 mg/kg, followed by 0.25 mg/kg every 6 h, and doses as high as 100 mg have been used in adults.). Since most patients have well-advanced malignancy resulting in this oncological emergency, surgery is uncommonly performed. Child's debility and relatively short life expectancy in majority of cases make neurosurgery not indicated. Radiotherapy administered without delay may be more feasible, less traumatic, and more available for such patients. There are no studies regarding efficacy of various radiotherapy schedules and doses in pediatric oncology; thus for SCC, radiation is usually administered based on data derived from studies in adult oncology practice (Prewett and Venkitaraman 2010; Wu et al. 2003). Since the accepted maximal dose for spinal cord is about 45 Gray, radiotherapy is given usually up to this limit. It is a common practice to give in such situation 30 Gray divided into 10 daily fractions 3 Gray each.

Conclusion

Alleviating physical distress caused by advanced cancer may be both benefiting for an ill child and rewarding for treating clinician. Meticulous attention to physical symptoms and signs allows their timely recognition and proper management. Applying principles of palliative care from the beginning of treatment of the child with cancer increases chances for successful management of physical distress during the entire course of disease, especially when cancer is less responsive to therapy, and during the end stage of a child's life.

Importantly non-pharmacologic techniques, such as play therapy, clown therapy, music therapy, pet therapy, hypnosis, aromatherapy, and many others, may be successfully incorporated into care of the child with advanced cancer. These non-pharmacologic therapies, when correctly applied, may lead to increase of efficacy of pharmacologic therapies and decrease in need of doses of opioids and other medications, thus potentially resulting in more effective and less toxic therapy in the context of palliative care. Although many have not been evaluated in randomized clinical studies, such non-pharmacologic approaches may have beneficial effects on anxiety, pain, mood, and quality of life in children with advanced cancer.

Proper management of physical distress allows the sick child and her family to maintain reasonable quality of life to the fullest extent possible, thus decreasing global suffering in a given situation. Pediatric oncologists and other involved medical providers should be duly educated in managing physical distress in children with advanced cancer and should see its alleviation as a professional duty in their everyday activity.

References

Wolfe J, Grier HE, Klar N, Levin SB, Ellenbogen JM, Salem-Schatz S, Emanuel EJ, Weeks JC (2000) Symptoms and suffering at the end of life in children with cancer. N Engl J Med 342:326–333

Pritchard M, Burghen E, Srivastava DK, Okuma J, Anderson L, Powell B, Furman WL, Hinds PS (2008) Cancer-related symptoms most concerning to parents during the last week and last day of their child's life. Pediatrics 121:e1301–e1309

Heath JA, Clarke NE, Donath SM, McCarthy M, Anderson VA, Wolfe J (2010) Symptoms and suffering at the end of life in children with cancer: an Australian perspective. Med J Aust 192:71–75

Theunissen JM, Hoogerbrugge PM, van Achterberg T, Prins JB, Vernooij-Dassen MJ, van den Ende CH (2007) Symptoms in the palliative phase of children with cancer. Pediatr Blood Cancer 49:160–165

Kreicbergs U, Valdimarsdóttir U, Onelöv E, Björk O, Steineck G, Henter JI (2005) Care-related distress: a nationwide study of parents who lost their child to cancer. J Clin Oncol 23:9162–9171

von Lützau P, Otto M, Hechler T, Metzing S, Wolfe J, Zernikow B (2012) Children dying from cancer: parents' perspectives on symptoms, quality of life, characteristics of death, and end-of-life decisions. J Palliat Care 28:274–281

Jalmsell L, Kreicbergs U, Onelöv E, Steineck G, Henter JI (2006) Symptoms affecting children with malignancies during the last month of life: a nationwide follow-up. Pediatrics 117:1314–1320

Mack JW, Hilden JM, Watterson J, Moore C, Turner B, Grier HE, Weeks JC, Wolfe J (2005) Parent and physician perspectives on quality of care at the end of life in children with cancer. J Clin Oncol 23:9155–9161

Wolfe J, Hammel JF, Edwards KE, Duncan J, Comeau M, Breyer J, Aldridge SA, Grier HE, Berde C, Dussel V, Weeks JC (2008) Easing of suffering in children with cancer at the end of life: is care changing? J Clin Oncol 26:1717–1723

Postovsky S, Ben Arush MW (2004) Care of a child dying of cancer: the role of the palliative care team in pediatric oncology. Pediatr Hematol Oncol 21:67–76
Schmidt P, Otto M, Hechler T, Metzing S, Wolfe J, Zernikow B (2013) Did increased availability of pediatric palliative care lead to improved palliative care outcomes in children with cancer? J Palliat Med 16:1034–1039
Cassel EJ (1982) The nature of suffering and the goals of medicine. N Engl J Med 306:639–645
Collins JJ, Byrnes ME, Dunkel IJ, Lapin J, Nadel T, Thaler HT, Polyak T, Rapkin B, Portenoy RK (2000) The measurement of symptoms in children with cancer. J Pain Symptom Manag 19:363–377
Wolfe J, Orellana L, Ullrich C, Cook EF, Kang TI, Rosenberg A, Geyer R, Feudtner C, Dussel V (2015) Symptoms and distress in children with advanced cancer: prospective patient-reported outcomes from the PediQUEST study. J Clin Oncol 33:1928–1935
Zhukovsky DS, Rozmus CL, Robert RS, Bruera E, Wells RJ, Chisholm GB, Allo JA, Cohen MZ (2015) Symptom profiles in children with advanced cancer: patient, family caregiver, and oncologist ratings. Cancer 121:4080–4087
Bower JE, Bak K, Berger A, Breitbart W, Escalante CP, Ganz PA, Schnipper HH, Lacchetti C, Ligibel JA, Lyman GH, Ogaily MS, Pirl WF, Jacobsen PB (2014) Screening, assessment, and management of fatigue in adult survivors of cancer: an American Society of Clinical oncology clinical practice guideline adaptation. J Clin Oncol 32:1840–1850
Ryan JL, Carroll JK, Ryan EP, Mustian KM, Fiscella K, Morrow GR (2007) Mechanisms of cancer-related fatigue. Oncologist 12(Suppl 1):22–34
Ullrich CK, Mayer OH (2007) Assessment and management of fatigue and dyspnea in pediatric palliative care. Pediatr Clin N Am 54:735–756
Ullrich CK, Dussel V, Hilden JM, Sheaffer JW, Moore CL, Berde CB, Wolfe J (2010) Fatigue in children with cancer at the end of life. J Pain Symptom Manag 40:483–494
Hockenberry MJ, Hooke MC, Gregurich M, McCarthy K (2009) Carnitine plasma levels and fatigue in children/adolescents receiving cisplatin, ifosfamide, or doxorubicin. J Pediatr Hematol Oncol 31:664–669
Graziano F, Bisonni R, Catalano V, Silva R, Rovidati S, Mencarini E, Ferraro B, Canestrari F, Baldelli AM, De Gaetano A, Giordani P, Testa E, Lai V (2002) Potential role of levocarnitine supplementation for the treatment of chemotherapy-induced fatigue in non-anaemic cancer patients. Br J Cancer 86:1854–1857
Cruciani RA, Zhang JJ, Manola J, Cella D, Ansari B, Fisch MJ (2012) L-carnitine supplementation for the management of fatigue in patients with cancer: an eastern cooperative oncology group phase III, randomized, double-blind, placebo-controlled trial. J Clin Oncol 30:3864–3869
Hooke MC, McCarthy K, Taylor O, Hockenberry MJ (2015) Fatigue and carnitine levels over multiple cycles of chemotherapy in children and adolescents. Eur J Oncol Nurs 19:7–12
Brown RL (2011) Tyrosine kinase inhibitor-induced hypothyroidism: incidence, etiology, and management. Target Oncol 6:217–226
Torino F, Corsello SM, Longo R, Barnabei A, Gasparini G (2009) Hypothyroidism related to tyrosine kinase inhibitors: an emerging toxic effect of targeted therapy. Nat Rev Clin Oncol 6:219–228
Olson K (2014) Sleep-related disturbances among adolescents with cancer: a systematic review. Sleep Med 15:496–501
Crabtree VM, Rach AM, Schellinger KB, Russell KM, Hammarback T, Mandrell BN (2015) Changes in sleep and fatigue in newly treated pediatric oncology patients. Support care cancer 23:393–401
Orsey AD, Wakefield DB, Cloutier MM (2013) Physical activity (PA) and sleep among children and adolescents with cancer. Pediatr Blood Cancer 60:1908–1913
Braam KI, van der Torre P, Takken T, Veening MA, van Dulmen-den Broeder E, Kaspers GJ (2013) Physical exercise training interventions for children and young adults during and after treatment for childhood cancer. Cochrane Database Syst Rev 4:CD008796
Reineke-Bracke H, Radbruch L, Elsner F (2006) Treatment of fatigue: modafinil, methylphenidate, and goals of care. J Palliat Med 9:1210–1214
Sharp V, Finlay F, Kevitiyagala D (2013) Question 1: is methylphenidate a useful treatment for cancer-related fatigue in children? Arch Dis Child 98:80–82
Hwang SS, Chang VT, Rue M, Kasimis B (2003) Multidimensional independent predictors of cancer-related fatigue. J Pain Symptom Manag 26:604e614
World Health Organization (2012). WHO guidelines on the pharmacological treatment of persisting pain in children with medical illnesses. Geneva: WHO. http://whqlibdoc.who.int/publications/2012/9789241548120_Guidelines.pdf. Accessed 15 Feb 2016
Zernikow B, Smale H, Michel E, Hasan C, Jorch N, Andler W (2006) Paediatric cancer pain management using the WHO analgesic ladder—results of a prospective analysis from 2265 treatment days during a quality improvement study. Eur J Pain 10:587–595
Friedrichsdorf S, Finney D, Bergin M et al (2007) Breakthrough pain in children with cancer. J Pain Symptom Manag 34:209–216
International Association for the Study of Pain (IASP) (n.d.) Taxonomy. http://www.iasp-pain.org/. Accessed 8 Feb 2016
Anghelescu DL, Faughnan LG, Popenhagen MP, Oakes LL, Pei D, Burgoyne LL (2014) Neuropathic pain referrals to a multidisciplinary pediatric cancer pain service. Pain Manag Nurs 15:126–131
Voepel-Lewis T, Merkel S, Tait AR et al (2002) The reliability and validity of the face, legs, activity, cry, consolability observational tool as a measure of pain in children with cognitive impairment. Anesth Analg 95:1224–12298
Visual Analog Scale (VAS) (n.d.) http://www.partners-againstpain.com/printout/A7012AS1.pdf. Accessed 12 Feb 2016

von Baeyer CL, Spagrud LJ, McCormick JC, Choo E (2009) Three new datasets supporting use of the Numerical Rating Scale (NRS-11) for children's self-reports of pain intensity. Pain 143:223–227
Face Pain Scale - Revised (n.d.) URL http://www.iasp-pain.org/fpsr. Accessed 24 Jan 2016
Hicks CL, von Baeyer CL, Spafford PA et al (2001) The Faces Pain Scale—Revised: toward a common metric in pediatric pain measurement. Pain 93:173–183
The Oucher Photographic Scale (n.d.) www.oucher.org . Accessed 10 Feb 2016
Beyer JE, Denyes MJ, Villarreal AM (1992) The creation, validation, and continuing development of the Oucher: a measure of pain intensity in children. J Pediatr Nurs 7:335–346
Marec-Berard P, Gomez F, Combet S, Thibault P, Bergeron PLMC (2015) HEDEN Pain Scale: a shortened behavioral scale for assessment of prolonged cancer or postsurgical pain in children aged 2 to 6 years. Pediatr Hematol Oncol 32(5):291–303
de Martino M, Chiarugi A (2015) Recent advances in pediatric use of oral paracetamol in fever and pain management. Pain Ther 4:149–168
Ceelie I, de Wildt SN, van Dijk M, van den Berg MM, van den Bosch GE, Duivenvoorden HJ, de Leeuw TG, Mathôt R, Knibbe CA, Tibboel D (2013) Effect of intravenous paracetamol on postoperative morphine requirements in neonates and infants undergoing major noncardiac surgery: a randomized controlled trial. JAMA 309:149–154
Heard K, Bui A, Mlynarchek SL, Green JL, Bond JR, Clark RF, Kozer E, Koff RS, Dart RC (2014) Toxicity from repeated doses of acetaminophen in children: assessment of causality and dose in reported cases. Am J Ther 21:174–183
Koling S, Hempel G, Lanvers C, Boos J, Würthwein G (2007) Monitoring paracetamol metabolism after single and repeated administration in pediatric patients with neoplastic diseases. Int J Clin Pharmacol Ther 45:496–503
Wong I, St John-Green C, Walker SM (2013) Opioid-sparing effects of perioperative paracetamol and nonsteroidal anti-inflammatory drugs (NSAIDs) in children. Paediatr Anaesth 23:475–495
Leese PT, Hubbard RC, Karim A, Isakson PC, Yu SS, Geis GS (2000) Effects of celecoxib, a novel cyclooxygenase-2 inhibitor, on platelet function in healthy adults: a randomized, controlled trial. J Clin Pharmacol 40(2):124–132
Schnabel A, Reichl SU, Meyer-Frießem C, Zahn PK, Pogatzki-Zahn E (2015) Tramadol for postoperative pain treatment in children. Cochrane Database Syst Rev (3):CD009574
Zernikow B, Michel E, Craig F, Anderson BJ (2009) Pediatric palliative care: use of opioids for the management of pain. Paediatr Drugs 11:129–151
Siden H, Naiewajek V (2003) high dose opioids in pediatric palliative care. J Pain Symptom Manag 25:397–399
Rasmussen VF, Lundberg V, Jespersen TW, Hasle H (2015) Extreme doses of intravenous methadone for severe pain in two children with cancer. Pediatr Blood Cancer 62:1087–1090
Nielsen LM, Olesen AE, Branford R, Chrirstrup LL, Sato H, Drewes AM (2015) Association between human pain-related genotypes and variability in opioid analgesia: an updated review. Pain Pract 15:580–594. See comment in PubMed Commons below
Morlion B, Clemens KE, Dunlop W (2015) Quality of life and healthcare resource in patients receiving opioids for chronic pain: a review of the place of oxycodone/naloxone. Clin Drug Investig 35:1–11
Kestenbaum MG, Vilches AO, Messersmith S, Connor SR, Fine PG, Murphy B, Davis M, Muir JC (2014) Alternative routes to oral opioid administration in palliative care: a review and clinical summary. Pain Med 15:1129–1153
Drake R, Longworth J, Collins JJ (2004) Opioid rotation in children with cancer. J Palliat Med 7:419–422
Kim HJ, Kim YS, Park SH (2015) Opioid rotation versus combination for cancer patients with chronic uncontrolled pain: a randomized study. BMC Palliat Care 14:41
Smith HS, Peppin JF (2014) Toward a systematic approach to opioid rotation. J Pain Res 7:589–608
Anghelescu DL, Faughnan LG, Oakes LL, Windsor KB, Pei D, Burgoyne LL (2012) Parent-controlled PCA for pain management in pediatric oncology: is it safe? J Pediatr Hematol Oncol 34:416–420
Howard RF, Lloyd-Thomas A, Thomas M, Williams DG, Saul R, Bruce E, Peters J (2010) Nurse-controlled analgesia (NCA) following major surgery in 10,000 patients in a children's hospital. Paediatr Anaesth 20:126–134
Anghelescu DL, Snaman JM, Trujillo L, Sykes AD, Yuan Y, Baker JN (2015) Patient-controlled analgesia at the end of life at a pediatric oncology institution. Pediatr Blood Cancer 62:1237–1244
Zernikow B, Michel E, Anderson B (2007) Transdermal fentanyl in childhood and adolescence: a comprehensive literature review. J Pain 8:187–207
James PJ, Howard RF, Williams DG (2010) The addition of ketamine to a morphine nurse- or patient-controlled analgesia infusion (PCA/NCA) increases analgesic efficacy in children with mucositis pain. Paediatr Anaesth 20:805–811
Anghelescu DL (2011) Methadone use in children and young adults at a cancer center: a retrospective study. J Opioid Manag 7:353–361
Friedrichsdorf S, Nugent A (2013) Management of neuropathic pain in children with cancer. Curr Opin Support Palliat Care 7:131–138
Haywood A, Good P, Khan S, Leupp A, Jenkins-Marsh S, Rickett K, Hardy JR (2015) Corticosteroids for the management of cancer-related pain in adults. Cochrane Database Syst Rev 4:CD010756
Korzeniewska-Eksterowicz A, Przysło Ł, Fendler W, Stolarska M, Młynarski W (2014) Palliative sedation at home for terminally ill children with cancer. J Pain Symptom Manag 48:968–974
Anghelescu DL, Faughnan LG, Baker JN, Yang J, Kane JR (2010) Use of epidural and peripheral nerve blocks

at the end of life in children and young adults with cancer: the collaboration between a pain service and a palliative care service. Paediatr Anaesth 20:1070–1077
Walker BJ, Long JB, De Oliveira GS et al (2015) Peripheral nerve catheters in children: an analysis of safety and practice patterns from the pediatric regional anesthesia network (PRAN). Br J Anaesth 115:457–462
Cooper MG, Keneally JP, Kinchington D (1994) Continuous brachial plexus neural blockade in a child with intractable cancer pain. J Pain Symptom Manag 9:277–281
Pacenta HL, Kaddoum RN, Pereiras LA, Chidiac EJ, Burgoyne LL (2010) Continuous tunneled femoral nerve block for palliative care of a patient with metastatic osteosarcoma. Anaesth Intensive Care 38:563–565
Fu J, Ngo A, Shin K, Bruera E (2013) Botulinum toxin injection and phenol nerve block for reduction of end-of-life pain. J Palliat Med 16:1637–1640
Chambers WA (2008) Nerve blocks in palliative care. Br J Anaesth 101:95–100
Sakamoto B, Kuber S, Gwirtz K, Elsahy A, Stennis M (2012) Neurolytic transversus abdominis plane block in the palliative treatment of intractable abdominal wall pain. J Clin Anesth 24:58–61
Hung JC, Azam N, Puttanniah V, Malhotra V, Gulati A (2014) Neurolytic transversus abdominal plane block with alcohol for long-term malignancy related pain control. Pain Physician 17:E755–E760
Gulati A, Shah R, Puttanniah V, Hung JC, Malhotra V (2015) A retrospective review and treatment paradigm of interventional therapies for patients suffering from intractable thoracic chest wall pain in the oncologic population. Pain Med 16:802–810
Sepsas E, Misthos P, Anagnostopulu M, Toparlaki O, Voyagis G, Kakaris S (2013) The role of intercostal cryoanalgesia in post-thoracotomy analgesia. Interact Cardiovasc Thorac Surg 16:814–818
Mercadante S, Nicosia F (1998) Celiac plexus block: a reappraisal. Reg Anesth Pain Med 23:37–48
Galloway K, Staats PS, Bowers DC (2000) Intrathecal analgesia for children with cancer via implanted infusion pumps. Med Pediatr Oncol 34:265–267
Aram L, Krane EJ, Kozloski LJ, Yaster M (2001) Tunneled epidural catheters for prolonged analgesia in pediatric patients. Anesth Analg 92:1432–1438
De Pinto M, Naidu RK (2015) Peripheral and neuraxial chemical neurolysis for the management of intractable lower extremity pain in a patient with terminal cancer. Pain Physician 18:E651–E656
Shimazaki M, Egawa H, Motojima F et al (2003) Intrathecal phenol block in a child with cancer pain–a case report. Masui 52:756–758
van der Geest IM, Darlington AS, Streng IC, Michiels EM, Pieters R, van den Heuvel-Eibrink MM (2014) Parents' experiences of pediatric palliative care and the impact on long-term parental grief. J Pain Symptom Manag 47:1043–1053
Liben S, Langner R, Bluebond-Langner M (2014) Pediatric palliative care in 2014: much accomplished, much yet to be done. J Palliat Care 30:311–316
Pianosi P, Smith CP, Almudevar A, McGrath PJ (2006) Dalhousie dyspnea scales: pictorial scales to measure dyspnea during induced bronchoconstriction. Pediatr Pulmonol 41:1182–1187
Craig F, Henderson EM, Bluebond-Langner M (2015) Management of respiratory symptoms in paediatric palliative care. Curr Opin Support Palliat Care 9:217–226
Heyse-Moore LH, Ross V, Mullee MA (1991) How much of a problem is dyspnoea in advanced cancer? Palliat Med 5:20–26
Drake R, Frost J, Collins JJ (2003) The symptoms of dying children. J Pain Symptom Manag 26:594–603
Blume ED, Balkin EM, Aiyagari R, Ziniel S, Beke DM, Thiagarajan R, Taylor L, Kulik T, Pituch K, Wolfe J (2014) Parental perspectives on suffering and quality of life at end-of-life in children with advanced heart disease: an exploratory study. Pediatr Crit Care Med 15:336–342
Ban Banzett RB, Mulnier HE, Murphy K, Rosen SD, Wise RJ, Adams L (2000) Breathlessness in humans activates insular cortex. Neuroreport 11:2117–2120
Booth S, Kelly M, Cox N, Adams L, Guz A (1996) Does oxygen help dyspnoea in patients with cancer. Am J Respir Crit Care Med 153:1515–1518
Evans KC, Banzett RB, Adams L, McKay L, Frackowiak RS, Corfield DR (2002) BOLD fMRI densifies limbic, paralimbic, and cerebellar activation during air hunger. J Neurophysiol 88:1500–1511
Frost JJ, Wagner HN Jr, Dannals RF, Ravert HT, Links JM, Wilson AA et al (1985) Imaging opiate receptors in the human brain by positron tomography. J Comput Assist Tomogr 9:231–236
Gaytan SP, Pasaron R (1998) Connections of the rostral ventral respiratory neuronal cell group: an anterograde and retrograde tracing study in the rat. Brain Res Bull 47:625–642
Clemens KE, Klaschik E (2011) Dyspnoea associated with anxiety—symptomatic therapy with opioids in combination with lorazepam and its effect on ventilation in palliative care patients. Support Care Cancer 19:2027–2033
Thomas JR, von Gunten C (2002) Clinical management of dyspnoea. Lancet Oncol 3:223–228
Escalante CP, Martin CG, Eiting LS, Cantor SB, Harle TS, Price KJ et al (1996) Dyspnea in cancer patients. Etiology, resource utilization, and survival—implications in a managed care world. Cancer 78:1314–1319
Philip J, Gold M, Milner A, Di Iulio J, Miller B, Spuryt O (2006) A randomized, double blind, crossover-trial of the effect of oxygen on dyspnoea in patients with advanced cancer. J Pain Symptom Manag 32:541–550
Bruera E, de Stoutz N, Velasco-Leiva A, Schoeller T, Hanson J (1993) Effect of oxygen on dyspnoea in hypoxaemic terminal cancer patients. Lancet 342:13–14
Bruera E, Scholler T, MacEachern T (1992) Symptomatic benefit of supplemental oxygen in hypoxemic patients with terminal cancer: the use of the N of 1 randomised controlled trial. J Pain Symptom Manag 7:365–368

Clemens KE, Quednau I, Klaschik E (2009) Use of oxygen and opioids in the palliation of dyspnoea in hypoxic and non-hypoxic palliative care patients: a prospective study. Support Care Cancer 17:367–377

Abernethy AP, McDonald CF, Frith PA, Clark K, Herndon JE 2nd, Marcello J et al (2010) Effect of palliative oxygen versus room air in relief of breathlessness in patients with refractory dyspnoea: a double-blind, randomised controlled trial. Lancet 376:784–793

Spathis A, Wade R, Booth S (2006) Oxygen in the palliation of breathlessness. In: Booth S, Dudgeon D (eds) Dyspnoea in advanced disease. Oxford University Press, Oxford, pp 205–236

Banzett RB, Adams L, O'Donnell CR, Gilman SA, Lansing RW, Schwartzstein RM. Using laboratory models to test treatment: morphine reduces dyspnea and hypercapnic ventilatory response. Am J Respir Crit Care Med 2011; 184: 920–927

Al J, Davies AN, Higgins JP, Gibbs JS, Broadley KE (2002) A systematic review of the use of opioids in the management of dyspnoea. Thorax 57:939–944

Clemens KE, Klaschik E (2007) Symptomatic therapy of dyspnoea with strong opioids and its effect on ventilation in palliative care patients. J Pain Symptom Manag 33:473–481

Clemens KE, Klaschik E (2008) Effect of hydromorphone on ventilation in palliative care patients with dyspnea. Support Care Cancer 16:93–99

Pauwels RA, Buist AS, Calverley PMA, Jenkins CR, Hurd SS (2001) Global strategy for the diagnosis, management, and prevention of chronic obstructive pulmonary disease: National Heart, Lung, and Blood Institute and World Health Organization Global Initiative For Chronic Obstructive Lung Disease (GOLD): executive summary. Respir Care 46:798–825

Barbour SJ, Vandebeek CA, Ansermino JM (2004) Increased tidal volume variability in children is a better marker of opioid-induced respiratory depression than decreased respiratory rate. J Clin Monit Comput 18:171–178

Thorns A, Sykes N (2000) Opioid use in last week of life and implications for end-of-life decision making. Lancet 3556:398–399

Clemens KE, Quednau I, Klaschik E (2008) Is there higher risk of respiratory depression in opioid naïve palliative care patients during symptomatic therapy of dyspnoea with strong opioids? J Palliat Med 11:204–216

Currow DC, McDonald C, Oaten S, Kenny B, Allcroft P, Frith P et al (2011) Once-daily opioids for chronic dyspnea: a dose increment and pharmacovigilance study. J Pain Symptom Manag 42:388–399

Zebraski SE, Kochenash SM, Raffa RB (2000) Lung opioid receptors: pharmacology and possible target for nebulized morphine in dyspnea. Life Sci 66:2221–2231

Charles MA, Reymond L, Israel F (2008) Relief of incident dyspnea in palliative cancer patients: a pilot, randomized, controlled trial comparing nebulized hydromorphone, systemic hydromorphone, and nebulized saline. J Pain Symptom Manag 36:29–38

Ben-Aharon I, Gafter-Gvili A, Paul M, Leibovici L, Stemmer SM (2008) Interventions for alleviating cancer-related dyspnea: a systematic review. J Clin Oncol 26:2396–2404

Penson RT, Joel SP, Roberts M, Gloyne A, Beckwith S, Slevin ML (2002) The bioavailability and pharmacokinetics of subcutaneous, nebulized and oral morphine-6-glucuronide. Br J Clin Pharmacol 53:347–354

Mitchell-Heggs P, Murphy K, Minty K, Guz A, Patterson SC, Minty PS, Rosser RM (1980) Diazepam in the treatment of dyspnea in the pink puffer syndrome. QJM 193:9–20

Stark RD, Gambles SA, Lewis JA (1981) Methods to assess breathlessness in healthy subjects: a critical evaluation and application to analyse the acute effects of diazepam and promethazine on breathlessness induced by exercise or by exposure to raised levels of carbon dioxide. Clin Sci 61:429–439

Woodcock AA, Gross ER, Geddes DM (1981) Drug treatment of breathlessness; contrasting effects of diazepam and promethazine in pink puffers. BMJ 283:343–346

Man GC, Hsu K, Sproule BJ (1986) Effect of alprazolam on exercise and dyspnea in patients with chronic obstructive pulmonary disease. Chest 90:832–836

Gililand HE, Prasad BK, Mirakhur RK, Fee J (1996) An investigation of the potential morphine-sparing effect of midazolam. Anesthesia 51:808–811

Navigante A, Cerchietti L, Cabalr M (2003) Morphine plus midazolam versus oxygen therapy in severe dyspnea management in the last week of life of patients with advanced cancer. Med Palliat 10:14–19

Dysart K, Miller TL, Wolfson MR, Shaffer TH (2009) Research in high flow therapy: mechanisms of action. Respir Med 103:1400–1405

Nava S, Ferrer M, Esquinas A, Scala R, Groff P, Cosentini R et al (2013) Palliative use of non-invasive ventilation in end-of-life patients with solid tumours: a randomised feasibility trial. Lancet Oncol 14:219–227

Hui D, Morgado M, Chisholm G, Withers L, Nguyen Q, Finch C, Frisbee-Hume S, Bruera E (2013) High-flow oxygen and bilevel positive airway pressure for persistent dyspnea in patients with advanced cancer: a phase II randomized trial. J Pain Symptom Manag 46:463–473

Gay PC (2009) Complications of noninvasive ventilation in acute care. Respir Care 54:246–257

Hoffer FA, Hancock ML, Hinds PS, Oigbokie N, Rai SN, Rao B (2007) Pleurodesis for effusions in pediatric oncology patients at end of life. Pediatr Radiol 37:269–273

MacRedmond R, O'Connell F (1999) Treatment of persistent dry cough: if possible, treat the cause; if not, treat the cough. Monaldi Arch Chest Dis 3:269–274

Morice AH, Menon MS, Mulrennan SA et al (2007) Opiate therapy in chronic cough. Am J Respir Crit Care Med 175:312–315

Wee B, Browning J, Adams A et al (2012) Management of chronic cough in patients receiving palliative care: review of evidence and recommendations by a task group of the Association for Palliative Medicine of Great Britain and Ireland. Palliat Med 26:780–787

Yancy WS, McCrory DC, Coeytaux RR et al (2013) Efficacy and tolerability of treatments for chronic cough: a systematic review and meta-analysis. Chest J 144:1827–1838

Molassiotis A, Bailey C, Caress A et al (2010) Interventions for cough in cancer. Cochrane Database Syst Rev (9):CD007881

Smith SM, Schroeder K, Fahey T (2014) Over-the-counter (OTC) medications for acute cough in children and adults in community settings. Cochrane Database Syst Rev (11):CD001831

Moroni M, Porta C, Gualtieri G et al (1996) Inhaled sodium cromoglycate to treat cough in advanced lung cancer patients. Br J Cancer 74:309–311

Choudry NB, Fuller RW, Anderson N et al (1990) Separation of cough and reflex bronchoconstriction by inhaled local anaesthetics. Eur Respir J 3:579–583

Ryan NM (2015) A review on the efficacy and safety of gabapentin in the treatment of chronic cough. Expert Opin Pharmacother 16:135–145

Gibson PG, Vertigan AE (2015) Management of chronic refractory cough. BMJ 351:h5590

Gibson P, Wang G, McGarvey L et al (2016) Treatment of unexplained chronic cough: CHEST guideline and expert panel report. Chest 149(1):27–44

Nannini LJ, Poole P, Milan SJ, Kesterton A (2013) Combined corticosteroid and longacting beta2-agonist in one inhaler versus inhaled corticosteroids alone for chronic obstructive pulmonary disease. Cochrane Library (8):CD006826

Kellett F, Robert NM (2011) Nebulised 7% hypertonic saline improves lung function and quality of life in bronchiectasis. Respir Med 105:1831–1850

Chatwin M, Ross E, Hart N et al (2003) Cough augmentation with mechanical insufflation/exsufflation in patients with neuromuscular weakness. Eur Respir J 21:502–508

Chatwin M, Simonds AK (2009) The addition of mechanical insufflation/exsufflation shortens airway-clearance sessions in neuromuscular patients with chest infection. Respir Care 54:1473–1479

Moran FC, Spittle A, Delany C et al (2013) Effect of home mechanical in-exsufflation on hospitalisation and life-style in neuromuscular disease: a pilot study. J Paediatr Child Health 49:233–237

Smith HS, Smith JM, Seidner P (2012) Opioid-induced nausea and vomiting. Ann Palliat Med 1:121–129

Baxter AL, Watcha MF, Baxter WV, Leong T, Wyatt MM (2011) Development and validation of a pictorial nausea rating scale for children. Pediatrics 127:e1542–e1549

Dupuis LL, Taddio A, Kerr EN, Kelly A, MacKeigan L (2006) Development and validation of the pediatric nausea assessment tool for use in children receiving antineoplastic agents. Pharmacotherapy 26:1221–1231

Roila F, Aapro M, Stewart A (1998) Optimal selection of antiemetics in children receiving cancer chemotherapy. Support Care Cancer 6:215–220

Roila F, Feyer P, Maranzano E, Olver I, Clark-Snow R, Warr D, Molassiotis A (2005) Antiemetics in children receiving chemotherapy. Support Care Cancer 13:129–131

Patel P, Robinson PD, Orsey A, Freedman JL, Langevin AM, Woods D, Sung L, Dupuis LL. Chemotherapy-induced nausea and vomiting prophylaxis: practice within the children's oncology group. Pediatr Blood Cancer. 63 (5), 887-892 2016

Jordan K, Roila F, Molassiotis A, Maranzano E, Clark-Snow RA, Feyer P, MASCC/ESMO (2011) Antiemetics in children receiving chemotherapy. MASCC/ESMO guideline update 2009. Support Care Cancer 19(Suppl 1):S37–S42

Kris MG, Tonato M, Bria E, Ballatori E, Espersen B, Herrstedt J, Rittenberg C, Einhorn LH, Grunberg S, Saito M, Morrow G, Hesketh P (2011) Consensus recommendations for the prevention of vomiting and nausea following high-emetic-risk chemotherapy. Support Care Cancer 19(Suppl 1):S25–S32

Vrabel M (2007) Is ondansetron more effective than granisetron for chemotherapy-induced nausea and vomiting? A review of comparative trials. Clin J Oncol Nurs 11:809–813

Bodge M, Shillingburg A, Paul S, Biondo L (2014) Safety and efficacy of aprepitant for chemotherapy-induced nausea and vomiting in pediatric patients: a prospective, observational study. Pediatr Blood Cancer 61:1111–1113

Kang HJ, Loftus S, Taylor A, DiCristina C, Green S, Zwaan CM (2015) Aprepitant for the prevention of chemotherapy-induced nausea and vomiting in children: a randomized, double-blind, phase 3 trial. Lancet Oncol 16:385–394

Currow DC, Quinn S, Agar M, Fazekas B, Hardy J, McCaffrey N, Eckermann S, Abernethy AP, Clark K (2015) Double-blind, placebo-controlled, randomized trial of octreotide in malignant bowel obstruction. J Pain Symptom Manag 49:814–821

Watanabe H, Inoue Y, Uchida K, Okugawa Y, Hiro J, Ojima E, Kobayashi M, Miki C, Kusunoki M (2007) Octreotide improved the quality of life in a child with malignant bowel obstruction caused by peritoneal dissemination of colon cancer. J Pediatr Surg 42:259–260

Davies DE, Wren T, MacLachlan SM (2012) Octreotide infusion for malignant duodenal obstruction in a 12-year-old girl with metastatic peripheral nerve sheath tumor. J Pediatr Hematol Oncol 34:e292–e294

Mercadante S, Porzio G (2012) Octreotide for malignant bowel obstruction: twenty years after. Crit Rev Oncol Hematol 83:388–392

Garcia MK, McQuade J, Haddad R, Patel S, Lee R, Yang P, Palmer JL, Cohen L (2013) Systematic review of acupuncture in cancer care: a synthesis of the evidence. J Clin Oncol 31:952–960

Richardson J, Smith JE, McCall G, Richardson A, Pilkington K, Kirsch I (2007) Hypnosis for nausea and vomiting in cancer chemotherapy: a systematic review of the research evidence. Eur J Cancer Care (Engl) 16:402–412

Santucci G, Mack JW (2007) Common gastrointestinal symptoms in pediatric palliative care: nausea, vomiting, constipation, anorexia, cachexia. Pediatr Clin N Am 54:673–689

Phillips RS, Gibson F (2008) A systematic review of treatments for constipation in children and young adults undergoing cancer treatment. J Pediatr Hematol Oncol 30:829–830

Constipation Guideline Committee of the North American Society for Pediatric Gastroenterology, Hepatology and Nutrition (2006) Evaluation and treatment of constipation in infants and children: recommendations of the North American Society for Pediatric Gastroenterology, Hepatology and Nutrition. J Pediatr Gastroenterol Nutr 43:e1–13

Pashankar FD, Season JH, McNamara J, Pashankar DS (2011) Acute constipation in children receiving chemotherapy for cancer. J Pediatr Hematol Oncol 33:e300–e303

Rowinsky EK, Donehower RC (1991) The clinical pharmacology and use of antimicrotubule agents in cancer chemotherapeutics. Pharmacol Ther 52:5–84

Fontana M, Bianchi C, Cataldo F, Conti Nibali S, Cucchiara S, Gobio Casali L, Iacono G, Sanfilippo M, Torre G (1989) Bowel frequency in healthy children. Acta Paediatr Scand 78:682–684

Fallon M, ONeill B (1997) ABC of palliative care. Constipation and diarrhoea. BMJ 315:1293–1296

Abrahm J (2000) A physician's guide to pain and symptom management in cancer patients. Johns Hopkins University Press, Baltimore, MD

Bradfield SM, Sandler E, Geller T, Tamura RN, Krischer JP (2015) Glutamic acid not beneficial for the prevention of vincristine neurotoxicity in children with cancer. Pediatr Blood Cancer 62:1004–1010

Mokhtar GM, Shaaban SY, Elbarbary NS, Fayed WA (2010) A trial to assess the efficacy of glutamic acid in prevention of vincristine-induced neurotoxicity in pediatric malignancies: a pilot study. J Pediatr Hematol Oncol 32:594–600

Author S (2014) Treatments for constipation: a review of systematic reviews. Rapid response report: summary with critical appraisal. Canadian Agency for Drugs and Technologies in Health, Ottawa (ON)

Gordon M, Naidoo K, Akobeng AK, Thomas AG (2013) Cochrane review: osmotic and stimulant laxatives for the management of childhood constipation (review). Evid Based Child Health 8:57–109

Feudtner C, Freedman J, Kang T, Womer JW, Dai D, Faerber J (2014) Comparative effectiveness of senna to prevent problematic constipation in pediatric oncology patients receiving opioids: a multicenter study of clinically detailed administrative data. J Pain Symptom Manag 48:272–280

Leppert W (2015) Emerging therapies for patients with symptoms of opioid-induced bowel dysfunction. Drug Des Devel Ther 9:2215–2231

Compendium of Pharmaceuticals and Specialities (2011) Methylnaltrexone product monograph. https://wwwe-therapeutics-ca.myaccess.library.utoronto.ca/cps

Rodrigues A, Wong C, Mattiussi A, Alexander S, Lau E, Dupuis LL (2013) Methylnaltrexone for opioid-induced constipation in pediatric oncology patients. Pediatr Blood Cancer 60:1667–1670

Flerlage JE, Baker JN (2015) Methylnaltrexone for opioid-induced constipation in children and adolescents and young adults with progressive incurable cancer at the end of life. J Palliat Med 18:631–633

Burness CB, Keating GM (2014) Oxycodone/naloxone prolonged-release: a review of its use in the management of chronic pain while counteracting opioid-induced constipation. Drugs 74:353–375

Leppert W (2014) Oxycodone/naloxone in the management of patients with pain and opioid-induced bowel dysfunction. Curr Drug Targets 15:124–135

Mercadante S, Casuccio A, Fulfaro F et al (2001) Switching from morphine to methadone to improve analgesia and tolerability in cancer patients: a prospective study. J Clin Oncol 19:2898–2904

Wirz S, Wittmann M, Schenk M et al (2009) Gastrointestinal symptoms under opioid therapy: a prospective comparison of oral sustained-release hydromorphone, transdermal fentanyl, and transdermal buprenorphine. Eur J Pain 13:737–743

Loeffen EA, Brinksma A, Tissing WJ (2015) Clinical implications of malnutrition in children with cancer. Support Care Cancer 23:2523–2524

Sala A, Pencharz P, Barr RD (2004) Children, cancer, and nutrition—a dynamic triangle in review. Cancer 100:677–687

Morley JE, Thomas DR, Wilson MM (2006) Cachexia: pathophysiology and clinical relevance. Am J Clin Nutr 83:735–743

Aoyagi T, Terracina KP, Raza A, Matsubara H, Takabe K (2015) Cancer cachexia, mechanism and treatment. World J Gastrointest Oncol 7:17–29

KCH F (1992) The mechanisms and treatment of weight loss in cancer. Proc Nutr Soc 51:251–265

Tisdale MJ (2009) Mechanisms of cancer cachexia. Physiol Rev 89:381–410

Tisdale MJ (2008) Catabolic mediators of cancer cachexia. Curr Opin Support Palliat Care 2:256–261

Brinksma A, Huizinga G, Sulkers E, Kamps W, Roodbol P, Tissing W (2012) Malnutrition in childhood cancer patients: a review on its prevalence and possible causes. Crit Rev Oncol Hematol 83:249–275

Common Terminology Criteria for Adverse Events (CTCAE) (2009) Version 4.0 (v4.03: June 14, 2010). U.S. Department of Health and Human Services. National Institutes of Health. National Cancer Institute

Tisdale MJ (2006) Clinical anticachexia treatments. Nutr Clin Pract 21:168–174

Veldhuijzen van Zanten SE, van Meerwijk CL, Jansen MH, Twisk JW, Anderson AK, Coombes L, Breen M, Hargrave OJ, Hemsley J, Craig F, Cruz O, Kaspers GJ, van Vuurden DG, Hargrave DR, SIOPE DIPG Network (2016) Palliative and end-of-life care for children with diffuse intrinsic pontine glioma: results from a London cohort study and international survey. Neuro Oncol 18(4):582–588

Postovsky S, Eran A, Weyl Ben Arush M (2008) Unusual case of leptomeningeal dissemination of a diffuse pontine high-grade astrocytoma in a child. Pediatr Neurosurg 44:208–211

Sethi R, Allen J, Donahue B, Karajannis M, Gardner S, Wisoff J, Kunnakkat S, Mathew J, Zagzag D, Newman K, Narayana A (2011) Prospective neuraxis MRI surveillance reveals a high risk of leptomeningeal dissemination in diffuse intrinsic pontine glioma. J Neuro-Oncol 102:121–127

Vallero SG, Lijoi S, Bertin D, Pittana LS, Bellini S, Rossi F, Peretta P, Basso ME, Fagioli F (2014) End-of-life care in pediatric neuro-oncology. Pediatr Blood Cancer 61:2004–2011

Kuhlen M, Hoell J, Balzer S, Borkhardt A, Janssen G (2016) Symptoms and management of pediatric patients with incurable brain tumors in palliative home care. Eur J Paediatr Neurol 20(2):261–269

Postovsky S, Moaed B, Krivoy E, Ofir R, Ben Arush MW (2007) Practice of palliative sedation in children with brain tumors and sarcomas at the end of life. Pediatr Hematol Oncol 24:409–415

Postovsky S, Ash S, Ramu IN, Yaniv Y, Zaizov R, Futerman B, Elhasid R, Ben Barak A, Halil A, Ben Arush MW (2003) Central nervous system involvement in children with sarcoma. Oncology 65:118–124

Kebudi R, Ayan I, Görgün O, Ağaoğlu FY, Vural S, Darendeliler E (2005) Brain metastasis in pediatric extracranial solid tumors: survey and literature review. J Neuro-Oncol 71:43–48

Paulino AC, Nguyen TX, Barker JL Jr (2003) Brain metastasis in children with sarcoma, neuroblastoma, and Wilms' tumor. Int J Radiat Oncol Biol Phys 57:177–183

Suki D, Khoury Abdulla R, Ding M, Khatua S, Sawaya R (2014) Brain metastases in patients diagnosed with a solid primary cancer during childhood: experience from a single referral cancer center. J Neurosurg Pediatr 14:372–385

Morris EC, Harrison G, Bailey CC, Hann IM, Hill FG, Gibson BE, Richards S, Webb DK, Medical Research Council Childhood Leukaemia Working Party (2003) Prognostic factors and outcome for children after second central nervous system relapse of acute lymphoblastic leukaemia. Br J Haematol 120:787–789

Wusthoff CJ, Shellhaas RA, Licht DJ (2007) Management of common neurologic symptoms in pediatric palliative care: seizures, agitation, and spasticity. Pediatr Clin N Am 54:709–733

Boyette-Davis JA, Walters ET, Dougherty PM (2015) Mechanisms involved in the development of chemotherapy-induced neuropathy. Pain Manag 5:285–296

Hurwitz CA, Relling MV, Weitman SD, Ravindranath Y, Vietti TJ, Strother DR, Ragab AH, Pratt CB (1993) Phase I trial of paclitaxel in children with refractory solid tumors: a Pediatric Oncology Group Study. J Clin Oncol 11:2324–2329

Pollono D, Tomarchia S, Drut R, Ibañez O, Ferreyra M, Cédola J (2003) Spinal cord compression: a review of 70 pediatric patients. Pediatr Hematol Oncol 20:457–466

Duong LM, McCarthy BJ, McLendon RE, Dolecek TA, Kruchko C, Douglas LL, Ajani UA (2012) Descriptive epidemiology of malignant and nonmalignant primary spinal cord, spinal meninges, and cauda equina tumors, United States, 2004-2007. Cancer 118:4220–4227

Fraser S, Roberts L, Murphy E (2009) Cauda equina syndrome: a literature review of its definition and clinical presentation. Arch Phys Med Rehabil 90:1964–1968

Prewett S, Venkitaraman R (2010) Metastatic spinal cord compression: review of the evidence for a radiotherapy dose fractionation schedule. Clin Oncol (R Coll Radiol) 22:222–230

Wu JS, Wong R, Johnston M, Bezjak A, Whelan T, Cancer Care Ontario Practice Guidelines Initiative Supportive Care Group (2003) Meta-analysis of dose-fractionation radiotherapy trials for the palliation of painful bone metastases. Int J Radiat Oncol Biol Phys 55:594–605

Easing Psychological Distress in Pediatric Cancer

8

Maru E. Barrera, Adam Rapoport, and Kim S. Daniel

8.1 Introduction

The diagnosis of childhood cancer is a life-threatening and changing major stressor not only for the child but also for the entire family and can cause severe psychological distress and suffering. Although medical advances in childhood cancer treatment have resulted in a survival rate beyond 80% (National Cancer Institute 2015), the cancer experience continues to be highly stressful for most children and their families, particularly during critical times such as at diagnosis and relapse, or for those who have a poor prognosis and reach end of life while receiving treatment. Evidence suggests that while most individuals psychologically affected by childhood cancer go on to recover, approximately 10–30% of survivors or family members will have long-term severe psychological distress (Kazak et al. 2012; Kwak et al. 2013; Long and Marsland 2011; Patenaude and Kupst 2005). Thus, it is at diagnosis when psychosocial support must begin as part of comprehensive cancer care for the child or adolescent and the family to prevent escalating distress and to enhance quality of life (Kwak et al. 2013). Minimizing psychological distress experienced by children with cancer and their families and maximizing their quality of life are also one of the central tenets of pediatric palliative care (Rapoport and Weingarten 2014). The primary aim of this chapter is to describe how we can help youth—children and adolescents—with cancer and their families reduce their psychological distress and improve their coping and quality of life.

To that aim, in this chapter, we have integrated several concepts. These include principles of palliative care, child-family-centered care, a preventive model of psychosocial assessment and intervention, and developmental principles applied to supportive psychological interventions.

When we refer to "family," we mean any or all of the multiple forms that the modern family takes. This broad and open definition of family is meant to be inclusive and to reflect the current social reality in society and children lives. Thus, parental figures in the child's life are referred to from hereon as caregivers. The focus on the child and family, is not only based on the obvious fact that in society children and adolescents are cared for and supported by their caregivers within the

M.E. Barrera, M.A., Ph.D., C.Psych. (✉) •
K.S. Daniel, M.Ed., Ph.D.
Hematology/Oncology Division and Psychology Department, Hospital for Sick Children,
555 University Ave., Toronto, ON, Canada
e-mail: maru.barrera@sickkids.ca; kim.daniel@sickkids.ca

A. Rapoport, M.D., F.R.C.P.C., M.H.Sc.
Paediatric Advanced Care Team (PACT), Hospital for Sick Children, 555 University Ave.,
Toronto, ON, Canada
e-mail: adam.rapoport@sickkids.ca

J. Wolfe et al. (eds.), *Palliative Care in Pediatric Oncology*, Pediatric Oncology,
https://doi.org/10.1007/978-3-319-61391-8_8

family, but because from the socio-ecological perspective, psychological distress in the child cannot be considered in isolation. How caregivers respond to the child's cancer diagnosis and treatment procedures influences how the child responds and behaves during these events. Similarly, a child's behavior during treatment impacts on their caregivers' behavior (Barrera et al. 2003, 2004a; Bearden et al. 2012; Caes et al. 2014; Fedele et al. 2013; Karlsson et al. 2014; Kazak and Baxt 2007; Kazak et al. 2011; Okado et al. 2014; Rodriguez et al. 2012). Moreover, these reciprocal influences impact on the overall psychological well-being of the entire family, even though each family member (the affected child, caregivers, and siblings) experiences cancer-related distress differently, depending on their different perspectives (Barrera et al. 2003, 2004a; Gerhardt et al. 2015; Kearney et al. 2015). This child and family perspective is supported by the recently published psychosocial standards in pediatric cancer and systematic reviews (Gerhardt et al. 2015; Kearney et al. 2015; Kazak et al. 2015a; Weaver et al. 2015).

Many pediatric cancer centers have adopted a child-family-centered model of care (MacKay and Gregory 2011; Wiener and Pao 2012). Child-family-centered care is defined as a partnership approach to healthcare decision-making between the child, the family, and the healthcare team, where each member of this partnership is considered an "expert" in his or her own perspective (Kuo et al. 2012). Thus, caregivers are considered the experts on their child's daily care and responses, the child as the expert of his/her preferences, and each healthcare provider (HCP) in the medical team is considered expert in his/her field of work. This model of care ensures that the voices of the patient and family are heard within the healthcare system (Kazak et al. 2015a) and that their cultural beliefs/values and their understanding of the healthcare system are considered. Sharing information between HCPs and family members is expected to take place in a respectful manner, honoring diversity, cultural and linguistic traditions, and care preferences. Consequently, medical decisions are expected to be made collaboratively in the best interest of the child and when developmentally feasible, with the child's involvement (Kuo et al. 2012).

Conducting early psychosocial screening and assessment and providing psychological support from diagnosis serve as a preventive intervention with the child and family to build capacity, to cope with the difficult cancer experience, and to build resilience to adversity (Gerhardt et al. 2015; Kearney et al. 2015; Kazak et al. 2015a; Weaver et al. 2015). Early psychosocial screening and assessment allow us to identify individual and family strengths, resources, and initial challenges. Psychosocial resources within the treating center can then address these issues with the family, fostering child/adolescent, parental, and sibling personal resources and resilience factors (e.g., improve emotional regulation, problem-solving). This can prevent further psychological adverse effects such as post-traumatic stress disorder (PTSD) or severe anxiety. To that aim, a number of psychological coping and intervention strategies are presented here that can address different levels of needs.

As children mature, it is important to maintain awareness of the child's development and abilities in all domains (physical, mental, or psychological—cognitive and emotional—and social domains) to guide the child's behavioral involvement in her/his own treatment, including decision-making, and parental management of the child's developing competence. Although for practical purposes the psychological and social domains are usually integrated into one—psychosocial—in this chapter we will focus mainly on the psychological aspect of distress and suffering.

Finally, we address psychological distress and suffering following a developmental family model, along three age/developmental periods: infants and preschoolers (roughly < 4 years), school-aged children (roughly 4–11 years), and adolescents (roughly 12–19 years) living at home and dependent on parents for treatment care and appointments. Take-home messages and recommendations are presented at the end of each developmental group, including Internet links and Quick Response (QR) codes for resources on easing psychological distress. Readers can scan the QR codes on their electronic device (e.g., smartphones) in order to get easy and immediate access to useful psychological Internet resources to support youth with cancer and their families.

8.2 Psychological Distress, Suffering, and Risk

All children, regardless of their health status, may experience fear, anxiety, and pain caused by medical procedures (Blount et al. 2003). Youth who are treated for cancer experience numerous stressful procedures, and their caregivers must suffer through them by proxy. While most adjust and learn to cope well with cancer and its treatment over time, a small but significant number experience psychological distress that can start at any stage of cancer: at diagnosis, during treatment (e.g., relapse), after completing treatment, as end of life approaches, and into survivorship (Patenaude and Kupst 2005; Vannatta et al. 2009). If patients are not screened psychosocially at regular intervals (e.g., at diagnosis, every significant treatment milestone), those with severe psychological distress (persistent feelings of intense sadness, fears) may develop more serious conditions such as severe behavior disturbances or mental health disorders such as anxiety disorder, depression, panic attacks, or post-traumatic stress disorder (PTSD).

Some youth, caregivers, or siblings may have preexisting mental health disorders, which place them and the family at increased risk for additional psychological distress. Thus, it is imperative that from the start children and adolescents with cancer, and their families, are screened for psychological distress and risk, to ensure that they are offered supports and interventions to enhance their coping. Given the unpredictability of the cancer trajectory, it is also important to conduct brief follow-up psychological distress screening at regular intervals, with standard tools, to adjust the psychosocial supports provided to the child with cancer and family.

8.2.1 Psychological Distress

The National Comprehensive Cancer Network defines psychological distress as a multifactorial, unpleasant, emotional experience of a psychological (feelings, worries, thoughts, behavior), social, and spiritual nature that may interfere with the ability to cope with cancer, its physical symptoms (and side effects) and treatment (National Comprehensive Cancer Network 2014). We conceptualize psychological distress on a continuum from normal feelings and thoughts of fear, sadness, anger, and vulnerability when anticipating or encountering an adverse, painful, or stressful event to a combination of distress responses that may persist with increased intensity and may lead to a mental health diagnosis if left untreated. The distress response may or may not be associated with painful responses; it can be discrete and disappear gradually or can be a reaction that becomes disabling and interferes with the medical treatment and effective coping in daily life. Brief psychological screening (see below for suggested tools) and a prompt intervention may reduce distress and prevent escalating behavioral problems.

Psychological distress in children and adolescents varies in how it is manifested, depending on the child's age or developmental level, personal characteristics, and external circumstances. See Table 8.1 for examples of distress responses in children. Generally, the first sign that the child is experiencing distress will be a change of typical behavior such as becoming irritable or feisty or perhaps more withdrawn. If caregivers notice these changes, acting sooner rather than later is

Table 8.1 Psychological distress responses in children

Lack of energy	Lack of appetite	Irritability
Fatigue	Nausea	Clinging behavior
Acting out	Crying easily	Fears
Fidgeting	Expressing excessive worries	Sadness
Inability to concentrate	Loss of interest in playing	Withdrawing from others

recommended before the behavior escalates or becomes more difficult to manage. Caregivers could explore what is going on with the child, in a calm and supportive manner, or they can consult with the treating team. As stated earlier, caregivers' reactions are critical in how the child's distress is expressed and what coping strategies are utilized. The importance of a calm, positive, and supportive approach to de-escalate distress cannot be emphasized enough; when all is calmed, then the child can be encouraged to chat about what is troubling him/her (see Box 8.1).

Box 8.1
Shawna*, a three-year-old quiet and shy girl, was diagnosed with acute lymphoblastic leukemia. Her parents described her as very compliant, brave, and soft-spoken. In fact, her parents reported that she never complained about feeling any pain or ask questions about her treatment. It wasn't until the middle course of Shawna's treatment where her parents noticed a significant change in her behaviors. As stated by Shawna's parents, she was becoming "defiant and oppositional" toward them. In fact, Shawna would drop to the floor, cry, kick, and shout at her parents when they brought her to the hospital for her chemotherapy. Shawna's parents became stressed and dreaded hospital visits because they anticipated Shawna's tantrums. Shawna's parents shared their frustrations with the treating team. After an initial assessment by a psychologist in the team, Shawna's parents learned that Shawna's behaviors were indicative of psychological distress (fear and anxiety) related to treatment. With counseling, they were able to sit calmly with their daughter, hold her, and provide comfort and understanding of her feelings instead of yelling "stop acting out" or "you need to behave." Shawna drew her fears when given the opportunity in a friendly and calm environment. What appeared as her being "oppositional" and "defiant" was actually her expressing her feelings of fear and anxiety about her cancer experience.*

8.2.2 Suffering

This is a term commonly used when referring to a holistic reaction to experiencing chronic or progressive disease or end of life in children and adults; it involves a combination of physical and psychological symptoms such as pain, fatigue, anxiety, fear, sadness, social responses, and spiritual pain (Krikorian et al. 2012; Montgomery et al. 2016). Cassell defined suffering as "a specific state of severe distress related to the imminent, perceived or actual, *threat to the integrity or existential continuity of the person*" (Krikorian et al. 2012; Cassell 1982). In this chapter we focus primarily on the psychological symptoms (distress) of suffering at any point in time throughout the cancer journey.

8.2.3 Psychological Risk and Resilience

Psychological risk is a term typically used when aiming to identify the psychological needs of patients and families. It is defined as "the vulnerability or likelihood" that atypical behavior or pattern of behaviors could become problematic when encountering a stressful, disruptive, or traumatic event or combination of events such as cancer diagnosis and treatment (Kazak et al. 2012, 2015b). The degree of psychological risk in a child and family is estimated based on their past experiences, history of typical, functioning (e.g., coping with difficult situations), and the personal and family/community resources available to manage or cope with the stressor. For example, a previous chronic or mental health condition in the child or a family member, or a caregiver's unemployment, could be considered psychological risk factors that make the family vulnerable to increased distress. Initial assessment of psychological risk can help the healthcare team explore further the family's specific needs and/or decide if other HCPs (e.g., psychologists, psychiatrists) should be involved for more in-depth assessment, psychological support, and intervention.

The alternative side of psychological risk is psychological resilience, which is defined as the ability to function well in the face of adversity, to overcome difficult situations, and to achieve personal goals under such circumstances (Masten 2001). Factors that promote resiliency include having strong supports and resources (e.g., available family members and friends that can help them under crisis, a supportive work environment) or a child's high level of functioning in a number of developmental domains (e.g., cognitive and social functioning, school performance) (Kazak et al. 2004; Rolland and Walsh 2006). It is important to identify both risk and resilient factors within the family that will help them cope more effectively with the demands that accompanies cancer and its treatment.

Kazak and her colleagues (Kazak et al. 2011, 2015b; Kazak 2006) have adapted a preventive risk model of health to childhood cancer, the Pediatric Psychosocial Preventative Health Model (PPPHM). This model integrates risk and resilient factors identified in the literature and provides a framework for healthcare providers to understand families' psychosocial needs for supportive care. The PPPHM proposes three levels of psychological risk: universal or low risk, medium or "targeted" risk, and high or clinical risk (see Fig. 8.1). *Universal or low risk* represents the majority of the families who are faced with childhood cancer; they experience distress but are able to function well using personal and external resources. These families may also be considered resilient. *Medium or "targeted" risk* refers to the second largest group of families. Families in this level

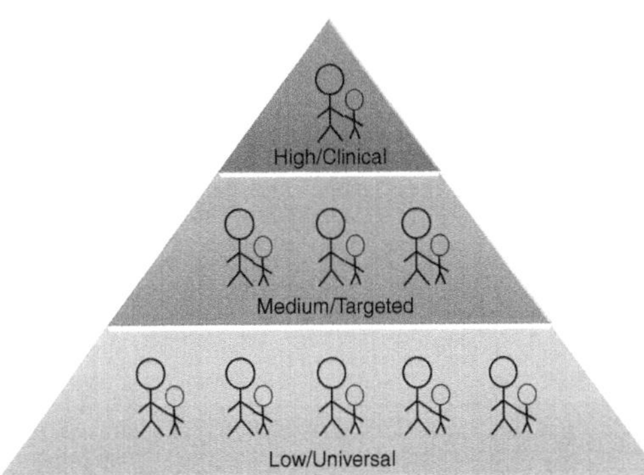

Fig. 8.1 Risk levels in the Pediatric Psychosocial Preventative Health Model (PPPHM) adapted from Kazak (2006)

experience acute distress related to the cancer diagnosis and treatment and have a number of risk factors (e.g., child has preexistent ADHD) but also have some resilient factors that allow them to function with some professional help. For example, the child and caregivers have available family and financial support; a family is receptive to early psychological support, which could prevent the development of chronic and more serious distress (see Box 8.1). The final level of risk, *clinical or high risk*, represents the smallest group of families. These families present with persistent and escalating distress, as well as several major risk factors such as mental health illness in the family and limited social and financial resources, all of which usually precede the diagnosis of childhood cancer. These families may have had or continue to have involvement with other health or community agencies for support and would require professional psychological help.

Initial psychological screening is essential to ensure that preexistent psychosocial stressors, and current services and supports, are identified to coordinate and plan for accessing additional services if needed. This tiered model of psychosocial risk is used below to describe psychological screening, assessment, and interventions to ease psychological distress.

8.3 Screening and Assessment for Psychological Risk and Distress in Pediatric Cancer

As part of standard care, early psychological screening and assessment need to be conducted and documented using brief, valid, and reliable tools (Kazak et al. 2015b). This should be the case whether one is interested in assessing psychological distress or risk. A diagnostic interview can follow to elaborate on current and past stressors, mental health issues, and coping strategies used by the youth and family. Follow-up brief assessments of psychological distress are necessary to recalibrate psychological supports for the youth and family (Kwak et al. 2013).

8.3.1 Distress Thermometer (DT)

The DT is a simple, valid, and reliable thermometer-like tool to assess distress, with a scale from 0 (no distress) to 10 (severe distress) (see Fig. 8.2). It has been widely used in adult oncology, along with a checklist of problem areas, with a high degree of success to triage for further psychological assessment and interventions (Carlson et al. 2012). The DT has also been used to assess parental psychological distress (Haverman et al. 2013) and has been adapted recently for children and adolescents who are undergoing cancer treatment (Patel et al. 2014; Zadeh 2015). The pediatric DT uses three faces (happy, neutral, and sad) for 2–4-year-old children and ten faces for 5–7-year-olds in a continuum from happy to sad, similar to that used to assess pain (see Fig. 8.2); for children 8 or older, the DT is similar to the one used with adults. A child under 7 years is typically asked to mark the face that best shows how worried, sad, or fearful he/she has been feeling (today, or in the last week, or since the last clinic visit). Older children are asked to circle the number (National Cancer Institute 2015; Caes et al. 2014) that best describes the level of distress they have been feeling (in the last week including today). The DT in children is also typically used along with a problem checklist of emotional, physical, and family problems. Reliability of the pediatric DT was found to improve with increasing age. Moderate validity was found compared to standard questionnaires of depression or emotional quality of life for children (Zadeh 2015). The DT is practical (brief) and useful to assess individual distress at one point in time but does not provide the broader scope of contextual familial factors that have been recognized to be important in children with cancer.

8.3.2 Psychosocial Assessment Tool

Using the PPPHM described above, Kazak and colleagues developed the Psychosocial Assessment Tool (PAT), a tool completed by a child's caregiver to screen for existent concerns and strengths (risk and resilient factors) in the patient, siblings (mood, worries, fears, attention, learning, problematic behavior), caregiver (mental health, worries, fears), and family (composition, size, support, financial burden) (Kazak et al. 2001; Pai et al. 2008). The PAT has been found to be reliable and valid and easy to complete by caregivers; it is now used in the United States, Canada, Australia, and Europe (Kazak et al. 2015b; Pai et al. 2008; Barrera et al. 2014a; McCarthy et al. 2009). The scoring of the PAT yields three levels of risk, based on the PPPHM described above: universal/low, targeted/medium, or clinical/high. External validity of the PAT with families in Canada, Australia, and the Netherlands indicates that 60–69% of families fall into the low-risk, 23–32% fall into the medium-risk, and 7–9% fall into the high-risk level of psychosocial distress.

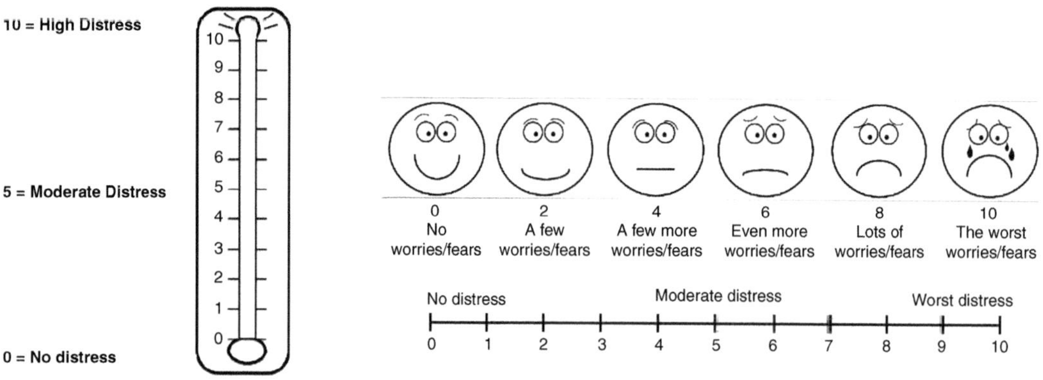

Fig. 8.2 Examples of distress thermometers used with children

8.3.3 Usefulness of Standard Psychosocial Screening

Screening for psychological risk and distress should be the first and necessary step for providing evidence-based psychosocial support for the youth and family (Kazak et al. 2011, 2015b). Psychosocial screening and assessment is now considered a standard part of psychosocial care in pediatric oncology (Kazak et al. 2015b). Documenting results from early screening and subsequent follow-up assessments can guide provision of psychological support and intervention (Patenaude et al. 2015). Although most clinicians may indeed conduct psychological assessments before intervening, evidence suggests that there is little documentation of early psychological assessment in the medical charts and even less evidence of the use of standard tools (Mitchell et al. 2005; Selove et al. 2012). Equally important, documentation can enhance communication among HCPs within the circle of care for the youth and family regarding not only the medical needs, but the psychosocial needs as well. This will increase the likelihood that all HCPs understand the unique relationship between the disease, the child, and family's psychosocial distress and facilitate mobilization of resources to help them cope.

There are a few emerging studies that support the utility of using PAT in the clinical setting (Kazak et al. 2011; Barrera et al. 2014b; Alderfer et al. 2009). Caregivers of children with cancer who completed the PAT received more psychosocial services (based on reports by social workers and child life specialists documented in medical charts) compared to medical charts of caregivers of children who were treated prior to conducting the study (Kazak et al. 2011; Alderfer et al. 2009). In another study, using a pilot randomized controlled trial, caregivers completed the PAT and were randomized to either the experimental group (EG, caring team received a summary of the PAT) or control group (CG, caring team did not receive a summary of the PAT). Six months later the EG showed a reduction in the high and medium psychosocial risk category and improvement in the pain-related quality of life of the child, compared to CG. These results suggest that early psychosocial screening may reduce family psychosocial risk and may lead to improved QoL (Barrera et al. 2014b).

After the initial psychological distress assessment, follow-up interviews with a psychosocial HCP are recommended to investigate further the nature of distress. Depending on the initial severity and nature of distress, standard instruments such as the ones listed below may be useful in getting further insight of the presenting psychosocial difficulties: the Brief Symptom Inventory-18 (Derogatis 2001) for adolescents or caregivers, the Hospital Anxiety and Depression Scale (Zigmond and Snaith 1983) or the equivalent scale for pediatrics, the Pediatric Index of Emotional Distress (Ferguson et al. 2010) or the Multidimensional Anxiety Questionnaire for Children (March et al. 1997). These are brief and well-validated instruments.

Evidence suggests that while children's and caregivers' psychological distress decreases over time, the sources of stress and caregiver burden may remain stable or increase based on the disease trajectory. Thus, the intensity of the psychological intervention would vary from case to case, but ongoing psychosocial support could bolster coping strategies and resources (Steele et al. 2003). It is important to know that high levels of psychological distress is typical in caregivers of a child with advanced cancer and is associated with a strong belief that the child is suffering severely (Rosenberg et al. 2013). Psychosocial support in these cases needs to be focused on "aligned prognostic understanding with concrete goals of care" (Rosenberg et al. 2013).

8.3.4 Challenges to Psychological Distress Screening and Care in Pediatric Cancer

Screening for psychological distress requires a clear goal of what has been screened for and the availability of a valid, reliable, and sensitive tool with predefined clinical level cutoff, to identify distress. There are, however, institutional, programmatic, and personal barriers to psychological distress or risk screening (Mitchell et al. 2005; Selove et al. 2012; Barrera 2015; Fagerlind et al. 2013). These include limited institutional policies supporting psychosocial care, inadequate funding for psychosocial resources, limited use of validated tools and documentation, time constraints to address psychosocial concerns, HCPs' perception of families' ability to complete instruments (English as a second language) or being interested in psychosocial assessment due to their values and beliefs (e.g., "what does this have to do with my child's cancer?", "I don't want to be stigmatized with mental illness"), and HCPs' personal attitudes and beliefs regarding the use of standardized tools ("there is no need for standard tools", "I don't think the rest of the healthcare team should read about the family problems"). These barriers need to be addressed at the various levels within each institution, the treating program, and within the individual HCPs and families, through dialogue and psychoeducation.

In summary, a strong mandate and acceptance by all stakeholders (HCPs, managers and administrators, youth, and their families) is needed in order to allocate adequate psychosocial resources for psychological screening, assessment, and treatment to families (Kazak et al. 2011; Barrera 2015; Holland 2010). In fact, a case can be made that given the increased survival rate in childhood cancer, we cannot afford not investing in psychosocial services (hiring providers who have the skills and training to adequately assess and intervene throughout the patients' and families' cancer journey) to prevent or reduce future social isolation, underachievement and underemployment, and mental illness difficulties, which are well-known long-term adverse effects in adult survivors of childhood cancer (Erickson et al. 2013; Lown et al. 2015; Nathan et al. 2011; Zebrack et al. 2014).

There are also developmental challenges. Considering that the majority of pediatric oncology patients are 5 years of age or younger at diagnosis, developmental challenges have been identified for self-reporting psychological distress and well-being, even when these children can report reliably on procedural pain (Altekruse et al. 2010; Cohen et al. 2008; Varni et al. 2007). Proxy reports by caregivers regarding psychosocial distress in young children (under school age) can be used, but may not be consistent with the child's self-report (when he/she is able to self-report) or a HCP's perception of the child's distress, particularly if a distress thermometer is used (Zadeh 2015). Thus, different perspectives of the child's psychosocial distress are useful to better understand distress contextually. On the other hand, the caregiver report may be the best proxy available for understanding the family's psychosocial risk prior to and during cancer treatment and trajectory.

8.4 Coping with Cancer-Related Stressors to Reduce Distress

Coping is generally defined as a person's strategies or effort to manage stressors or stressful thoughts or situations in order to reduce or alleviate distress. How a person copes with stress depends on his/her personal characteristics, past experience, the circumstances, and the type and severity of the stressor. There are a number of conceptual models for coping strategies that have emerged since Lazarus and Folkman's early work (Folkman and Lazarus 1988; Lazarus and Folkman 1984). In the context of coping with psychological distress related to childhood cancer diagnosis and treatment, problem-focused strategies, emotion-focused strategies, and engagement versus disengagement are considered here.

8.4.1 Problem-Focused Strategies

Problem-focused strategies deal with the cause of the problem and how to manage it, change it, or eliminate it to reduce distress (e.g., learning new skills, seeking more information about the problem to eliminate or control the problem). Since children and caregivers cannot control cancer as a stressor directly (e.g., whether or not the medical treatment will work or the child will develop complications of treatment), problem-focused coping alone may not be a useful coping strategy for reducing distress in this context (Barrera et al. 2004a).

8.4.2 Emotion-Focused Strategies

Emotion-focused strategies refer to changing or releasing one's own emotional reactions (sadness, fear, anger, hostility) that are triggered by the perceived stressor to gain personal control (Brannon and Feist 2009). There are numerous emotion-focused strategies that can be used to manage emotional distress related to pediatric cancer. These include systematic relaxation techniques, cognitive behavioral therapy strategies, and problem-solving strategies. Some of these strategies are described below.

8.4.3 Control-Based or Engagement Strategies

Based on the concepts of perceived control of illness-related stress, Compas et al. (2012, 2014) proposed three control-based types of coping strategies: primary control engagement, secondary engagement control, and disengagement. *Primary control coping* referred to (a) strategies aimed directly at changing the source of stress, as in the problem-focused coping strategy described above or (b) changing or modulating the emotional reaction or expression to the stressor, which is similar to the emotion-focused coping strategy described above. *Secondary control coping* refers to efforts to adapt to the stressor after reappraising it, accepting personal limitations to control the stressor (e.g., how the disease responds to medical treatment), and engaging in positive thinking. The key to these strategies is acceptance of having little or no control over the stressor. Mindfulness practice described below is a good example of secondary control coping.

Finally, *disengagement* coping refers to efforts to move or orient attention away from (ignore) the sources of stress (e.g., caregivers who may choose not to come to the treating center to reduce distress) or one's reaction to the stressor (e.g., refusing to take pills which makes the child vomit). Empirical evaluations of this coping model are emerging, with secondary control coping being found to be associated with reductions of anxiety and depression symptoms in adolescents (Compas et al. 2014). These findings support the use of secondary control coping strategies which are reflected in intervention strategies such as CBT, mindfulness, and progressive relaxation, described below.

8.5 Psychological Intervention to Ease Psychological Distress

A recent systematic review of the psychological intervention research to help youth with cancer and their caregivers manage distress indicates a drastic "paradigm shift" in the last 20 years due to changes in standard of care. These changes include the use of local and general anesthesia during the most painful and stressful procedures, such as lumber punctures or bone marrow aspirations (Flowers and Birnie 2015). Although the experience for youth undergoing cancer treatment currently may differ from the experience of youth in previous decades, psychological distress is generated not only by procedure but also by uncertainty of outcomes in general and fears of death specifically. These issues continue to be sources of distress for children undergoing cancer treatment and their caregivers.

The psychological intervention strategies described below aim to help youth and their caregivers develop positive and constructive coping strategies to manage distress. However, there is little research assessing what kinds of psychotherapeutic techniques are most effective and when during the cancer trajectory (Steele et al. 2015).

8.5.1 Psychoeducation

All families who have a youth diagnosed with cancer should receive developmentally appropriate psychoeducation and anticipatory guidance, in a timely manner, regarding the nature of the medical diagnosis. This should include information regarding the impact these experiences can have on behavior and feelings and the resources available to youth and their caregivers. Psychoeducation aims "to empower them, assist with day-to-day management of the disease and decision making, relieve uncertainty, and enhance psychosocial adaptation to the illness" (Thompson and Young-Saleme 2015). Psychoeducation is the foundation of any psychosocial service and needs to be routinely integrated as part of the comprehensive care in pediatric oncology.

Anticipatory guidance refers to the general pediatric practice of proactively providing information regarding expected patterns and events that accompany normal child growth and development (e.g., child's health and behavior, normal milestones). This information is shared with families to help them appreciate what can be expected as their child grows, how to best support normal behavior, and to help them identify abnormal behaviors. Providing youth and caregivers with developmentally appropriate information, psychoeducation, and anticipatory guidance, in a timely fashion throughout the cancer trajectory, has been accepted as a psychosocial standard of care (Thompson and Young-Saleme 2015).

In this chapter, psychoeducation is used to refer to provision of relevant information to family members regarding what to expect at various phases during the cancer trajectory, including examples of possible behavioral reactions in the youth with cancer during different stages of treatment (e.g., when taking steroids), what are the common complaints during treatment (e.g., changes in mood, appetite, nausea, headaches), what are the common issues with healthy siblings, (e.g., feeling sad but resentful, being distracted at school when the brother or sister is hospitalized), and how to prevent or minimize these reactions. Information about a variety of resources, within the treating center and community or on the Internet, are also critical to enhance coping and reduce distress. Some of these resources are provided here.

Although rigorous evidence on the impact of psychoeducation on pediatric cancer health outcomes is relatively limited, existent evidence suggests that providing psychoeducation and anticipatory guidance to youth, caregivers, and other family members such as siblings can reduce psychological distress and can increase trust in the healthcare system (Thompson and Young-Saleme 2015; Barlow and Ellard 2004). Evidence also suggests that psychoeducation is most effective with children and adolescents when it is interactive and individualized (Barlow and Ellard 2004; Bradlyn et al. 2003). Some computer games, videos, or web-based formats to provide psychoeducation have been found to be effective and accepted by youth and families, but low utilization of these available resources is a major concern (Ewing et al. 2009).

In summary, regardless of their psychosocial risk and distress level (universal, medium, or high risk), all youth who are diagnosed and treated for cancer, and their families, must be provided with psychoeducation throughout the cancer trajectory. Psychoeducation should be extended to the community of the child and family (e.g., school) to ensure that their community supports them. While some of this information may be generic, efforts should be made to tailor information to the specific needs, preferences, and cultural values of the child and family. Psychoeducation should be a priority in every pediatric cancer center as it empowers youth and families; it may prevent the development of severe psychological distress and fosters trust in the healthcare system.

8.5.2 Psychological Support

Psychological support involves therapeutic, empathic listening, that is, of a nonjudgmental nature. It validates and empowers those who are experiencing psychological distress and helps them meet the challenges they encounter at any of the states of the illness. Psychological support has been found to be helpful to youth undergoing cancer treatment and their families (Askins and Moore 2008) and has been reported to be used shortly after cancer diagnosis or during crisis intervention (Steele et al. 2015).

Like psychoeducation, psychological support is considered the basis for any effective preventive intervention as it fosters the development of trusting relationships with the professionals on the

HCT. Psychological support and psychoeducation may be all that is needed for families considered to have universal psychosocial risk. Its effectiveness alone, however, has not been investigated.

8.5.3 Behavioral Approaches and Distraction Techniques

A number of behavioral approaches have been used to help youth and their caregivers manage procedural pain and distress related to cancer (Birnie et al. 2014). These include progressive muscle relaxation techniques (refer to https://www.youtube.com/watch?v=aaTDNYjk-Gw), systematic desensitization either using imagery or "in vivo" exposure, belly or diaphragmatic breathing exercises with bubbles or party blowers, (refer to https://www.youtube.com/watch?v=Uxbdx-SeOOo), guided imagery, (refer to https://www.youtube.com/watch?v=GIJn5XhqPN8), hypnosis training, and numerous distraction techniques (Blount et al. 2003; Uman et al. 2013). Distraction techniques refer to those coping strategies that take the attention away from the stressor or painful procedure and can involve activities such as blowing bubbles, playing video games, watching a favorite video or movie, or listening to music (refer to https://www.youtube.com/watch?v=EKh4ApbDsHw).

Child life specialists, therapeutic clowns, and play or music therapists typically engage hospitalized children with or without their caregivers in these activities to reduce boredom while providing distraction during painful or stressful procedures to reduce distress (Rapoport and Weingarten 2014). Distraction techniques can be used at any age for discrete and temporary reduction of distress and increase in coping with stressors, but they may not be effective for more severe, chronic, or persistent distress.

8.5.4 Cognitive Behavioral Therapy (CBT)

CBT is an evidence-based treatment that supports individuals to change their negative and anxious thoughts so they can feel and function better in order to improve their quality of life. Its main premise capitalizes on the relationships of mind (thoughts) emotions (that need to be regulated) and behavior or action to cope with stressors or distorted thinking (see Box 8.3).

Notably, intrusive or distorted thinking can lead to dysfunctional emotions or behaviors. Thus, reconstructing the child's, and/or caregiver's maladaptive thoughts to more balanced thoughts, may change how they feel and behave. It is important to consider the child's developmental level and his/her ability for symbolic thinking, which are necessary factors for CBT to be effective. Nonetheless, CBT is the most widely used psychotherapeutic-behavioral technique in pediatrics for managing conditions such a depression and anxiety disorder (Otto et al. 2004).

CBT techniques, however, may not be warranted to reduce distress in patients who relapse or are contemplating end of life because their intrusive and distressing negative thought patterns of fear of disease progression and death are warranted and realistic (Greer et al. 2010). Similarly, caregivers of children with progressive disease may best benefit from psychological support that helps them align prognostic understanding with concrete goals for quality of life and care (Rosenberg et al. 2013).

8.5.5 Mindfulness

Since the introduction of mindfulness intervention to the western world by Kabat-Zinn in 1979, his program known as mindfulness-based stress reduction (MBSR) has been widely used as complimentary treatment for adults with cancer, cardiovascular disease, fibromyalgia, and chronic pain (Kabat-Zinn 1990). Segal and colleagues adapted MBSR for the treatment of mental health adult patients, particularly for relapse prevention of depression, creating mindfulness-based cognitive therapy (MBCT) (Segal et al. 2013). Other mindfulness-based interventions have been adapted as lifestyle prevention in education, parenting, the workplace, and other settings (Rouleau et al. 2015).

Mindfulness in general is referred to the awareness that develops by paying purposeful attention to an event or situation, how it is in the present moment, with nonjudgment and acceptance with compassion. Mindfulness teaches individuals how to live in the present, rather than being lost in their thoughts about the past or worry about the future. A person can be mindful of any and all aspects of his/her experiences, sensations in their bodies, thinking, feeling, smelling, seeing, touching, and tasting. Mindfulness supports people to step out of "autopilot" so they can be more purposeful in their day-to-day actions and choices. Being mindful helps people concentrate on their direct experiences with full awareness (body sensations, emotions, thoughts) whether they are pleasant, unpleasant, or neutral.

In MBCT, the emphasis is on changing individual's relationship with their negative thoughts and feelings and becoming more aware of early warning signals indicating changes or deterioration in the pattern of their thoughts (Segal et al. 2013). Thus, the individual learns to pay attention to those early signs as they come and go and return to the present moment, such as focusing on the breath, getting attentional control as a prevented approach to relapse of depression. Mindfulness practice teaches individuals how to respond, rather than react or avoid difficulties or stressors (Brown and Ryan 2003). Lastly, the practice of mindfulness helps individuals relate to themselves and others with kindness, warmth, respect, and compassion (Wood et al. 2015).

Although this technique is just beginning to be systematically evaluated with children and adolescents with cancer or their caregivers, it has the potential to reduce distress by accepting the present reality of the diagnosis. Given its reliance on higher intellectual processes for examining one's own thoughts and feelings to manage psychological distress, this technique is more accessible to adolescents and their caregivers. However, with specific clinical modifications, mindfulness best practices may be useful even with preschoolers (Khaddouma et al. 2015). A recent systematic review and meta-analysis of mindfulness-based interventions in healthcare with adults and adolescents concluded that MBSR and MBCT as complimentary therapy can be effective in alleviating mental and physical symptoms, of cancer, cardiovascular disease, chronic pain, depression, and anxiety disorders and as preventive measures in healthy adults and children (Gotink et al. 2015). Moreover, two recent systematic reviews of mindfulness-based programs exclusively for adolescents concluded that these interventions can be effective in adolescents with mental health symptoms. There are, however, significant methodological limitations in the existent studies (Kallapiran et al. 2015; Tan 2016).

A recently published feasibility randomized controlled trial assessing an adapted mindfulness-based intervention in adolescent females with chronic pain found the program feasible (acceptable); participants reported positive changes in coping with pain, but no changes were observed on the standardized measures of quality of life, depression, anxiety, pain perception, and psychological distress (Chadi et al. 2016). More rigorous research is needed to determine the effectiveness of these interventions in children and adolescents with cancer and other chronic conditions.

Finally, the practice of mindfulness-based interventions can be used by individuals who have progressive disease and are at the end of life. These individuals can learn how to witness and perhaps accept their pain and fears by participating in activities that bring their conscious awareness to their bodily sensations and identify somatic symptoms in a nonjudgmental manner (Rouleau et al. 2015) (see guided video for youth https://www.youtube.com/watch?v=yYQKF-9poLM).

8.5.6 Other Interventions and Programs Used in Pediatric Oncology

8.5.6.1 Expressive Therapies

These are intervention strategies that can be used with youth with cancer by a variety of HCPs including art, play, music, dance, clown, and pet therapy (Kaminski et al. 2002; Linge 2013; Rhondali et al. 2013; Treurnicht Naylor et al. 2011; Wikström 2005; Wilson 2006). These therapies can be particularly helpful for expressing feelings related to cancer and reducing distress at any stage of the disease, including end of life (Sourkes 1995). Art in particular (drawing, painting) can be useful for establishing rapport with the youth, communicating and helping youth regulate their emotions and possibly resolve trauma (see Fig. 8.3). However, there is limited systematic assessment of the effectiveness of these techniques in pediatric oncology (Treurnicht Naylor et al. 2011). These strategies can be combined with CBT to facilitate acquisition of additional strategies to manage emotional reactions and regulate behavior related to cancer and its treatment.

There are also specific programs that have been developed for youth with cancer, for siblings, or for the entire family, such as summer or weekend camps and adventure therapy (Epstein 2004). The primary focus of these programs is to provide enjoyable, positive experiences. Although most of these programs do not have direct therapeutic focus, they may help to reduce distress in the participants as they improve their quality of life (Stevens et al. 2004).

The following are some specific therapeutic programs designed to reduce distress in either children or their caregivers or both.

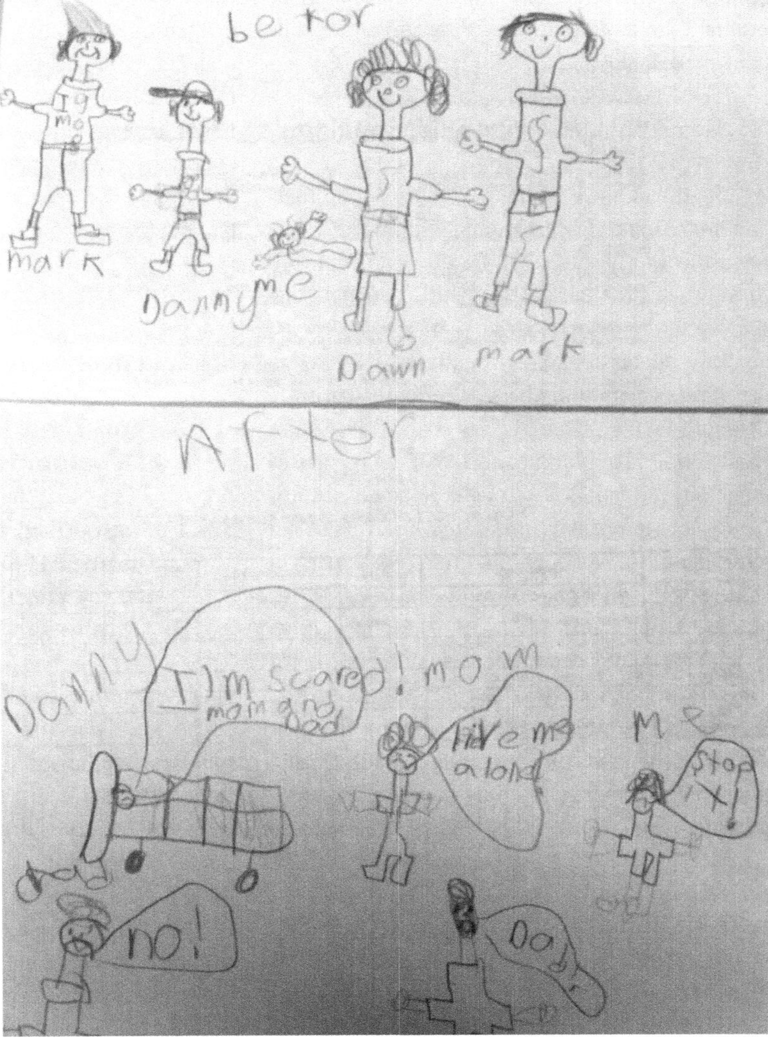

Fig. 8.3 A family before and after a child was diagnosed with cancer, drawn by a 10-year-old boy

8.5.6.2 Surviving Cancer Competently Intervention Program (SCCIP)

SCCIP is a program that integrated principles of CBT and family therapy and was developed for families (the affected child caregivers and siblings) who have a child recently diagnosed with cancer (Kazak et al. 1999, 2005). SCCIP consists of four 45-min sessions focusing on distress reduction. Sessions 1 and 2 consist of separate sessions for adolescent patients, caregivers, and siblings to address "how cancer has affected me and my family"; session 3 consists of multiple family discussion groups that included all family members in a group of six to eight families; and session 4 consists of a family therapy-oriented session, which included all family members (Kazak et al. 1999). This intervention has been evaluated in a pilot study with promising results (Kazak et al. 2005).

8.5.6.3 Problem-Solving Skills Training (PSST)

Adapted from the original problem-solving therapy for adults (D'Zurilla and Goldfried 1971; D'Zurilla and Nezu 2007), PSST was developed to improve problem-solving skills and personal growth and to reduce "negative affectivity" (e.g., anxiety, depression, post-traumatic distress) in caregivers (mainly mothers) of children recently diagnosed with cancer (Askins et al. 2009; Sahler et al. 2005, 2013; Varni et al. 1999). It consists of eight 1-h individual sessions conducted according to a comprehensive manual. Caregivers select a problem to work on the following "Bright IDEAS": Bright signifies optimism and positive attitude to problem-solving; I is for *i*dentify a problem; D is for *d*etermine the options; E is for *e*valuate the options; A is for *a*ct on the option; and S is for see if it works. PSST has been extensively evaluated using rigorous randomization methodology and found to be beneficial to caregivers (Askins et al. 2009; Sahler et al. 2005, 2013).

8.5.6.4 Siblings Coping Together (SibCT) Program

This intervention program was designed exclusively to address psychological distress in siblings of children who have been diagnosed and treated for cancer (Barrera et al. 2002, 2004b; Salavati et al. 2014). SibCT consists of eight weekly 2-h group sessions where principles of CBT, problem-solving, and family systems as well as expressive therapies and psychoeducation are integrated to address difficult situations for siblings within the family and at school. Each session has a specific theme: the first two sessions focus on introducing their family and learning about cancer; the following two sessions address school and family issues concerning the sibling, following by specific issues related to the relationship with the child with cancer. The final sessions are focused all about the sibling's present and future goals, ending with a graduation ceremony during the last session. Preliminary evaluation of this program indicated reduction of distress and acceptability of the intervention (Barrera et al. 2002, 2004b; Salavati et al. 2014). Rigorous evaluation of SibCT has recently been conducted using randomized controlled methodology, and the preliminary results indicate positive outcomes (Rokeach et al. 2014; Barrera et al. 2017).

8.6 Psychological Distress and Interventions for Youth and Their Families at Various Developmental Stages

8.6.1 Psychological Distress in Infants and Preschoolers (0 to < 4 years) and Their Families

There is little research on the psychological impact of cancer on children under 4 years of age, despite the fact that a high percentage of childhood malignancies are diagnosed during the first 4 years of life (Greenberg et al. 2015). Healthy and secure caregiver-infant relationships are the foundation for healthy social and emotional development and for future trusting relationships with others (Sameroff and Emde 1989; Schneider-Rosen 1990). A diagnosis of childhood cancer during this important period may disrupt the development of such relationships by adding unpredictability, distress, and changes in daily routines. Combined with having little understanding of why invasive and painful procedures are done to their bodies, infants and preschool-aged children are at risk for developing post-traumatic distress disorder (PTSD) or symptoms (PTSS) (Kazak and Baxt 2007; Graf et al. 2013; Roy and Russell 2000; Vernon et al. 2016).

In fact, children from 18 to 48 months have been identified to be particularly vulnerable to reexperiencing traumatic experiences, including traumatic medical procedures (Graf et al. 2013; Scheeringa and Zeanah 1995). As well, when the young child has cancer and is hospitalized, emotional bonding between the child and the primary caregiver becomes stronger, and the caregiver typically "surrenders to care for the child" to the detriment of her/his own personal needs and the needs of healthy siblings (Quirino and Collet 2012). Consequently, the child may become irritable and clingier to one caregiver than the other, a situation that could aggravate distress in the family.

Within this age period, caregivers have reported higher acting out and aggressive behaviors (e.g., kicking, hitting, refusing to cooperate with procedures) compared to school-aged children and adolescents (Barrera et al. 2003) (see Box 8.1). The child's limited communication abilities and emotional regulation, their self-centered view of the world, magical thinking, and difficulties separating reality from imagined world, all make it difficult for HCPs to communicate with the child. Thus, it is through the universal language of playing, and the help of their trusted caregivers, that we can best engage with them.

Although caregivers of children in this age group may be relieved that their child is too young and perhaps will not remember the cancer experience, they may suffer severely for seeing their child, who has hardly lived life, go through cancer treatment and fear for their young child's life. Combined with the practical demands and impact of the cancer diagnosis and treatment, fear of death and uncertainty of treatment outcomes place caregivers at risk for developing PTSD or PTSS (Roy and Russell 2000). Caregivers' severe distress may interfere with the child's treatment, impact parenting and their ability to support the affected child and healthy siblings, and ultimately threaten family function and stability (Kearney et al. 2015). Ongoing assessment of caregivers' psychological distress will facilitate access to appropriate interventions for their mental health needs. The strong evidence of adverse impact of childhood cancer on caregivers has resulted in a psychosocial standard of assessment and intervention for parents of children with cancer (Kearney et al. 2015). Finally, mothers of healthy infants who also have an older child with cancer experience more psychological distress compared to mothers of infants with cancer and healthy older children (Vernon et al. 2016). This study supports the importance of considering the family psychological risk when a child is diagnosed with cancer, particularly when the child is an infant.

8.6.2 Psychological Intervention to Reduce Distress in Infants and Preschoolers and Their Families

Psychological interventions during this period need to be especially aimed at the child-caregiver dyad, as responses of one member of the dyad can directly influence the responses of the other. Initial psychological assessment in this age group will identify the nature of the child-caregiver relationship; preexisting family concerns, including caregiver anxiety; and strengths in the youngster and family. Additionally, early psychological assessment should aim to identify children and caregivers at risk not only for distress but also for mental health, including PTSD. Below, we list a number of recommendations and tips for interventions with this age group.

- *Psychoeducation, anticipatory guidance, and psychological support* must be the first line of intervention regardless of the child's developmental level but is of particular importance for this group age, given their risk for PTSS or PTSD in both, children and caregivers.

- Efforts should be made to *support the child-caregiver relationship* both during hospitalizations and outpatient visits and at home (see Box 8.1).
- *Simple communication.* Communicating with children under 4 years of age should involve simple words through play, or drawings, in short segments, e.g., "you have a lump in your chest; let's draw a person with a lump in the chest"; "medicine will make it go away; let's draw the medicine making the lump go away."
- During this age period, *distraction techniques* such as listening to music, blowing bubbles, or watching a favorite video can be useful in helping the child and caregiver manage stressful and painful procedures such as access to an internal line for chemotherapy or drawing blood.
- When a child is hospitalized, caregivers should be encouraged to *create* "a home away from home" or a "second home" to facilitate the child's adjustment to the unfamiliar environment. Caregivers should be encouraged to bring pictures, favorite toys, and bedding.
- During hospitalizations, efforts should also be made to *provide special support to the primary caregiver*, typically the mother, to ensure that she takes time to attend to her personal needs.
- Also during hospitalizations, when possible, HCPs should encourage caregivers *sharing responsibilities for caring* of the young child to allow the primary caregiver to spend time at home with healthy siblings and practicing self-care. This will reduce physical and mental fatigue and help prevent strain on the family relationships.
- Encourage caregivers and children to *engage with available psychosocial services* in the center such as therapeutic clowns, recreational activities, child life specialists, and music or art therapists, to help the child adjust to the new environment, build positive experiences and relationships, and improve quality of life. This will also facilitate engagement with psychosocial HCPs if more serious difficulties develop.
- When distress is severe, *involve behavior experts* in CBT or mindfulness strategies that can be taught to youth and caregivers to improve coping and reduce psychological distress.
- Encourage family life to *return to daily routines* as soon as possible, to avoid developing the role of the "sick," "fragile," or "cancer child" (a child who is inactive or disengaged after he/she is able to become somewhat active and engaged); professional help may be needed to help the young child (and caregivers) resume regular family life as much as possible.
- Ensure that *healthy siblings receive* needed attention from the caregivers and other trusted adults.
- Ensure that routines are in place, even if they need to be adjusted during the child's treatment process.
- Ensure that *basic but flexible discipline and expectations remain in place*, adjusted to the child's health and disease trajectory. For example, kicking, hitting, or destroying objects (toys, medical equipment) should be unacceptable, and consequences (e.g., reducing the use of electronics) need to be implemented. This will prevent the development of more serious problems.
- Ensure that when possible, the *child remains in contact with other family members*, e.g., siblings and grandparents. This will benefit all involved.
- If *the child's behavior becomes unmanageable* or interferes with treatment (e.g., refusal to take medication), referral to a behavior specialist (e.g., psychologist) is recommended.

8.7 Psychological Distress in School-Aged Children (4–11 Years) and Their Families

Most children in this age group are attending school, from junior kindergarten to Grade 6. Consequently, for this age group, school has become the hub for the child's cognitive, social, and emotional development. During this period of their lives, children develop rapidly, gaining verbal and social skills, emotional regulation, and intellectual abilities that allow them to learn and adapt to new situations quicker than younger children. They have the abilities to expand their interests and knowledge of the world outside their home and enjoy interacting with peers. Thus, when a child in this age group is diagnosed with cancer, they may want to know all about it and ask many questions. Playing a more active role in the process of managing a cancer diagnosis and treatment along with their caregivers depends on the child's developmental age, personality, and cultural background. For some school-aged children, missing school because of cancer treatment may become a major issue, perhaps an even bigger issue than the disease itself. These children typically have done well in school, both academically and socially, and being separated from their peers is a major stressor and loss (see Box 8.2).

Box 8.2

Jonny *was a typical fun-loving and active 10-year-old boy before he was diagnosed with a brain tumor. He loved attending school, learning, and especially socializing with his peers. Due to Jonny's treatment, he was not able to attend school. As a result, Jonny became depressed, irritable, and stressed. When questioned, Jonny noted that he was not sad about having cancer, but very sad that he was missing school and falling behind in class. He was also worried that his friends would eventually forget about him. Being among his peers has helped Jonny cope with his past feelings of loneliness as he was the only child and reared solely by his grandmother. Understanding the importance of school and peer relationships has on his overall well-being Jonny's healthcare providers (e.g., psychologist, oncologist, interlink nurse, and child life specialists) arranged with his school and grandmother for a way that he can stay connected with his classmates. Jonny was reassured by his teacher that she will provide him with supplemental homework assignments so he will not fall behind and arranged to have video chats with his classmates on a weekly basis so he can stay in the "loop" with his peers. After these arrangements were implemented, Jonny's mood began to elevate and he became less worried and sad but more hopeful and happy.*

For other children whose experience at school may not have been as positive (e.g., they were struggling socially or/and academically), missing school may not be a major problem initially. Whatever the case may be, an early psychological screening will bring these issues to the surface and will alert the HCT of the child's interests, socio-emotional and cognitive competencies, and academic functioning.

Many pediatric cancer centers offer school in the hospital for children who are hospitalized for prolonged periods of time (e.g., more than 2 weeks). Children can have "school" in their room or in a classroom, depending on their wellness, usually for an hour a day (Knaul et al. 2006). This is important for children as it gives them a sense of normalcy. With the caregiver's and child's consent, teachers or members of the HCT will connect with the school system sooner rather than later to ensure that there is continuity of contact with the school community for both academic and socio-emotional purposes. This ongoing contact will facilitate school reentry when the child is ready to resume school attendance and may reduce anxiety in children that are concerned about falling behind or fear being rejected or not accepted by peers. The importance of this aspect of the child's life is emphasized by the recognition of academic continuity and school reentry support as standard of psychosocial care in pediatric oncology (Thompson and Young-Saleme 2015).

Although children within this age range are typically interested in learning new things and usually are cooperative, in the early stages of treatment, caregivers may notice changes in their typical behavior and possibly developmental regression. For example, children may start bedwetting even though the child might have been toilet trained long ago; or the child may become more irritable and become tearful easily, as might be expected in younger children. These are not uncommon occurrences and are clear signs that the child needs additional psychological support.

Caring for children with cancer during this age period has its own challenges; these children are typically able to communicate their needs and wants verbally and are eager to please their caregivers. I remember a 9-year-old girl walking into my office (MB) announcing "I'm here because I have an anger management problem." With therapy, this little girl became busy making a cartoonlike character whose anger energy was transformed and used to build houses for people in poor countries.

When a child in this age group is diagnosed with cancer, however, caregivers may struggle with what to tell and how much, given their own feelings and fears related to the disease, cultural beliefs and personal/family resources. Because children usually take their psychological clues from their caregivers, it is important that caregivers acknowledge their own emotional distress and seek professional help if they feel overwhelmed or highly distressed. This will benefit not only the caregivers but also the child with cancer and the whole family. During this age period, most children can understand the meaning of their diagnosis and communicate their own thoughts and feelings when given the opportunity.

Importantly, children during this age period can think in concrete terms, and many of them can understand the relation between body and mind, an important concept that will be helpful in understanding their emotional states, and how their emotions relate with thoughts and behavior. Consequently, behavioral techniques and CBT problem-solving strategies can be used to help them and their caregivers manage behavioral issues and fears. Psychological interventions for managing distress have been found effective in improving coping and reducing distress in children, adolescents, and parents. Methodological limitations in these studies, however, reduce the validity of these interventions (Pai et al. 2006; Flowers and Birnie 2015). Early psychological screening and assessment could identify the child's and family's distress and risk as well as the child's competencies and previous experiences with medical procedures such as vaccination. This information will be useful for mobilizing psychosocial resources to help the child and family to cope with the cancer.

8.7.1 Psychological Interventions and Tips to Reduce Distress in School-Aged Children and Their Families

The following are suggestions for psychological interventions for this age group:

- *Psychological support, anticipatory guidance, and psychoeducation* would include specific recommendations to help calm the child and family and gain some control over their emotional state.
- Meeting with a psychosocial professional (e.g., social worker) to *discuss caregivers' concerns regarding changes in the child's behavior* may help to normalize the child's behavior given the circumstances.
- Efforts should be made to create as *predictable an environment* as possible for medical diagnostic and treatment procedures. Knowing what to expect will reassure children and caregivers alike. Caregivers could then prepare the child for clinic visits or specific procedures, which may foster a collaborative relationship to care.
- HCPs should *support and encourage youth and caregivers to utilize available resources in the treatment center or the community* at every stage of the illness and treatment.
- *Foster normal behavior and expectations*, with flexibility, depending on the child's personality, competencies, and wellness. This is important to ensure that the child with cancer continues to develop competently, and unrealistic expectations and entitlements are not fostered during treatment, for example, expecting that other family members continue to do things for them when they are now able to do

them for themselves (i.e., "bring me a glass of water").

- Age-appropriate, *open, and direct communication* is recommended. Some children in this age group may prefer to express their feelings by drawing, which would be a good way to open conversation for further psychological support (see Figs. 8.3 and 8.4). However, it is important to spend time listening to the caregivers' views, beliefs, and concerns regarding sharing information about cancer as they may have different cultural beliefs on this matter. A compromised approach is advisable to foster collaboration with the family, ensuring the best interest of the child.
- *Communication* with children from 4 to 11 years *should be direct*, making sure that the child has the opportunity to ask questions and express his/her views. They need to have the opportunity to be involved as much or as little as possible given the specific procedure and their preferences and the surrounding circumstances.
- As with younger children, it is important to *gain the trust of the child* as soon as possible; this will improve cooperation and facilitate reduction of distress. Art and playing are excellent vehicles to communicate and to maintain the child's interest.
- *Distraction techniques* such as listening to music, blowing bubbles, or watching a favorite video or electronic game are effective distraction techniques for this age group.
- Age-appropriate art and craft materials are also popular with this age group. Making things for other family members or their classmates will *keep them positively involved* and busy during hospitalizations or treatment-related visits, depending on their general energy level and wellness.
- *Light physical activities* (depending on the child's condition) should be encouraged on a daily basis to maintain the body physically active also.
- During this age period, the *child can play a more active role* in selecting what will help him/her with stressful treatment procedures or situations. This can be addressed with or without the caregiver, depending on the child's preferences, and the distress level of both the child and the caregiver during procedures.
- Electronic gadgets or video games could be used either to *keep the child in contact with friends*, classmates, and family members or *to distract the child during painful or stressful procedures*. However, caregivers are encouraged to maintain some "rules" regarding the use of electronics or entertainment (e.g., when, for how long) to minimize abuse of "screen time" (see Box 8.2).
- For most children, like for most caregivers, *the greatest fear* is: "am I going to die" or "is my child going to die?" Children may ask this question, and caregivers need to be prepared to answer it. Depending on the child's disease progression and response to treatment, caregivers need to be able to reassure the child in an honest but positive manner. For example,

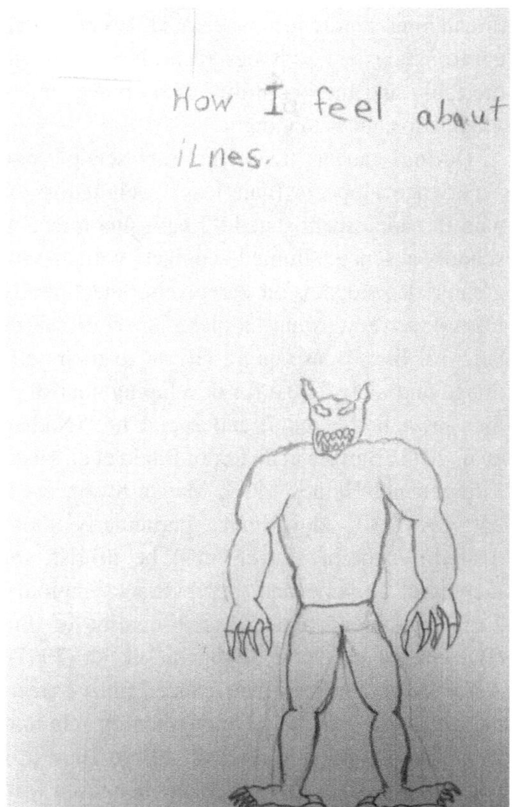

Fig. 8.4 Feelings about cancer, by a 12-year-old boy

they can be told "You are being treated to make the disease go away" or "We are here with you to help you go through treatment." Talking with an HCP (e.g., social worker, psychologist, or palliative care nurse) on the team would help caregivers and the child address this question.

- *Siblings of kids in this age group* can become involved with the affected child by playing, watching videos, or simply spending time together during hospital visits or at home. This will help both the child with cancer and the healthy sibling who will feel included in the patient's life. This will also give everyone a sense of normalcy.
- If possible, if more than one caregiver is available, caregivers should be encouraged to *share care of the child with cancer* to allow the child to continue to develop a trusting relationship with other caregivers, to allow the primary caregiver to spend time at home with healthy siblings if they have other children, and to practice self-care to reduce physical and mental fatigue.
- It is essential to *conduct an assessment of the child's academic and social support* needs initially and during treatment and after treatment to ensure successful school and community reintegration.
- A *school reentry plan* must be part of the comprehensive plan of care, and it should be carefully developed with the HCT, child, caregivers, and school staff and tailored to the child's specific needs. The plan should start shortly after diagnosis to ensure that teachers are informed of the child's condition and progress and to encourage peer support and contact with the ill child throughout the cancer treatment. This will provide the child with a sense of normalcy, social support, and hope for a normal life.
- Encourage family *to return to daily life routines* as soon as possible to avoid developing the role of the "cancer" child. The affected child can be helped to gradually reintegrate to family life; healthy siblings can gradually receive more needed attention from the caregivers, e.g., resuming some chores such as setting the table.
- If behavior and emotional difficulties in the child or family become a serious concern, a *referral to a behavior specialist* who may use CBT, mindfulness, or other strategies for distress reduction.

8.8 Psychological Distress in Adolescents (12–19 Years) and Their Families

There are many changes youth experience when they reach adolescence. These include physiological (hormonal), physical appearance, mental (abstract thinking), emotional (intense and shifting emotions), and social changes (self-image, self-confidence, independence from caregivers, peer group acceptance, romantic relationships, sense of social responsibility). Thus, a cancer diagnosis during this developmentally difficult period can be particularly stressful for the adolescent and his/her family. Given the life-threatening nature of cancer, adolescents also confront existential issues regarding their own mortality and the possibility of becoming infertile due to cancer treatment.

During cancer treatment adolescents may experience alopecia (hair loss), weight loss or gain (an adolescent stated: "I have moon face"), school absence, limited contact with peers, greater dependency on caregivers, and literally loss of privacy. Many adolescents with cancer perceive the disease as an affront to their self-image and a challenge for developing control of their own body, mind, and social life (Nathan et al. 2011; Barrera et al. 2006; Bauld et al. 1998; Ettinger and Heiney 1993; Madan-Swain et al. 2000). These adolescents, particularly those treated for brain cancer, may be at risk for increased anxiety and depression symptoms, social isolation, and reduced quality of life (Barrera et al. 2008; Vannatta et al. 2007). Adolescents also see their cancer and its treatment as a hindrance to develop romantic relationships and dating (Stinson et al. 2015). Thus, it is not surprising that this age group diagnosed with cancer has emerged as especially vulnerable for psychosocial distress and educational and vocational attainment (Erickson et al. 2013; Lown et al. 2015; Nathan et al. 2011; Zebrack et al. 2014; Barrera et al. 2006).

Reports of the Childhood Cancer Survivor Study (CCSS) and the Canadian Childhood Survivor Study described symptoms of psychological distress in the majority of survivors that were equivalent to those of the general population. However, high level of distress and poor academic and social outcomes were associated with a diagnosis of brain cancer, female gender, low household income, treatment with cranial irradiation, and poor physical health status (Barrera et al. 2005; Hudson et al. 2003; Zebrack et al. 2004; Zeltzer et al. 2009). In a recent prospective report examining psychological distress and unmet needs for psychosocial support in adolescents and young adults (AYA) with cancer during the first year of diagnosis, substantially higher clinically significant chronic distress rates were found in AYA with cancer compared to healthy AYA. Additionally, 57% reported unmet needs for information and 41% reported unmet needs for counseling, and these unmet needs were associated with distress overtime (Zebrack et al. 2014). One identified challenge with this population is the poor utilization of existent psychosocial services, which was attributed to AYA being fearful (a) of being stigmatized if they access mental health services or (b) of being perceived as being different from their peers (Zebrack et al. 2014). These findings make the case for better psychoeducation and support of AYA. They also raise concerns regarding the psychological well-being of AYA. Importantly, there are also reports of adolescent survivors of childhood cancer feeling more emotionally mature than their healthy peers (Christiansen et al. 2015).

Caregivers are caught in the middle of their child's transition from childhood to adolescence. Sharing control and decision-making with the adolescent regarding treatment can be a source of conflict in the adolescent-caregiver relationship. In addition to psychological distress, an initial psychological screening can explore the maturity, competencies, and preferences of the adolescent, the adolescent-caregiver relationship, and the family cultural patterns and resources. This initial assessment will help to develop a collaborative and supportive relationship with both, adolescent and caregivers, to support them accordingly. Follow-up psychological screening and assessment will ensure that emerging distress along the course of treatment is addressed adequately.

8.8.1 Psychological Interventions and Tips to Reduce Distress in Adolescents and Their Families

- *Psychological support, anticipatory guidance, and psychoeducation* tailored to adolescents with specific malignancies are recommended. This will help them to understand their condition better, adjust their expectations, and normalize their physiological and distress reactions. Preparing adolescents for treatment and addressing commonly asked questions such as "can I go on dates during treatment?" will contribute to reduction of their distress. When possible, these questions are best addressed with HCPs involved in the adolescent treatment, as the answers can be tailored to the specific adolescent.
- It is recommended that *communication with adolescents and caregivers be open, direct, and private.* Initially, some adolescents may feel more comfortable communicating with the HCPs with their caregivers present. However, they should be given the option of discussing certain issues (e.g., questions about sexuality) privately. Whether they communicate with the HCPs alone or with caregivers present, they should be encouraged to ask questions, express their views, and actively participate in decision-making (see Box 8.3).
- *Communication with adolescents,* as with younger children, some adolescents may need icebreakers initially and may feel more comfortable, for example, drawing how they feel about their disease (see Fig. 8.4). Drawings could be conversation starters. Finding what interests the youth (sports, games, etc.) would help to "break the ice" and to begin establish-

Box 8.3

***Kayla**, a bright and intelligent 17-year-old girl, was recently diagnosed with Hodgkin lymphoma. Shortly after diagnosis, Kayla was convinced that she was "actively dying"; therefore, she didn't see why she should keep receiving chemotherapy. Kayla was regularly experiencing rapid breathing, heart palpitations, dizziness, muscle tension, and abdominal pain. She was referred to psychology because of her inability to cope with her treatment process. After an initial assessment by a psychologist from the team, Kayla was informed that the physical symptoms she was experiencing were not indicative that she was "actively dying," but she was experiencing symptoms of severe anxiety disorder induced by her medical condition. Kayla responded well to initial psychoeducation regarding how she responds to anxiety (physically, cognitively, and behaviorally). As well, Kayla was eager to learn about CBT to assist her in managing her thoughts, feelings, and behaviors. As part of CBT, Kayla was asked to keep a log of her automatic thoughts. Her thought records revealed that she experienced much anxiety and worry about not only her thoughts of "actively dying" but also her inability to finish tasks and projects that she was once engaged in (e.g., fundraiser for animal shelter). Automatic thoughts included concern about how her family, teachers, and friends would perceive her now. Using cognitive restructuring techniques, Kayla became aware of the cognitive distortions she engaged in, such as "jumping to conclusions" and "all-or-nothing thinking." Kayla was given the tools to challenge her cognitive distortions by examining evidence that lead her to develop a more balanced way of thinking. Kayla received information from her oncologist that if she adheres to treatment she has an excellent chance of recovery. Kayla also received evidence from her family, teachers, and friends that they are not disappointed in her inability to lead projects now. Kayla began to express that her cancer diagnosis is a temporary "setback," and although she has cancer, she can still be active and live fully in the present moment.*

ing rapport. It is important, however, to allow youth and caregivers to address their concerns at their own pace to foster trust, ensure the best interest of the adolescent, and support their family relationships.

- As with young children, *the greatest fear* for adolescents is fear of dying; hence, it is important they have the opportunity of addressing the question: "am I going to die?" Depending on the child's disease progression and response to treatment, talking with an HCP (e.g., social worker or psychologist, palliative care physician, or nurse) is recommended if the adolescent does not feel comfortable speaking about this subject with his/her caregivers.
- *Fertility preservation* is an issue that needs to be addressed with youth shortly after diagnosis (Crawshaw et al. 2009). This is a sensitive issue that the adolescent may or may not want to discuss with caregivers present. Thus, it is essential that the adolescent is asked in private, what his or her wishes are. Trained fertility counselors are recommended to adequately deal with this issue and fully answer the adolescent's questions.
- *Age-appropriate art and craft materials* may be of interest for some adolescents, particularly when they spend long periods of time hospitalized. This will serve as distraction from distress and boredom.
- Behavioral or psychosocial experts can help adolescents and caregivers to *explore what they can control*, or what they can do to help with treatment, and to *accept what they cannot change* as they move forward with their "new normal."
- Today, the *use of the Internet* is an integral part of life. This cannot be truer than when we talk about adolescents who typically use social networks like Facebook, Instagram, Snapchat,

FaceTime, and Twitter to keep connected with friends and peers. When an adolescent is undergoing cancer treatment, the social network provided by the Internet can be very helpful, almost a lifeline that can keep him/her connected with friends, peers, and family members. Thus, online communication may reduce access barriers and provide emotional support to the adolescent. This can make a big difference in how well the adolescent, siblings, and caregivers can cope with cancer and the related life disruptions.

- There are *numerous organizations* that have been created specifically *to serve the childhood and AYA community*. Examples of these organizations are the American Childhood Society (www.acs.org) and the Pediatric Oncology Group of Ontario (www.pogo.ca). Most of these organizations use blogs, YouTube, Facebook, and Twitter and can provide links to other platforms that can help youth and their caregivers address specific issues or concerns. For example, Look Good Feel Better for Teens (www.lookgoodfeelbetter.org) provides tips for adolescents dealing with physical appearance; another useful site for adolescents is 2 Be Me (www.2beme.org), a site for adolescents with cancer that provides helpful information regarding their personal care. Starbright World (www.starbrightworld.org) is a virtual hangout where seriously ill adolescents and their siblings can connect with each other via moderated chat rooms, games, bulletin boards, and videos.
- Access to *psychosocial support through adolescent-friendly, face-to-face, by phone, or a safe and private online chat* forum such as "VSee," the world's largest video telemedicine platform. VSee is a HIPAA-compliant telehealth app that aims to make telemedicine simple and secure for healthcare users and their patients around the world (see https://vsee.com for more information).
- Despite the benefits of Internet access, *caution is recommended when using online sources* of information regarding disease and treatment or for support. Adolescents and caregivers are strongly recommended to check whether or not their sources are reputable and to share the information with a treating HCP. Additionally, when blogging or sharing private-personal information (including pictures and videos) online, it is important that privacy protection is checked carefully.
- Using *electronic gadgets or video games could also be helpful as distracting strategies* for coping during painful or stressful procedures. However, HCPs, adolescents, and caregivers need to be aware of the potential negative effect of the abuse of "screen time" (e.g., disruption of sleep patterns, addiction to video games). Thus, adolescents and caregivers are encouraged to negotiate some "rules" regarding the use of electronics (e.g., when, for how long) to minimize abuse of screen time.
- While online contact is helpful, meeting with a *psychosocial professional face to face*, or even by phone, to address psychological distress (mood and behavioral changes, fears) is a valuable option for both, adolescent and caregivers. Normalizing their distress responses and tailoring recommendations for coping with specific stressor or circumstance can be invaluable (see Box 8.3).
- There are a number of *cancer-specific camps* available in many communities, which could be helpful for children and adolescents with cancer and their siblings. Camps provide opportunities for interacting with other youth with cancer in a "normal" fun setting and for sharing information and support. Camps can also help the youth regain self-confident and improve quality of life (Epstein et al. 2005) (see http://www.ooch.org/camp/news--media https://www.youtube.com/watch?v=ew6RIbLmDCM).
- *Siblings usually feel excluded* from the family circle when they have a brother or sister who is undergoing cancer treatment. As with younger children, it is important that siblings become involved with the affected youth. The best way to get siblings involved is by encouraging them to play, watch videos, or simply spend time with the youth with cancer. Some of the camps mentioned above also offer programs for siblings (Epstein et al. 2005) (see http://www.ooch.org/camp/news--media).

These experiences can have beneficial effects for siblings.

- Some treatment centers offer special activities or programs for siblings of children with cancer (see SinCT described above (Barrera et al. 2002, 2004b; Salavati et al. 2014)). Effort should be made to ensure that siblings are provided with the available resources.
- As with younger children, caregivers should be encouraged to *share care of the affected adolescent* if another caregiver is available. This will allow the primary caregiver to spend time with healthy siblings at home and to practice self-care.
- Also as caregivers with younger children, *caregivers* of adolescents should also be provided with *psychological support to manage their distress.*
- *Adventure therapy* has become popular for adolescents with cancer or other chronic illnesses and is offered in many pediatric cancer centers (Epstein 2004; Chung et al. 2014). Although the effectiveness of adventure therapy has not been adequately tested, there are suggestions that it can help participants restore self-esteem and strengthen social connections (Stevens et al. 2004) (see https://www.youtube.com/watch?v=WW20hrIMRsU).
- A *school reentry plan* must be part of comprehensive care for adolescents, and it should be carefully developed in collaboration with the adolescent, caregivers, and school staff.
- Some adolescents may be involved in *romantic relationships* prior to the cancer diagnosis. This relationship can potentially provide strong moral support to the youth. The youth may have questions such as "can I go on dating during treatment?" It is important that caregivers and HCPs are aware and supportive of the adolescent's need for privacy, as he/she integrates the demands of treatment and limitations of the disease into the romantic relationship. Open and direct communication is recommended to ensure that both the adolescent and partner are aware of the limitations related to cancer treatment and well-being of the affected adolescent.

Conclusions

Recent medical advances to improve childhood cancer survivorship have not eliminated the psychological distress in the child and family that inevitably begins at diagnosis. Although psychological distress varies in severity from individual to individual and depends on the disease trajectory, personal characteristics, and contextual family factors, it is at diagnosis when its screening, assessment, and psychological support and intervention must begin for the child or adolescent, caregivers, and siblings. The goals of implementing early assessment and psychological interventions are to prevent escalating psychological distress and to enhance coping and quality of life. There is also evidence of resilience in this population that can be enhanced by targeted interventions. Ongoing periodic assessment of psychological distress and strengths is necessary to allow for recalibration of the psychosocial support for the family, based on need. The degree of psychological support and intervention to ease or prevent psychological distress can vary from minimal to intense and must to be tailored to the needs of the affected child and family. Psychological supports can come from within the family or their social network in the community, the treating center, community organizations, or a combination of all. The success of this process depends on the quality of communication between the family and healthcare providers, based on trusting and respectful relationships. The ultimate aim for youth with cancer and his/her family is to experience minimal psychological distress and maximal quality of life so that they can not only survive cancer, but thrive both during and after treatment.

Acknowledgments We thank the organizations listed in this chapter for granting us permission for publishing their QRs, Dr. Anne Kazak for her inspiration and support of our work, and Kelly Hancock and Alexandra Neville for their assistance in the preparation of this manuscript.

References

Alderfer MA, Mougianis I, Barakat LP, Beele D, DiTaranto S, Hwang WT, Reilley AT, Kazak AE (2009) Family psychosocial risk, distress, and service utilization in pediatric cancer. Cancer 115(S18):4339–4349

Altekruse SF, Kosary CL, Krapcho M, Neyman N, Aminou R, Waldron W, et al. (2010) SEER cancer statistics review, 1975–2007, National Cancer Institute. Bethesda, MD, http://seer.cancer.gov/csr/1975_2007/, based on November 2009 SEER data submission, posted to the SEER web site

Askins MA, Moore BD (2008) Psychosocial support of the pediatric cancer patient: lessons learned over the past 50 years. Curr Oncol Rep 10(6):469–476

Askins MA, Sahler OJZ, Sherman SA, Fairclough DL, Butler RW, Katz ER, Dolgin MJ, Varni JW, Noll RB, Phipps S (2009) Report from a multi-institutional randomized clinical trial examining computer-assisted problem-solving skills training for English-and Spanish-speaking mothers of children with newly diagnosed cancer. J Pediatr Psychol 34(5):551–563

Barlow JH, Ellard DR (2004) Psycho-educational interventions for children with chronic disease, parents and siblings: an overview of the research evidence base. Child Care Health Dev 30(6):637–645

Barrera M (2015) Early warning signs of psychosocial risk in children with cancer and their families. Invited keynote at the Pediatric Oncology Group of Ontario, psychosocial education day, Toronto, ON.Canada; www.pogo.ca

Barrera M, Chung JY, Greenberg M, Fleming C (2002) Preliminary investigation of a group intervention for siblings of pediatric cancer patients. Children's Health Care 31(2):131–142

Barrera M, Wayland LA, D'Agostino NM, Gibson J, Weksberg R, Malkin D (2003) Developmental differences in psychological adjustment and health-related quality of life in pediatric cancer patients. Children's Health Care 32(3):215–232

Barrera M, Hancock K, Rokeach A, Cataudella D, Atenafu E, Johnston D, Punnett A, Nathan PC, Bartels U, Cassidy M, Silva M, Jansen P, Shama W, Greenberg C (2014a) External validity and reliability of the Psychosocial Assessment Tool (PAT2) among Canadian parents of children newly diagnosed with cancer. Pediatr Blood Cancer 61(1):165–170

Barrera M, Hancock K, Rokeach A, Atenafu E, Cataudella D, Punnett A, Johnston D, Cassidy M, Zelcer S, Silva M, Jansen P, Bartels U, Nathan PC, Shama W, Greenberg C (2014b) Does the use of the revised Psychosocial Assessment Tool (PATrev) result in improved quality of life and reduced psychosocial risk in Canadian families with a child newly diagnosed with cancer? Psychooncology 23(2):165–172

Barrera M, Shaw AK, Speechley KN, Maunsell E, Pogany L (2005) Educational and social late effects of childhood cancer and related clinical, personal, and familial characteristics. Cancer 104(8):1751–1760

Barrera M, Damore-Petingola S, Fleming C, Mayer J (2006) Support and intervention groups for adolescents with cancer in two Ontario communities. Cancer 107(S7):1680–1685

Barrera M, Schulte F, Spiegler B (2008) Factors influencing depressive symptoms of children treated for a brain tumor. J Psychosoc Oncol 26(1):1–16

Barrera M, Hancock K, Rokeach A, Cataudella D, Atenafu E, Johnston D et al (2014a) External validity and reliability of the Psychosocial Assessment Tool (PAT2) among Canadian parents of children newly diagnosed with cancer. Pediatr Blood Cancer 61(1):165–170

Barrera M, Hancock K, Rokeach A, Atenafu E, Cataudella D, Punnett A et al (2014b) Does the use of the revised Psychosocial Assessment Tool (PATrev) result in improved quality of life and reduced psychosocial risk in Canadian families with a child newly diagnosed with cancer? Psycho-Oncology 23(2):165–172

Barrera M, Schulte F, Atenafu E, Hancock K, Saleh A, Nathan P (2017) Improvements in symptoms of depression and quality of life in siblings of children with cancer after group intervention participation: a randomized control trial (under review)

Bauld C, Anderson V, Arnold J (1998) Psychosocial aspects of adolescent cancer survival. J Paediatr Child Health 34(2):120–126

Bearden DJ, Feinstein A, Cohen LL (2012) The influence of parent preprocedural anxiety on child procedural pain: Mediation by child procedural anxiety. J Pediatr Psychol 37(6):680–686

Birnie KA, Noel M, Parker JA, Chambers CT, Uman LS, Kisely SR, McGrath PJ (2014) Systematic review and meta-analysis of distraction and hypnosis for needle-related pain and distress in children and adolescents. J Pediatr Psychol 39(8):783–808

Blount RL, Piira T, Cohen LL (2003) Management of pediatric pain and distress due to medical procedures. In: Roberts MC (ed) Handbook of pediatric psychology. The Guilford Press, New York, NY, pp 216–233

Bradlyn AS, Beale IL, Kato PM (2003) Psychoeducational interventions with pediatric cancer patients: part I. Patient information and knowledge. J Child Fam Stud 12(3):257–277

Brannon L, Feist J (2009) Personal coping strategies. In: Health psychology: an introduction to behavior and health, 7th edn. Wadsworth Cengage Learning, Belmont, CA

Brown KW, Ryan RM (2003) The benefits of being present: mindfulness and its role in psychological well-being. J Pers Soc Psychol 84(4):822–848

Caes L, Vervoort T, Devos P, Verlooy J, Benoit Y, Goubert L (2014) Parental distress and catastrophic thoughts about child pain: Implications for parental protective

behavior in the context of child leukemia-related medical procedures. Clin J Pain 30(9):787–799
Carlson LE, Waller A, Mitchell AJ (2012) Screening for distress and unmet needs in patients with cancer: review and recommendations. J Clin Oncol 30(11):1–20
Cassell EJ (1982) The nature of suffering and the goals of medicine. N Engl J Med 306(11):639–645
Chadi N, McMahon A, Vadnais M, Malboeuf-Hurtubise C, Djemli A, Dobkin PL et al (2016) Mindfulness-based intervention for female adolescents with chronic pain: a pilot randomized trial. J Can Acad Child Adolesc Psychiatry 25(3):159–168
Christiansen HL, Bingen K, Hoag JA, Karst JS, Velázquez-Martin B, Barakat LP (2015) Providing children and adolescents opportunities for social interaction as a standard of care in pediatric oncology. Pediatr Blood Cancer 62(S5):S674–S699
Chung OKJ, Li HCW, Chiu SY, Ho KY, Lopez V (2014) Sustainability of an integrated adventure-based training and health education program to enhance quality of life among Chinese childhood cancer survivors: a randomized controlled trial. Cancer Nurs 38(5):366–374
Cohen LL, Lemanek K, Blount RL, Dahlquist LM, Lim CS, Palermo TM, McKenna KD, Weiss KE (2008) Evidence-based assessment of pediatric pain. J Pediatr Psychol 33(9):939–955
Compas BE, Jaser SS, Dunn MJ, Rodriguez EM (2012) Coping with chronic illness in childhood and adolescence. Annu Rev Clin Psychol 8:455–480
Compas BE, Desjardins L, Vannatta K, Young-Saleme T, Rodriguez EM, Dunn M, Bemis H, Snyder S, Gerhardt CA (2014) Children and adolescents coping with cancer: self-and parent reports of coping and anxiety/depression. Health Psychol 33(8):853–861
Crawshaw MA, Glaser AW, Hale JP, Sloper P (2009) Male and female experiences of having fertility matters raised alongside a cancer diagnosis during the teenage and young adult years. Eur J Canc Care 18(4):381–390
Derogatis LR (2001) Brief Symptom Inventory (BSI)-18. Administration, scoring and procedures manual. NCS Pearson, Inc., Minneapolis
D'Zurilla TJ, Goldfried MR (1971) Problem solving and behavior modification. J Abnorm Psychol 78(1):107–126
D'Zurilla TJ, Nezu AM (2007) Problem-solving therapy: A positive approach to clinical intervention, 3rd edn. Springer Publishing, New York, NY
Epstein I (2004) Adventure therapy: a mental health promotion strategy in pediatric oncology. J Pediatr Oncol Nurs 21(2):103–110
Epstein I, Stinson J, Stevens B (2005) The effects of camp on health-related quality of life in children with chronic illnesses: a review of the literature. J Pediatr Oncol Nurs 22(2):89–103
Erickson JM, MacPherson CF, Ameringer S, Baggott C, Linder L, Stegenga K (2013) Symptoms and symptom clusters in adolescents receiving cancer treatment: A review of the literature. Int J Nurs Stud 50(6):847–869
Ettinger RS, Heiney SP (1993) Cancer in adolescents and young adults. Psychosocial concerns, coping strategies, and interventions. Cancer 71(S10):3276–3280
Ewing LJ, Long K, Rotondi A, Howe C, Bill L, Marsland AL (2009) Brief report: a pilot study of a web-based resource for families of children with cancer. J Pediatr Psychol 34(5):523–529
Fagerlind H, Kettis Å, Glimelius B, Ring L (2013) Barriers against psychosocial communication: oncologists' perceptions. *J Clin Oncol* 31(30):3815–3822
Fedele DA, Hullmann SE, Chaffin M, Kenner C, Fisher MJ, Kirk K, Eddington AR, Phipps S, McNall-Knapp RY, Mullins LL (2013) Impact of a parent-based interdisciplinary intervention for mothers on adjustment in children newly diagnosed with cancer. J Pediatr Psychol 38(5):531–540
Ferguson E, O'Connor S, Caldwell F, Knowles S, Carney T, House E, O'Connor R (2010) The Paediatric Index of Emotional Distress (PI-ED): A new index for 8–16 years olds. Psychol Health 25:32–33
Flowers SR, Birnie KA (2015) Procedural preparation and support as a standard of care in pediatric oncology. Pediatr Blood Cancer 62(S5):S668–S697
Folkman S, Lazarus RS (1988) The relationship between coping and emotion: Implications for theory and research. Soc Sci Med 26(3):309–317
Gerhardt CA, Lehmann V, Long KA, Alderfer MA (2015) Supporting siblings as a standard of care in pediatric oncology. Pediatr Blood Cancer 62(S5):S678–S732
Gotink RA, Chu P, Busschbach J, Benson H, Fricchione GL, Hunink M (2015) Standardised mindfulness-based interventions in healthcare: an overview of systematic reviews and meta-analyses of RCTs. PLoS ONE 10(4):1–17
Graf A, Bergstraesser E, Landolt MA (2013) Posttraumatic stress in infants and preschoolers with cancer. Psycho-Oncology 22(7):1543–1548
Greenberg ML, Barnett H, Williams J (2015) Atlas of childhood cancer in Ontario 1985–2004. Pediatric Oncology Group of Ontario. http://www.pogo.ca/wp-content/uploads/2015/09/POGO_CC-Atlas-1985-2004_Full-Report-2015.pdf. Accessed 26 May 2016
Greer JA, Park ER, Prigerson HG, Safren SA (2010) Tailoring cognitive-behavioral therapy to treat anxiety comorbid with advanced cancer. J Cogn Psychother 24(4):294–313
Haverman L, van Oers HA, Limperg PF, Houtzager BA, Huisman J, Darlington AS, Maurice-Stamm H, Grootenhuis MA (2013) Development and validation of the distress thermometer for parents of a chronically ill child. J Pediatr 163(4):1140–1146
Holland JC (2010) Psycho-oncology. Oxford University Press, New York, NY
Hudson MM, Mertens AC, Yasui Y, Hobbie W, Chen H, Gurney JG, Yeazel M, Recklitis CJ, Marina N, Robison LR, Oeffinger KC (2003) Health status of adult long-term survivors of childhood cancer: a report from the Childhood Cancer Survivor Study. JAMA 290(12):1583–1592

Kabat-Zinn J (1990) Full catastrophe living: using the wisdom of your body and mind to face stress, pain, and illness. Dell Publishing, New York, NY

Kallapiran K, Koo S, Kirubakarn R, Hancock K (2015) Review: effectiveness of mindfulness in improving mental health symptoms of children and adolescents: a meta-analysis. Child Adolesc Mental Health 20(4):182–194

Kaminski M, Pellino T, Wish J (2002) Play and pets: the physical and emotional impact of child-life and pet therapy on hospitalized children. Children's Health Care 31(4):321–335

Karlsson K, Englund ACD, Enskär K, Rydström I (2014) Parents' perspectives on supporting children during needle-related medical procedures. Int J Qualitative Stud Health Well-being 9(1):23063

Kazak AE (2006) Pediatric Psychosocial Preventative Health Model (PPPHM): research, practice, and collaboration in pediatric family systems medicine. Families Systems Health 24(4):381–395

Kazak AE, Baxt C (2007) Families of infants and young children with cancer: a post-traumatic stress framework. Pediatr Blood Cancer 49(S7):1109–1113

Kazak AE, Simms S, Barakat L, Hobbie W, Foley B, Golomb V, Best M (1999) Surviving Cancer Competently Intervention Program (SCCIP): a cognitive-behavioral and family therapy intervention for adolescent survivors of childhood cancer and their families. Family Process 38(2):176–191

Kazak AE, Prusak A, McSherry M, Simms S, Beele D, Rourke M, Alderfer M, Lange B (2001) The Psychosocial Assessment Tool (PAT)©: pilot data on a brief screening instrument for identifying high risk families in pediatric oncology. Fam Syst Health 19(3):303

Kazak AE, Alderfer M, Rourke MT, Simms S, Streisand R, Grossman JR (2004) Posttraumatic stress disorder (PTSD) and posttraumatic stress symptoms (PTSS) in families of adolescent childhood cancer survivors. J Pediatr Psychol 29(3):211–219

Kazak AE, Simms S, Alderfer MA, Rourke MT, Crump T, McClure K, Jones P, Rodriguez A, Boeving A, Hwang WT, Reilly A (2005) Feasibility and preliminary outcomes from a pilot study of a brief psychological intervention for families of children newly diagnosed with cancer. J Pediatr Psychol 30(8):644–655

Kazak AE, Barakat LP, Hwang WT, Ditaranto S, Biros D, Beele D, Kersun L, Hocking MC, Reilly A (2011) Association of psychosocial risk screening in pediatric cancer with psychosocial services provided. Psychooncology 20(7):715–723

Kazak AE, Brier M, Alderfer MA, Reilly A, Fooks Parker S, Rogerwick S, Ditaranto S, Barakat LP (2012) Screening for psychosocial risk in pediatric cancer. Pediatr Blood Cancer 59(5):822–827

Kazak AE, Abrams AN, Banks J, Christofferson J, DiDonato S, Grootenhuis MA, Kabour M, Madan-Swain A, Patel SK, Zadeh S, Kupst MJ (2015a) Psychosocial assessment as a standard of care in pediatric cancer. Pediatr Blood Cancer 62(S5):S426–S459

Kazak AE, Schneider S, Didonato S, Pai ALH (2015b) Family psychosocial risk screening guided by the pediatric psychosocial preventative health model (PPPHM) using the Psychosocial Assessment Tool (PAT). Acta Oncol 54(5):574–580

Kearney JA, Salley CG, Muriel AC (2015) Standards of psychosocial care for parents of children with cancer. Pediatr Blood Cancer 62(S5):S632–S683

Khaddouma A, Gordon KC, Bolden J (2015) Mindful M&M's mindfulness and parent training for a preschool child with disruptive behavior disorder. Clinical Case Studies 14(6):407–421

Knaul FM, Ortega SX, Fernández CJ, Suárez VM (2006) Inclusión Educativa Para Niños, Niñas Y Jóvenes Hospitalizados: Un Análisis Basado En El Programa Nacional De México. Imprenta Nacional, Mexico, DF.

Krikorian A, Limonero JT, Maté J (2012) Suffering and distress at the end-of-life. Psycho-Oncology 21(8):799–808

Kuo DZ, Houtrow AJ, Arango P, Kuhlthau KA, Simmons JM, Neff JM (2012) Family-centered care: current applications and future directions in pediatric health care. Matern Child Health J 16(2):297–305

Kwak M, Zebrack BJ, Meeske KA, Embry L, Aguilar C, Block R et al (2013) Trajectories of psychological distress in adolescent and young adult patients with cancer: a 1-year longitudinal study. J Clin Oncol 31(17):2160–2166

Lazarus RS, Folkman S (1984) Stress, appraisal, and coping. Springer Publishing Company, New York, NY

Linge L (2013) Joyful and serious intentions in the work of hospital clowns: a meta-analysis based on a 7-year research project conducted in three parts. Int J Qual Studies Health Well-being 8:1–8

Long KA, Marsland AL (2011) Family adjustment to childhood cancer: a systematic review. Clin Child Fam Psychol Rev 14(1):57–88

Lown EA, Phillips F, Schwartz LA, Rosenberg AR, Jones B (2015) Psychosocial follow-up in survivorship as a standard of care in pediatric oncology. Pediatr Blood Cancer 62(S5):S531–S601

MacKay LJ, Gregory D (2011) Exploring family-centered care among pediatric oncology nurses. J Pediatr Oncol Nurs 28(1):43–52

Madan-Swain A, Brown RT, Foster MA, Vega R, Byars K, Rodenberger W, Bell B, Lambert R (2000) Identity in adolescent survivors of childhood cancer. J Pediatr Psychol 25(2):105–115

March JS, Parker JD, Sullivan K, Stallings P, Conners CK (1997) The Multidimensional Anxiety Scale for Children (MASC): factor structure, reliability, and validity. J the Am Acad Child Adolesc Psychiatr 36(4):554–565

Masten AS (2001) Ordinary magic: resilience processes in development. Am Psychol 56(3):227–238

McCarthy MC, Clarke NE, Vance A, Ashley DM, Heath JA, Anderson VA (2009) Measuring psychosocial risk in families caring for a child with cancer: the psychosocial assessment tool (PAT2. 0). Pediatr Blood Cancer 53(1):78–83

Mitchell W, Clarke S, Sloper P (2005) Survey of psychosocial support provided by UK paediatric oncology centres. Arch Dis Child 90(8):796–800

Montgomery K, Sawin KJ, Hendricks-Ferguson VL (2016) Experiences of pediatric oncology patients and their parents at end of life: A systematic review. J Pediatr Oncol Nurs 33(2):85–104

Nathan PC, Hayes-Lattin B, Sisler JJ, Hudson MM (2011) Critical issues in transition and survivorship for adolescents and young adults with cancers. Cancer 117(S10):2335–2341

National Cancer Institute (2015) A snapshot of pediatric cancers. http://www.cancer.gov/research/progress/snapshots/pediatric. Accessed 23 June 2016

National Comprehensive Cancer Network (2014) NCCN clinical practice guidelines in oncology: distress management. http://williams.medicine.wisc.edu/distress.pdf. Accessed 24 May 2016

Okado Y, Long AM, Phipps S (2014) Association between parent and child distress and the moderating effects of life events in families with and without a history of pediatric cancer. J Pediatr Psychol 39(9):1049–1060

Otto MW, Smits JA, Reese HE (2004) Cognitive-behavioral therapy for the treatment of anxiety disorders. J Clin Psychiatry 65:34–41

Pai AL, Drotar D, Zebracki K, Moore M, Youngstrom E (2006) A meta-analysis of the effects of psychological interventions in pediatric oncology on outcomes of psychological distress and adjustment. J Pediatr Psychol 31(9):978–988

Pai AL, Patiño-Fernández AM, McSherry M, Beele D, Alderfer MA, Reilly AT, Hwang WT, Kazak AE (2008) The Psychosocial Assessment Tool (PAT2. 0): psychometric properties of a screener for psychosocial distress in families of children newly diagnosed with cancer. J Pediatr Psychol 33(1):50–62

Patel SK, Fernandez N, Wong AL, Mullins W, Turk A, Dekel N, Smith M, Ferrell B (2014) Changes in self-reported distress in end-of-life pediatric cancer patients and their parents using the pediatric distress thermometer. Psychooncology 23(5):592–596

Patenaude AF, Kupst MJ (2005) Psychosocial functioning in pediatric cancer. J Pediatr Psychol 30(1):9–27

Patenaude AF, Pelletier W, Bingen K (2015) Communication, documentation, and training standards in pediatric psychosocial oncology. Pediatr Blood Cancer 62(S5):S870–S895

Quirino DD, Collet N (2012) Cancer among infants: adjustments in family life. *Texto & Contexto-Enfermagem 21*(2):295–303

Rapoport A, Weingarten K (2014) Improving quality of life in hospitalized children. Pediatr Clin N Am 61(4):749–760

Rhondali W, Lasserre E, Filbert M (2013) Art therapy among palliative care inpatients with advanced cancer. Palliat Med 27(6):571–572

Rodriguez EM, Dunn MJ, Zuckerman T, Vannatta K, Gerhardt CA, Compas BE (2012) Cancer-related sources of stress for children with cancer and their parents. J Pediatr Psychol 37(2):185–197

Rokeach A, Hancock K, Schulte F, Atenafu E, Nathan P, Barrera M (2014) Reduction of anxiety level in parents and siblings of children with cancer after sibling participation in a psychosocial group intervention: a randomized controlled trial. In: Oral Presentation at the 46th Congress of the International Society of Paediatric Oncology. ON, Toronto

Rolland JS, Walsh F (2006) Facilitating family resilience with childhood illness and disability. Curr Opin Pediatr 18(5):527–538

Rosenberg AR, Dussel V, Kang T, Geyer JR, Gerhardt CA, Feudtner C, Wolfe J (2013) Psychological distress in parents of children with advanced cancer. JAMA Pediatr 167(6):537–543

Rouleau CR, Garland SN, Carlson LE (2015) The impact of mindfulness-based interventions on symptom burden, positive psychological outcomes, and biomarkers in cancer patients. Cancer Manag Res 7:121–131

Roy CA, Russell RC (2000) Case study: possible traumatic stress disorder in an infant with cancer. J Am Acad Child Adolesc Psychiatry 39(2):257–260

Sahler OJZ, Fairclough DL, Phipps S, Mulhern RK, Dolgin MJ, Noll RB, Katz ER, Varni JW, Copeland DR, Butler RW (2005) Using problem-solving skills training to reduce negative affectivity in mothers of children with newly diagnosed cancer: report of a multisite randomized trial. J Consult Clin Psychol 73(2):272–283

Sahler OJZ, Dolgin MJ, Phipps S, Fairclough DL, Askins MA, Katz ER, Noll RB, Butler RW (2013) Specificity of problem-solving skills training in mothers of children newly diagnosed with cancer: results of a multisite randomized clinical trial. J Clin Oncol 31(10):1329–1335

Salavati B, Seeman MV, Agha M, Atenafu E, Chung J, Nathan PC, Barrera M (2014) Which siblings of children with cancer benefit most from support groups? Children's Health Care 43(3):221–233

Sameroff AJ, Emde RN (1989) Relational disturbances in early childhood: A developmental approach. Basic Books, New York, NY

Scheeringa MS, Zeanah CH (1995) Symptom expression and trauma variables in children under 48 months of age. Infant Ment Health J 16(4):259–270

Schneider-Rosen K (1990) The developmental reorganization of attachment relationships. In: Greenberg MT, Cicchetti D, Cummings EM (eds) Attachment in the preschool years: theory, research and intervention. The University of Chicago Press, Chicago, IL, pp 185–220

Segal Z, Williams M, Teasdale J (2013) Mindfulness-based cognitive therapy for depression. The Guilford Press, New York, NY

Selove R, Kroll T, Coppes M, Cheng Y (2012) Psychosocial services in the first 30 days after diagnosis: results of a web-based survey of children's oncology group (COG) member institutions. Pediatr Blood Cancer 58(3):435–440

Sourkes BM (1995) Armfuls of time: the psychological experience of the child with a life-threatening illness. University of Pittsburgh Press, Pittsburgh, PA
Steele RG, Long A, Reddy KA, Luhr M, Phipps S (2003) Changes in maternal distress and child-rearing strategies across treatment for pediatric cancer. J Pediatr Psychol 28(7):447–452
Steele AC, Mullins LL, Mullins AJ, Muriel AC (2015) Psychosocial interventions and therapeutic support as a standard of care in pediatric oncology. Pediatr Blood Cancer 62(S5):S585–S618
Stevens B, Kagan S, Yamada J, Epstein I, Beamer M, Bilodeau M, Baruchel S (2004) Adventure therapy for adolescents with cancer. *Pediatr Blood Cancer 43*(3):278–284
Stinson JN, Jibb LA, Greenberg M, Barrera M, Luca S, White ME, Gupta A (2015) A qualitative study of the impact of cancer on romantic relationships, sexual relationships, and fertility: perspectives of Canadian adolescents and parents during and after treatment. J Adolesc Young Adult Oncol 4(2):84–90
Tan L (2016) A critical review of adolescent mindfulness-based programmes. Clin Child Psychol Psychiatry 21(2):193–207
Thompson AL, Young-Saleme TK (2015) Anticipatory guidance and psychoeducation as a standard of care in pediatric oncology. Pediatr Blood Cancer 62(S5):S684–S693
Treurnicht Naylor K, Kingsnorth S, Lamont A, McKeever P, Macarthur C (2011) The effectiveness of music in pediatric healthcare: a systematic review of randomized controlled trials. Evid Based Complementary Altern Med 2011:464759
Uman LS, Birnie KA, Noel M, Parker JA, Chambers CT, McGrath PJ, Kisely SR (2013) Psychological interventions for needle-related procedural pain and distress in children and adolescents. Cochrane Database Syst Rev 10:1–135
Vannatta K, Gerhardt C, Wells R, Noll R (2007) Intensity of CNS treatment for pediatric cancer: predictors of social outcomes in survivors. Pediatr Blood Cancer 49:716–722
Vannatta K, Salley CG, Gerhardt CA (2009) Pediatric oncology: progress and future challenges. In: Roberts MC, Steele RG (eds) Handbook of pediatric psychology. The Guilford Press, New York, NY, pp 319–333
Varni JW, Sahler OJ, Katz ER, Mulhern RK, Copeland DR, Noll RB (1999) Maternal problem-solving therapy in pediatric cancer. J Psychosoc Oncol 16(3–4):41–71
Varni JW, Limbers CA, Burwinkle TM (2007) How young can children reliably and validly self-report their health-related quality of life? An analysis of 8,591 children across age subgroups with the PedsQL™ 4.0 Generic Core Scales. Health Qual Life Outcomes 5(1):1
Vernon L, Eyles D, Hulbert C, Bretherton L, McCarthy MC (2016) Infancy and pediatric cancer: an exploratory study of parent psychological distress. Psycho-Oncology 26(3):361–368
Weaver MS, Heinze KE, Kelly KP, Wiener L, Casey RL, Bell CJ, Wolfe J, Garee AM, Watson A, Hinds PS (2015) Palliative care as a standard of care in pediatric oncology. Pediatr Blood Cancer 62(S5):S829–S833
Wiener L, Pao M (2012) Comprehensive and family-centered psychosocial care in pediatric oncology: Integration of clinical practice and research. In: Kreitler S, Ben-Arush MW, Martin A (eds) Pediatric psycho-oncology: psychosocial aspects and clinical interventions, 2nd edn. John Wiley & Sons, Ltd., Chichester, UK, pp 7–17
Wikström BM (2005) Communicating via expressive arts: The natural medium of self-expression for hospitalized children. Pediatr Nurs 31(6):480–485
Wilson JM (2006) Child life services. Pediatrics 118(4):1757–1763
Wood AW, Gonzalez J, Barden SM (2015) Mindful caring: using mindfulness-based cognitive therapy with caregivers of cancer survivors. J Psychosoc Oncol 33(1):66–84
Zadeh S (2015) The development of a pediatric screen: next generation distress thermometer? Presented at the 2015 World Congress of Psycho-Oncology, Washington, Washington, DC
Zebrack BJ, Gurney JG, Oeffinger K, Whitton J, Packer RJ, Mertens A, Terk N, Castleberry R, Dreyer Z, Robison LL, Zeltzer LK (2004) Psychological outcomes in long-term survivors of childhood brain cancer: a report from the childhood cancer survivor study. J Clin Oncol 22(6):999–1006
Zebrack BJ, Corbett V, Embry L, Aguilar C, Meeske KA, Hayes-Lattin B, Block R, Zeman DT, Cole S (2014) Psychological distress and unsatisfied need for psychosocial support in adolescent and young adult cancer patients during the first year following diagnosis. Psychooncology 23(11):1267–1275
Zeltzer LK, Recklitis C, Buchbinder D, Zebrack B, Casillas J, Tsao JC, Lu Q, Krull K (2009) Psychological status in childhood cancer survivors: a report from the Childhood Cancer Survivor Study. J Clin Oncol 27(14):2396–2404
Zigmond AS, Snaith RP (1983) The hospital anxiety and depression scale. Acta Psychiatr Scand 67(6):361–370

Easing Existential Distress in Pediatric Cancer Care

9

Jennifer Currin-McCulloch, Tullio Proserpio, Marta Podda, and Carlo Alfredo Clerici

Key Points

Spiritual care providers should conduct activities with patients, family members, the people close to them, visitors, and staff, for the purposes of:

1. Affirming and defending the value and dignity of every person
2. Discussing the spiritual dimension of suffering, illness, and death
3. Highlighting the power of spiritual healing and growth
4. Helping to determine the spiritual needs of all faith traditions
5. Endeavoring to protect patients and their families from undue spiritual distress
6. Offering spiritual accompaniment
7. Ensuring religious worship when requested
8. Offering a service when requested
9. Organizing and participating in teaching programs
10. Promoting mediation and reconciliation
11. Supporting and participating in research programs about spiritual care
12. Assessing the efficiency and effectiveness of spiritual care

J. Currin-McCulloch (✉)
University of Texas at Austin, Austin, TX, USA
e-mail: jcurrinmcculloch@utexas.edu

T. Proserpio
Cappellania Ospedaliera, Fondazione IRCCS Istituto Nazionale Tumori di Milano, Milan, Italy

Methodist Research Institute, Houston, TX, USA
e-mail: Tullio.Proserpio@istitutotumori.mi.it

M. Podda
SC Pediatria, Fondazione IRCCS Istituto Nazionale Tumori, Milano, Milan, Italy

C.A. Clerici
SS Psicologia, Fondazione IRCCS Istituto Nazionale Tumori, Milano, Milan, Italy

Dipartimento di Oncologia e Ematologia, Università degli Studi di Milano, Milan, Italy

9.1 The Integration of Spirituality into Healthcare

Awareness of the need for global care of those facing a serious illness is widely acknowledged, and even expected, but up until a few decades ago, these aspects were not routinely considered. The emphasis on assessment and care of patients' spiritual well-being in palliative care settings emerged during the early 1990s (Puchalski et al. 2009). Healthcare teams began to recognize the implications of spiritual crises on both the patient and family system and began to integrate spiritual assessments, care plans, and spiritual care providers into the multidisciplinary care of patients and families (Astrow et al. 2001; Puchalski et al. 2009). In palliative care, spiritual care providers play an integral role at the bedside in supporting patients and families with their spiritual and existential concerns while also

J. Wolfe et al. (eds.), *Palliative Care in Pediatric Oncology*, Pediatric Oncology,
https://doi.org/10.1007/978-3-319-61391-8_9

advocating for spiritual care needs within multidisciplinary teams (Proserpio et al. 2011).

It is important to recognize that spirituality and religiosity hold different meanings and values for individuals. To clarify the terminology and use in this chapter, the authors provide definitions for each concept. The consensus conference defined spirituality as "the aspect of humanity that refers to the way individuals seek and express meaning and purpose and the way they experience their connectedness to the moment, to self, to others, to nature, and to the significant or sacred" (Puchalski et al. 2009, p 887). According to Puchalski et al. (2009), each of us has a spiritual history that may or may not include religious traditions but, rather, may include significant experiences of philosophical principles. Religion can be seen as "differentiated by particular beliefs and practices, requirements of membership, and modes of social organization" (Miller and Thoresen 2003). The authors have chosen to utilize the word spirituality throughout the chapter to describe an individual's overall approach to finding meaning in the world since it promotes the broadest context of meaning and also encompasses the domains of religion and faith.

Spirituality, in the broadest sense of the term, has gained acceptance and received significant attention within the practice of pediatric palliative care and in social science research. Recent studies and reviews (Meireles et al. 2015; Purow et al. 2011; Kamper et al. 2010; Petersen 2014) have confirmed the benefits of addressing spiritual concerns. In periods of great stress, spirituality can provide comfort as well as hope (Kamper et al. 2010). Defining the precise meaning of the construct of hope is anything but easy (Proserpio et al. 2014), but hope is described here as a protective factor that can sustain resilience, in addition to upholding the dignity of life, particularly among people with cancer (Hendricks-Ferguson 2006; Haase et al. 2014). Spirituality also offers families comfort, peace, and a sense of control when facing the whirlwind of challenges that a life-threatening illness creates (Hexem et al. 2011; Schneider and Mannell 2006; Knapp et al. 2011; McSherry et al. 2007).

Spiritual care providers operate in a culture of evidence-based medical care, which can present challenges to provision of spiritual care. In many health settings and hospitals, spiritual care providers, who have received specialized training in the spiritual and existential care of patients and families, oversee this aspect of patients' and families' well-being (Koenig 2012). However, many barriers stand in the way of these spiritual care providers in meeting the needs of their patients. A survey of pastoral care providers in a large pediatric hospital (Feudtner et al. 2003) portrayed three main barriers that prevented them from providing care to children and their families: inadequate numbers of spiritual care staff to cover the hospital; a lack of specialized training to detect children and families' needs within a hospital setting; and delayed referrals to visit children and their families, often not until the very last moments of life. The same study shared spiritual care providers' concerns that staffing limitations only allowed them to see families in the intensive care units or in acute crises. The spiritual care providers highlight the benefits of meeting with patients and families earlier in their care trajectory to foster relationships and to screen for potential existential and spiritual crises (Feudtner et al. 2003).

Spiritual care providers may also face barriers in collaborating within their team or the healthcare system. Although the benefits of incorporating spiritual and religious care in healthcare systems are known, there are often barriers to integrating different specialties and perspectives. Knowledge and perspectives do not necessarily oppose each other, because they all aim to benefit the patient and family, but sometimes, obstacles arise in collaboration. Greater dialogue between multiple professionals can enhance spiritual care. Ideally, the spiritual care provider collaborates with the behavioral health specialists on the team and with the patient and family's spiritual support system outside of the healthcare system. Thus, the interdisciplinary team can work together to assess and respond to these needs to provide exceptional patient and family-centered spiritual care.

The notion of a genuine integration between disciplines for mental health (psychology, social work, and psychiatry) and spiritual and religious practices is complex. Robinson et al. (2006) described the role of non-trained individuals on the healthcare team as spiritual generalists and those with specialized spiritual care training as spiritual care specialists. One easy way for spiritual generalists to open dialogues about spiritual history with children and families is by introducing a simple question such as, "Is spirituality or religion a part of your life?" Doctors, nurses, social workers, and psychologists can gather spiritual histories from families that identify their spiritual/religious practices, their sources of strength, and how to nourish those resources; however, trained spiritual care providers should perform more extensive spiritual assessments (Puchalski et al. 2009). The detailed spiritual assessments, unlike the survey-like measures of spiritual histories, require specialized training and listening skills aimed at soliciting stories about the person's life, spirituality or religion, and its place in their lives (Puchalski et al. 2009). Other reasons for referral to a trained spiritual care provider include requests for prayer and sacraments; perspectives of faith to support medical decisions; or when patient or family demonstrate signs of spiritual distress or have interfaith family disagreements (Robinson et al. 2006; Purow et al. 2011).

9.2 Spiritual and Psychosocial Issues in Pediatric Palliative Care

Joann, a 16-year-old girl, learned that she had osteosarcoma, a cancer of the bone, after having a fall on her arm during a high school softball tournament. She had been feeling some pain and fatigue but assumed it was from the hours of training in preparation for the upcoming tournament. Since they lived in a rural community with limited healthcare access, her care was transferred to a specialty children's hospital 4 h away from their home. Her mother left her job and came to the hospital to be with her daughter, leaving at home a 13-year-old son and husband. After the many tests, scans, and doctor's assessments, Joann and her mother learned that her cancer was terminal, having spread throughout both lungs. Joann and her mom set up temporary residence in an apartment by the hospital and started an intensive treatment course of surgery, chemotherapy, and radiation. For several months, Joann struggled with pain, fatigue, sadness about her lost arm, and being away from her friends from school and softball. She knew that she would never be able to play softball again, shattering her visions of the future. Her mom expressed her fears to the medical team that Joann's health appeared to be declining rapidly. She missed her husband and worried about their son since he is having trouble in school, missed his sister tremendously, and started raising questions about what would happen when his sister died. Four months into treatment, the doctors told Joann and her mom that the treatments did not work as hoped and that they did not have any more treatments to stop the growth of her cancer. Joann shared with the hospital chaplain that she could sense what was happening and had accepted her future; however, she worried that her mom, dad, and little brother would have trouble with her death and asked for the medical teams' guidance in preparing her family for her death.

The diagnosis of cancer or other life-threatening conditions places families in a world of uncertainty, grasping for knowledge, comfort, and security. When a child enters the hospital with a serious illness, both children and their family members must quickly embrace the medical system, learn about treatment options, and navigate relationships with multiple healthcare providers while also attempting to keep stability and hope within their family system (Jones 2006). In addition to the enormity of their healthcare crisis, families spend extended periods of time away from home, therefore, losing connection with the social and spiritual support systems that usually provide solace (Jones 2012). Even families with many resources and resilient coping mechanisms may experience existential and spiritual crises as they attempt to adapt and explore resilience amidst the new challenges placed before them (Jones and Weisenfluh 2003).

When faced with the uncertainty of a serious illness, one's beliefs about the world and their health are challenged, often leaving them questioning the reason for their illness, the outlook for their future, and even their faith (McSherry et al. 2007; Mishel 1988). As a child or adolescent and their family attempt to assimilate the knowledge of their illness into their cognitive schema, they may struggle to find meaning in their illness and experience spiritual or existential distress. Common spiritual aspects of existential distress revolve around meaning-making, loss of purpose, and questions seeking understanding such as "Why me?" or "What am I meant to do with my life?" (Boston et al. 2011). Non-spiritual existential concerns emphasize a personal sense of hopelessness, isolation, and identity confusion (Boston et al. 2011). Through the process of discovering meaning and transcendence through challenging experiences, individuals may feel a diminishing sense of burden from their suffering (Cassel 1982).

Early studies on existential meaning-making started with the research of Viktor Frankl. As a psychologist and survivor of the holocaust, he transformed his experiences into theories of how survivors of trauma can find meaning from crises. The basic premise of Frankl's logotherapy claims that man's primary motivational force is his drive to discover meaning in life (Frankl 1992). He believed that incurable diseases, such as inoperable cancer, require individuals to face a challenge and adjust their cognitive schema to adapt to their illness.

Within pediatric palliative care, variance exists between institutions in how they assess and deliver spiritual care to their patients and families. Petersen (2014) performed a review of research in this field and identified six main themes in the provision of spiritual care for children at the end of life: "assessing the child's spiritual needs; assisting the child to express feelings and concerns; guiding the child in strengthening relationships; helping the child be remembered; aiding the child to find hope; and assisting the child to find meaning and purpose" (p 1246). Other pediatric health literature describes the incorporation of the BELIEF mnemonic as a way of assisting pediatric providers in opening conversations with youth about their spiritual well-being. The aspects of the mnemonic include: "B-Belief System; E-Ethics; L-Lifestyle; I-Involvement in a Spiritual Community; E-Education; and F-Future Events" (McEvoy 2000, p 217). By engaging children and adolescents around these six realms of spiritual life, providers can gather a better understanding of whether and how spirituality affects their daily lives.

Many of the concerns of children with life-threatening illnesses revolve around their worries about their family's well-being. They worry about how their parents or siblings will react to their loss or that once they have died, will they be remembered (Jones and Weisenfluh 2003). They may fear the physical symptoms associated with end of life such as pain or dying alone. It is important that the child is reassured with respect to these fears and the parents and those dear to the child can be close to them at the moment of death (Meert et al. 2005).

Spiritual distress can manifest itself in various ways. Some children are very clear about the origin of their feelings, while others, due to development abilities or psychosocial reasons, may be unaware or questioning the emotional and/or spiritual dimensions of their experience of the illness. Often the greatest sign of spiritual suffering is the constant feeling of despair, questioning, or spiritual restlessness (McSherry et al. 2007). The multidisciplinary expertise of the healthcare team can help to determine whether the unease is a result of physical, emotional, social, or spiritual origin. These needs may be addressed by mental health experts as well as spiritual experts, but only by working together can teams constructively help the patient and family.

Most of the studies of children's spiritual well-being incorporate qualitative research methods. Bull et al. (2007) showed children with life-threatening conditions cards with scenes of youth with physical impairments in medical settings to gather their descriptions about the children's lives and listen for their expressions of spirituality. From these storytelling interactions, children depicted the youth on the cards, who seemingly were in similar situations, with words like anxiety, pain, hell, and being scared. Kamper et al. (2010) utilized findings from within another qualitative study of children with advanced cancer to gather further understanding of what brings meaning and spiritual quality of life to children with advanced cancer. Children reported that knowing someone cares and playing a video game on the computer makes them happy. More than half of the children stated physical impairments or not having hospital visitors made them feel bad or unhappy. When these same children were asked if they did anything to feel closer to God, 78% of the children reported that they did activities such as pray or asked others to pray for them. Topics of prayer requests included feeling normal, stronger, being able to go home, having less pain, and seeking positive treatment results. Of those that prayed, 77% felt that the prayers worked.

Survey research on hope and spirituality in adolescents with cancer revealed that girls reported more hopeful feelings and higher spiritual well-being than boys (Hendricks-Ferguson 2006). Middle adolescent youth experienced more religious well-being than later adolescents. Girls experienced both more emotional and religious well-being than boys. Boys in early adolescence experienced the least hope, while girls in early adolescence experienced the most hope (Hendricks-Ferguson 2006). Children and adolescents long to dream and continue to think about what they would like to accomplish and appreciate when healthcare providers ask them about their achievements in life, their personal connections, and what they have yet to accomplish (Champagne 2008).

Factors that influence children's coping include their ability to communicate their feelings, their family's willingness and capability to nurture their child through suffering, and the healthcare team's infrastructure to support existential and spiritual distress. Even though children face significant symptom burden from their illnesses, they still often long to be a child, to play, and to enjoy the love of their family (McSherry et al. 2007). The child may need to talk, to ask questions, and to understand, but if the adult is silent or redirects the conversation, the child may feel that they cannot explore their concerns, leaving them isolated with difficult feelings (Purow et al. 2011).

Parents often wonder about the best way to communicate with their child about their illness and how much to involve them in the decision-making processes involved with treatment. Children, in their attempts to make sense of their illness and their future, may develop numerous questions that may be difficult for parents to answer. Common concerns of children arise through questions such as "What does heaven look like?" "Will my grandparents be waiting for me when I get there?" "Is it going to hurt when I die?" In starting communications with children about their health and future, discussions should be geared toward age-appropriate understanding of the body and its functions. Child life specialists and social workers can guide parents about ways to initiate conversations and inform children about their illness. Honest discussions with children about their illness allow them to have an understanding about their bodies and more control to make informed decisions about their healthcare (Jones and Weisenfluh 2003). Therefore, whenever possible, children should be a part of the decision-making process for their care (Jones and Weisenfluh 2003). This method of open communication works well in reducing worries and also helps to build trust within the family during a time of great uncertainty.

9.3 Child and Adolescent Development and Understanding of Their Illness

Children, regardless of their age, may experience a spiritual or existential crisis when living with a life-threatening condition. Their reactions to their physical and psychosocial changes and life within the hospital setting vary based upon their cognitive and emotional development (Jones and Weisenfluh 2003; Petersen 2014). As children grow up, they may embrace a personal faith as a mechanism for finding comfort and strength. Faith development parallels emotional and cognitive development and biological maturation (Fowler and Dell 2006). Table 9.1 portrays children's spiritual development, cognitive under-

Table 9.1 Children's spiritual development, understanding of death, and supportive interventions for expression of feelings and worries

Age range	Children's spiritual development	Children's developmental understanding of the death	Supportive interventions for expression of children's feelings and worries
1–4	The child models spirituality based on their loved ones' beliefs. Religious symbols bring forth feelings of love and companionship or terror and guilt	The child has a very limited understanding of the concrete aspects of death. They view death as temporary and reversible	Play activities assist children in expressing their emotional or spiritual concerns. Medical toys such as puppets, coloring books, and play therapy dolls help encourage expression of concerns
5–10	The child's development of spiritual beliefs arises through fantasy and stories of good and evil	They can think concretely and have imaginative belief systems. However, they lack the ability to understand the intricacies of death. Children may be afraid of going to sleep and not waking. They fear that they may have done something wrong to cause their illness and feel guilt for bringing suffering to the family	The incorporation of drama, play therapy, and drawings helps children express their worries about their illness. Discussions about symbols in their play create opportunities for children to discuss their fears and guilt
10–13	They begin to understand the larger meanings of punishment and rewards. They may question God about their illness and wonder why they must suffer	They can grasp the permanence of death. They fear the specifics of what will happen as they approach death and after they die	Discussions with youth about their worries may help in the processing of emotions and release of existential and spiritual distress. They may wish to talk with family and friends about dying, their fears, and to gather comfort knowing family will eventually heal after their death. Games and time with friends foster therapeutic distractions for children
14–18	The adolescent ponders existential concerns about the meaning of life, what they hope to become, and how they want to be remembered. They may see God through qualities such as understanding, acceptance, loyalty, and as a guide during difficult times	Adolescents typically have a clear understanding of their illness and grasp the realities of their life-threatening condition. However, they may lack the emotional maturity to cope with the enormity of their situation	Support groups, teen play rooms, and flexible visitation rules help to promote socialization and adolescent development. Allowing adolescents to participate in their medical decisions enhances their sense of control and self-efficacy

standing of death, and suggested interventions to ease existential and spiritual suffering. Not until children reach mid-adolescence do they begin to understand the existential aspects of life and death (Hurwitz et al. 2004).

Before 5 years of age, children focus on play, being able to leave the hospital and avoiding separation from their parents, especially during scary medical procedures (McSherry et al. 2007). The attachment that infants feel with their caregivers influences their sense of trust or mistrust with others (Fowler and Dell 2006). They have very little understanding of death or temporality and view death as a temporary, reversible event (Jones and Weisenfluh 2003). Preschool children express their worries through crying, temper tantrums, or regressive behaviors (Jones and Weisenfluh 2003). At this stage, children model beliefs from those around them. They may settle on images of religious symbols as bringing forth terror or guilt or positive aspects such as companionship and love. The best way to support preschoolers with physical and spiritual crises is to provide outlets for them to express their feelings through medical play with activities such as puppets, coloring books, or play therapy dolls (Jones and Weisenfluh 2003).

During elementary school years, children are concrete thinkers and are not able to fully understand the intricacies of death. They begin to think concretely and develop imaginative belief systems, relate through fantasy and story, and see religion through symbolism and stories of good and evil (Fowler and Dell 2006). Elementary-aged children may fear that something that they did wrong may have caused their illness or have guilt about the impact of their illness on their family (McSherry et al. 2007). They may fear going to sleep and not waking up (McSherry et al. 2007). Increased exposure to death from trauma like murder, war, or illness may expedite children's understanding of death (Jones and Weisenfluh 2003). They also feel protective over their parents and siblings and feel guilt for bringing this burden on their family and listen for clues from parents about when it is ok to die (Jones and Weisenfluh 2003). Common behavioral reactions in this age group include crying and screaming, and when closer to death, they may withdraw or express tremendous peace (Jones and Weisenfluh 2003). The way in which children live out their own impending death can be expressed through the symbolic language present in their drawings and in the games they play. Observing them allows adults to get in touch with their reality more intimately.

As children begin to approach their teen years, they experience more maturity in their cognitive and emotional understanding of their illness and faith. Around age 10, children will begin to fully grasp the permanence of death (Jones and Weisenfluh 2003). They may have more fears and questions about what will happen to their bodies and what happens as they approach or experience death. They may also begin to interpret larger meanings of rewards and punishments for behaviors and can discern that not all bad behaviors receive punishment. These children may temporarily question God based upon this unjust "moral retribution" (Fowler and Dell 2006).

Creating open safe environments for children this age to share their worries helps them in processing their emotions. They may need time to talk with their families to share their love and to ensure that they are going to be ok after they die (Jones and Weisenfluh 2003). Children at this age find great comfort in play and spending time with their friends. Game sharing can also help people find the emotional closeness that facilitates dialogue. Being with other kids, socialization, and support groups also engenders environments for children to explore their feelings and seek normalization.

Developmental objectives in adolescents are traditionally described in a psychological context as structuring identity, personality, and peer relationships, leading to the possibility of stable and intimate relationships (Abrams et al. 2007). The search for meaning is typical in teenagers, and they may ponder key questions related to existential dimensions such as "Who am I?" "What do I want to do with my life?" As they face their life-threatening illness, additional existential and spiritual concerns may develop such as "Why did this cancer happen to me?" "Is there life after death and what is this like?" "Will I ever feel like myself again?" Adolescents typically have a clear understanding of their illness and grasp the realities of their life-threatening condition. However, they may not have the emotional maturity to cope with the enormity of their situation. Spiritual and psychosocial connection with these youth will support them in discovering how to express these feelings of confusion and frustration (Jones and Weisenfluh 2003).

The crisis of relationships with adult figures needed for individuation is a developmental milestone for adolescents, which can be challenging when the disease and treatments require cohabitation with parents and dependence on them as caregivers. They may become isolated from their peer support network and display anger relating to the social activities and developmental milestones they miss due to their illness (Jones and Weisenfluh 2003). In some contexts, the peer group originates in the context of religion, and when a large portion of a teen's time is spent attending to their medical needs, it becomes difficult to participate in community worship (Fowler and Dell 2006). Perhaps, the youth may feel they have abandoned those who were central in their life before their illness.

Adolescents can incorporate operational thinking that allows them to reason and conceive in the abstract (Fowler and Dell 2006). They also develop attachments to their own personal visions of the world and values that may conform with friends, parents, teachers, or other significant people in their lives. Adolescents may see God through qualities such as understanding, acceptance, loyalty, and as a guide during difficult times (Fowler and Dell 2006). By encouraging adolescents to participate in their care decisions and prepare for their health trajectory, they may feel more in control of their present day and the unknowns of their future. Discussions about advanced directives and wishes for their healthcare at the end of life also provide adolescents opportunities to reflect on their lives, their achievements, and the legacies that they would like to leave behind for their loved ones.

Even though they may have a clear understanding of their physical decline, adolescents still long to participate in developmental milestones and to focus on fun events like prom, graduation, and hanging out with friends (McSherry et al. 2007). Connecting adolescents with others undergoing similar medical experiences may help to normalize their experiences and reduce isolation (Jones and Weisenfluh 2003). Additionally, for adolescents that have a love interest, family and the medical team should provide opportunities for them to nurture these connections, even at the end of life (Jones and Weisenfluh 2003.

9.4 Spiritual Care for Families of Children with Life-Threatening Illnesses

9.4.1 Parental Spiritual Well-Being

Parents who have a child with a life-threatening illness often turn to their spirituality to find comfort and peace (Proserpio et al. 2014; Meert et al. 2005; Schneider and Mannell 2006; Hexem et al. 2011). One study (Schneider and Mannell 2006) of parents of children who were hospitalized for a life-threatening illness revealed that parents desire guidance from their spiritual advisors and consider them an essential aspect of family support. These parents described the key religious aspect of spirituality as their faith (Schneider and Mannell 2006). Parents received great strength from prayer and reading the bible, recognizing that it provides them with a concrete task that they can do to cope with their feelings of helplessness (Hexem, et al. 2011; Schneider and Mannell 2006; Robinson et al. 2006). Some parents experienced questioning of their faith and wondered why God would bring such suffering on their families; however, most parents eventually returned to their faithfulness (Hexem et al. 2011; Schneider and Mannell 2006). Many parents attended a place of worship and found that this environment offered a place of serenity and a feeling that they were not alone. Parents also found tremendous peace through time spent in nature seeing animals and walking among the trees (Schneider and Mannell 2006).

Several studies explored the experiences of peace and meaning-making in parents of children with cancer and life-threatening conditions utilizing a survey developed to assess adult cancer patient's spirituality, the Functional Assessment of Chronic Illness Therapy—Spiritual Well-Being (FACIT-Sp) (Peterman et al. 2002). Mack et al. (2009) tested FACIT-Sp with parents of children with cancer and found that parents were indeed able to find feelings of peace during their child's illness. Those who had trust in their child's physician and who learned of their child's prognosis were more likely to have peace (Mack et al. 2009). A study of parents of children receiving state-funded palliative care services in Florida (Knapp et al. 2011) explored parental spiritual well-being in pediatric palliative care utilizing FACIT-Sp to discover that parents who were unmarried, living in single-parented homes, and from lower educational backgrounds were more likely to disagree with a statement of feeling at peace during their child's illness. The same study looked at race/ethnicity and parent's spiritual coping and found that white non-Hispanic parents were more likely to disagree with the statement that their child's illness strengthened their faith or spiritual beliefs. Black parents were more likely to incorporate spirituality and faith into their coping processes than Whites.

Parents also felt that their spirituality helped them to keep their child's illness within perspective. Spiritual care providers and community congregations provided parents opportunity to ventilate when they felt overwhelmed by their situations (Hexem et al. 2011) and provided practical support such as meals, cards, and moral guidance when they were angry. Parents felt tremendous comfort knowing that they could place their worries in God's hands and peace in knowing that their child would be safe and cared for in the afterlife (Hexem et al. 2011; Robinson et al. 2006). Another perspective that their spirituality offered was an understanding of why their child had to suffer. Some believed that their child was a gift from God brought to families for a special reason (Hexem et al. 2011).

Kylmä and Juvakka (2007) investigated factors that endanger and engender hope in parents of children with cancer. They described hope for these parents as offering them the ability to envision possibilities in life, a sense of connection with one's own and other's spiritual beliefs, and desires for something positive in life such as their child's return to normal or improved quality of life. Endangering of hope occurred when parents saw their child's health decline and had negative experiences with healthcare providers or when parents' resources for financial, emotional, or psychosocial support became limited. Positive influences in engendering hope included their child's positive presence; their child's health improvement; quality of healthcare; strong foundation of emotional, spiritual, and peer resource networks; and their child's return to a normal life. The authors recommended supporting parents by increasing their ability to continue normal aspects of life that bring them joy; helping them develop a future-oriented focus; and assisting them in nurturing their social and spiritual support systems.

Parents who had a child die from a life-threatening condition reflected that through their child's illness and their connection with other parents in similar situations, they could develop wisdom, hope, trust, and love (Robinson et al. 2006). Some examples of these spiritual strengths included being about to learn to have some acceptance about what is happening, knowing that time will help in their healing while acknowledging that there will always be a void when their child is gone. Parents also felt comfort in recognizing that they had done all that they could for their child and knew when to stop intensive medical treatments. A sense of hope, even when things felt unsurmountable, was vital for these parents. And lastly, parents stated that their continuous expression of love to their child gave parents great comfort.

There are limited protocols for the spiritual care of parents of children with life-threatening conditions. However, similar to the BELIEF (McEvoy 2000) mnemonic for initiating spiritual dialogues with children and adolescents, nursing literature (Puchalski et al. 2009, p 893) reports the use of SPIRIT (Maugans 1996), HOPE (Anandrajah and Hight 2001), and FICA (Puchalski 2006; Puchalski and Romer 2000) as mechanisms for discussing spiritual histories with adults. Table 9.2 displays tools for initiating spiritual history discussions. These are not

Table 9.2 Tools for initiating spiritual history discussions

F:	Faith/beliefs	H:	Hope
I:	Importance	O:	Organized religion
C:	Community	P:	Personal spirituality
A:	Address in care	E:	Effects of care and decisions
S:	Spiritual belief system	B:	Belief system
P:	Personal spirituality	E:	Ethics
I:	Integration with a spiritual community	L:	Lifestyle
R:	Ritualized practices and restrictions	I:	Involvement in a spiritual community
I:	Implications for medical care	E:	Education
T:	Terminal events planning	F:	Future events

assessment forms, per se, but mnemonics for ways to approach spiritual care of adults. Of note, implementation of these mechanisms for opening conversations about adult spirituality was created for adults with medical conditions; therefore, adaptations may be necessary to best address the spiritual concerns of parents of children with life-threatening medical conditions.

9.4.2 Spiritual Well-Being in Siblings

Siblings of a child who has a life-threatening condition frequently encounter psychosocial distress. They experience difficulties in trying to understand their sister or brother's health decline and often spend extended time away from their parents who are at the hospital caring for their sick child (Sloper 2000). Since parents aren't around to ask questions, siblings often create images of what might be happening from the small pieces of information that they are able to overhear. Siblings' psychosocial distress is often fueled by uncertainty, unknown futures, and limited control over life (Murray 2002; Nolbris et al. 2007). Most challenges appear for siblings during acute phases of their sister or brother's illness at the time of diagnosis, during treatment, and at relapse or end of life (Sloper 2000). If the child with the life-threatening illness reaches end of life, the presence of physical symptoms and distress may foster increased fear, uncertainty, and anxiety in siblings (Bluebond-Langner 2000). The more regular families can keep their day-to-day schedule and important people in siblings' lives, the better chances siblings have to feel that their world may again resemble something approximating normal (Murray 2002). Bringing siblings to the hospital and allowing them to be a part of the healthcare experience may also help reduce feelings of uncertainty and prevent feelings of isolation. While at the hospital, the supportive care services team can meet with siblings to assess their needs and watch for potential signs of distress and provide access to play activities and support groups (Contro et al. 2002; Murray 2002).

Providing information to siblings helps to increase their awareness of their brother or sister's health condition and may aid in their ability to create a vision of what their future might look like. A study of bereaved siblings' reflections of hospital encounters revealed that they felt left out of hospital communications and often spoke down to as if they were ignorant, even though they strongly desired inclusion in conversations (Steele et al. 2013). Studies show that with increased knowledge, siblings better understood their brother or sisters' illness and treatment (Gaab et al. 2014; Humphrey et al. 2015; Sloper 2000). Members of the healthcare team can help increase a sibling's understanding of their brother or sister's illness and therefore, reduce some of the unknowns and worries (Steele et al. 2013; Murray 2002). Child life specialists are experts in helping siblings gather information about their brother or sister's illness, treatments, and procedures that may occur. They incorporate medical play to help siblings visualize what their sister or brother may encounter at the hospital or clinic. Providing this outlet for children to ask questions of the medical team may open opportunities for them to ask questions of an adult without worry of creating family tension.

The level of severity of a child's illness often presents varying impacts on siblings' well-being. When a child or adolescent's condition reaches end of life, siblings are exposed to multiple distressing situations (Bluebond-Langner 2000). This time may include extended hospital stays, increased healthcare providers in the home, and an overall tension in the home. During this time, healthcare providers need to closely monitor siblings and answer questions about physical symptoms and prepare them for future changes or for the death of their sibling (Bluebond-Langner 2000).

9.5 Future Directions

Other factors to consider in providing an initial assessment with families are to determine the influence of their family and culture on their interpretation of illness and on their personal coping abilities and support networks. Families come to their healthcare crisis with cultural interpretations of illness and with a range of expectations or desires for help from healthcare providers. Families may choose to rely on their families and social networks to help them in coping with their illnesses. Other families may have religious beliefs that have parameters on the amount and types of medical care that individuals may receive. Talking with families around the time of diagnosis about their familial values, religious beliefs, and social supports will help in discovering the family's needs and to best support their wishes and values.

There is a need for education for all healthcare providers on the importance of paying attention to spiritual and existential needs. Knowing how to perceive and recognize the spiritual dimension creates an additional tool with which to care for the patient and family. Some studies demonstrate that an appropriate course of spiritual training by practitioners brings benefit to team members, in terms of a greater empathetic capacity, less frustration in the workplace, and improved teamwork (Wasner et al. 2005; Cerra and Fitzpatrick 2008). Training may begin in their respective university programs and advance throughout their career with continuing education opportunities. It does not call for an additional workload for practitioners, but the acquisition of a greater sensitivity in these areas.

The need to protect the rights of patients in a broad sense, as required by the Joint Commission International (2011), renders support for integrated multidisciplinary spiritual care. Objectives must move toward a thorough assessment of needs and provision of support that fosters communication, relationship building, and spiritual care planning that engenders trust and hope. This may place new demands on healthcare systems, including specialized training for hospital chaplains and other spiritual care providers who work within multidisciplinary teams. It is important to retain the role of a specially trained spiritual care provider as an integral part of the pediatric palliative care team for care of children, siblings, and parents. Additionally, the spiritual care provider should also support the spiritual and existential needs of the multidisciplinary team as personal struggles often arise when caring for children with life-threatening illnesses and their families (Purow et al. 2011).

Clinical experience has shown that the continuous and active presence of a spiritual care provider in healthcare settings, as part of the multidisciplinary team, can respond to needs of a spiritual nature, in close collaboration with psychosocial providers. In accordance with the Joint Commission International (2011), the spiritual care provider should be introduced as early as possible, as an additional resource within the team to support the spiritual and existential well-being of children and families.

While the importance of the influence of spirituality on the health and well-being of children with life-threatening illnesses and their families is beginning to be addressed, there are many areas for future growth. Most studies on the spiritual life of children and adolescents with life-threatening conditions and their families published in the United States include a predominantly white Christian sample. Recognizing that spirituality may be something that individuals choose to keep private, attempts to extend research to include samples that better reflect the multiple spiritual practices of the patient population may allow spiritual care providers to extend their understanding of the needs and ways to enter into dialogue with families from many spiritual backgrounds. There remains a continued need for the development and testing of tools that appropriately assess spirituality/religiosity in ways that match children's cognitive, physical, and emotional developmental abilities. There is a need to implement longitudinal studies to observe the child with a life-threatening condition along the entire trajectory of the illness or condition. Longitudinal studies may help identify pathways and support mechanisms for understanding how spirituality can impact both the child and family's quality of life.

To briefly summarize, it is recommended that:

Spiritual care providers should conduct activities with patients, family members, friends, visitors, and staff, for the purposes of:

1. Affirming and defending the infinite value and dignity of every person
2. Discussing the existential and spiritual dimension of suffering, illness, and death
3. Highlighting the power of faith, support, guidance, and reconciliation
4. Helping to ensure that the spiritual needs of all religious and cultural traditions are addressed while respecting the beliefs of each
5. Endeavoring to protect patients from undue spiritual intrusion
6. Offering spiritual accompaniment via empathic listening and showing an understanding of those who are in anguish
7. Ensuring religious worship, rituals, and sacraments depending on the religious tradition of everyone
8. Offering spiritual support to members of the multidisciplinary team
9. Organizing and participating in teaching programs for professionals in the world of health
10. Promoting mediation and reconciliation
11. Supporting and participating in research programs about spiritual care

References

Abrams AN, Hazen EP, Penson RT (2007) Psychosocial issues in adolescents with cancer. Cancer Treat Rev 33(7):622–630

Anandrajah G, Hight E (2001) Spirituality and medical practice: using the HOPE questions as a practical tool for spiritual assessment in office practice. Am Fam Physician 63(1):81–88

Astrow AB, Puchalski CM, Sulmasy DP (2001) Religion, spirituality, and health care: social, ethical, and practical considerations. Am J Med 110(4):283–287

Bluebond-Langner M (2000) In the shadow of illness: parents and siblings of the chronically ill child. Princeton University Press, Princeton, NJ

Boston P, Bruce A, Schreiber R (2011) Existential suffering in the palliative care setting: an integrated literature review. J Pain Symptom Manag 41(3):604–618

Bull A, Gillies M, Division Y (2007) Spiritual needs of children with complex healthcare needs in hospital. Paediatr Nurs 19(9):34–38

Cassel EJ (1982) The nature of suffering and the goals of medicine. N Engl J Med 306:639–645

Cerra A, Fitzpatrick JJ (2008) Can in-service education help prepare nurses for spiritual care? J Christ Nurs 25(4):204–209

Champagne E (2008) Living and dying: a window on (Christian) children's spirituality. Int J Child Spirituality 13(3):253–263

Contro N, Larson J, Scofield S, Sourkes B, Cohen H (2002) Family perspectives on the quality of pediatric palliative care. Arch Pediatr Adolesc Med 156(1):14–19

Feudtner C, Haney J, Dimmers MA (2003) Spiritual care needs of hospitalized children and their families: a national survey of pastoral care providers' perceptions. Pediatrics 111(1):e67–e72. https://doi.org/10.1542/peds.111.1.e67

Fowler JW, Dell ML (2006) Stages of faith from infancy through adolescence: reflections on three decades of faith development theory. In: The handbook of spiritual development in childhood and adolescence, pp 34–45

Frankl V (1992) Man's search for meaning: an introduction to logotherapy, 4th edn. Beacon Press, Boston, MA

Gaab EM, Owens GR, MacLeod RD (2014) Siblings caring for and about pediatric palliative care patients. J Palliat Med 17(1):62–67

Haase JE, Kintner EK, Monahan PO, Robb SL (2014) The resilience in illness model (rim) part 1: exploratory evaluation in adolescents and young adults with cancer. Cancer Nurs 37(3):E1–E12

Hendricks-Ferguson V (2006) Relationships of age and gender to hope and spiritual well-being among adolescents with cancer. J Pediatr Oncol Nurs 23(4):189–199

Hexem KR, Mollen CJ, Carroll K, Lanctot DA, Feudtner C (2011) How parents of children receiving pediatric palliative care use religion, spirituality, or life philosophy in tough times. J Palliat Med 14(1):39–44

Humphrey LM, Hill DL, Carroll KW, Rourke M, Kang TI, Feudtner C (2015) Psychological well-being and family environment of siblings of children with life threatening illness. J Palliat Med 18(11):981–984

Hurwitz CA, Duncan J, Wolfe J (2004) Caring for the child with cancer at the close of life: "there are people who make it, and I'm hoping I'm one of them". J Am Med Assoc 292(17):2141–2149

Joint Commission International (2011) Joint commission international accreditation standards for hospitals, 4th edn. Ringgold Inc, Portland, OR
Jones BL (2006) Caregivers of children with cancer. Hum Behav Soc Environ 14(1/2):221–239
Jones BL (2012) The challenge of quality care for family caregivers in pediatric cancer care. Semin Oncol Nurs 28(4):213–220
Jones B, Weisenfluh S (2003) Pediatric palliative and end-of-life care: developmental and spiritual issues of dying children. Smith Coll Stud Soc Work 73(3):423–443
Kamper R, Van Cleve L, Savedra M (2010) Children with advanced cancer: responses to a spiritual quality of life interview. J Spec Pediatr Nurs 15(4):301–306
Knapp C, Madden V, Wang H, Curtis C, Sloyer P, Shenkman E (2011) Spirituality of parents of children in palliative care. J Palliat Med 14(4):437–443
Koenig HG (2012) Role of the chaplain on the medical-surgical team. Assoc Operating Room Nurses J 96(3):330–332
Kylmä J, Juvakka T (2007) Hope in parents of adolescents with cancer: factors endangering and engendering parental hope. Eur J Oncol Nurs 11(3):262–271
Mack JW, Wolfe J, Cook EF, Grier HE, Cleary PD, Weeks JC (2009) Peace of mind and sense of purpose as core existential issues among parents of children with cancer. Arch Pediatr Adolesc Med 163(6):519–524
Maugans TA (1996) The SPIRITual history. Arch Fam Med 5(1):11–16
McEvoy M (2000) An added dimension to the pediatric health maintenance visit: the spiritual history. J Pediatr Health Care 14(5):216–220
McSherry M, Kehoe K, Carroll JM, Kang TI, Rourke MT (2007) Psychosocial and spiritual needs of children living with a life-threatening illness. Pediatr Clin North Am 54(5):609–629. https://doi.org/10.1016/j.pcl.2007.08.002
Meert KL, Thurston CS, Briller SH (2005) The spiritual needs of parents at the time of their child's death in the pediatric intensive care unit and during bereavement: a qualitative study. Pediatr Crit Care Med 6(4):420
Meireles CB, Maia LC, Miná VAL, Novais MDSMC, Peixoto JAC, Cartaxo MABS, de Lima JMF, dos Santos FAV, de Matos Cassiano JJ, Pinheiro PG, Neto MLR (2015) Influence of spirituality in pediatric cancer management: a systematic review. Int Arch Med 8. https://doi.org/10.3823/1634
Miller WR, Thoresen CE (2003) Spirituality, religion, and health: an emerging research field. Am Psychol 58(1):24–35. https://doi.org/10.1037/0003-066X.58.1.24
Mishel MH (1988) Uncertainty in illness. Image J Nurs Sch 20(4):225–232
Murray JS (2002) A qualitative exploration of psychosocial support for siblings of children with cancer. J Pediatr Nurs 17(5):327–337
Nolbris M, Enskär K, Hellström A (2007) Experience of siblings of children treated for cancer. Eur J Oncol Nurs 11(2):106–112. https://doi.org/10.1016/j.ejon.2006.10.002
Peterman AH, Fitchett G, Brady MJ, Hernandez L, Cella D (2002) Measuring spiritual well-being in people with cancer: the functional assessment of chronic illness therapy—Spiritual Well-being Scale (FACIT-Sp). Ann Behav Med 24(1):49–58
Petersen CL (2014) Spiritual care of the child with cancer at the end of life: a concept analysis. J Adv Nurs 70(6):1243–1253
Proserpio T, Piccinelli C, Clerici CA (2011) Pastoral care in hospitals: a literature review. Tumori 97(5):666–671
Proserpio T, Ferrari A, Lo VS, Massimino M, Clerici CA, Veneroni L, Bresciani C, Casali PG, Ferrari M, Bossi P, Galmozzi G, Pierantozzi A, Licitra L, Marceglia S, Mariani L (2014) Hope in cancer patients: the relational domain as a crucial factor. Tumori 101(4):447–454
Puchalski C (2006) Spiritual assessment in clinical practice. Psychiatr Ann 36(3):150–155
Puchalski C, Romer AL (2000) Taking a spiritual history allows clinicians to understand patients more fully. J Palliat Med 3(1):129–137. https://doi.org/10.1089/jpm.2000.3.129
Puchalski C, Ferrell B, Virani R, Otis-Green S, Baird P, Bull J, Chochinov H, Handzo G, Nelson-Becker H, Prince-Paul M, Pugliese K, Sulmasy D (2009) Improving the quality of spiritual care as a dimension of palliative care: the report of the Consensus Conference. J Palliat Med 12(10):885–904
Purow B, Alisanski S, Putnam G, Ruderman M (2011) Spirituality and pediatric cancer. South Med J 104(4):299–302. https://doi.org/10.1097/SMJ.0b013e3182083f40
Robinson MR, Thiel MM, Backus MM, Meyer EC (2006) Matters of spirituality at the end of life in the pediatric intensive care unit. Pediatrics 118(3):e719–e729
Schneider MA, Mannell RC (2006) Beacon in the storm: an exploration of the spirituality and faith of parents whose children have cancer. Issues Compr Pediatr Nurs 29(1):3–24
Sloper P (2000) Experiences and support needs of siblings of children with cancer. Health Social Care Community 8(5):298–306
Steele AC, Kaal J, Thompson AL, Barrera M, Compas BE, Davies B, Fairclough DL, Foster TL, Gilmer MJ, Hogan N, Vannatta K, Gerhardt CA (2013) Bereaved parents and siblings offer advice to healthcare providers and researchers. J Pediatr Hematol Oncol 35(4):253
Wasner M, Longaker C, Fegg MJ, Borasio GD (2005) Effects of spiritual care training for palliative care professionals. Palliat Med 19(2):99–104

Easing Social Distress in Pediatric Cancer

10

Wendy Pelletier, Ilaria Ripamonti, and Kira Bona

10.1 Introduction

Despite advances in pediatric cancer treatment, nearly 20% of children will die of their disease, and a majority of children will experience distressing symptoms throughout the course of illness, regardless of whether that illness culminates in cure or death (American Cancer Society 2012; Howlader et al. 2011; Pui et al. 2012; Wolfe et al. 2000a, b). The impact of a child's life-threatening illness on families extends beyond the physical, psychological, and emotional to include frequent disruptions to the concrete social fabric of day to day life. As providers seek to optimize communication with families and enhance quality of life throughout the illness trajectory, attention to domains of social distress and potential disparities in access to care can augment the quality of care provided. In this chapter, we will focus on three domains of parental social distress in the context of pediatric cancer which should be considered as targets for intervention during the provision of high-quality interdisciplinary palliative care: employment, financial hardship, and social supports. We will draw on current literature and expert opinion to highlight the prevalence of social distress in these domains, identify potential disparities in receipt of high-quality palliative care, and offer practical recommendations for incorporation of these domains into the practice of pediatric palliative care. Consideration of the impact of pediatric cancer on the child and siblings is addressed in Chap. 2, and the psychological impact of pediatric cancer is addressed in Chap. 7.

10.1.1 Employment

Employment for many parents represents more than financial necessity. Being engaged in satisfying and fulfilling employment is associated with psychological benefits such as improved self-esteem and life satisfaction and decreased depression (Wakefield et al. 2014). Furthermore,

W. Pelletier, M.S.W., R.S.W. (✉)
Pediatric Hematology/Oncology/Transplant Program, Alberta Children's Hospital, Calgary, AB, Canada
e-mail: wendy.pelletier@albertahealthservices.ca

I. Ripamonti, B.S.W., R.S.W.
Pediatric Onco-Hematology, Blood & Marrow Transplant Program, University of Milano-Bicocca, Monza's Hospital San Gerardo/Fondazione MBBM, Monza, Italy

K. Bona, MD, M.P.H.
Department of Medicine, Boston Children's Hospital, Boston, MA, USA

Department of Pediatric Oncology and Division of Population Sciences, Dana-Farber Cancer Institute, Boston, MA, USA

Harvard Medical School, Boston, MA, USA

Center for Outcomes and Population Research, Dana-Farber Cancer Institute, Boston, MA, USA

J. Wolfe et al. (eds.), *Palliative Care in Pediatric Oncology*, Pediatric Oncology,
https://doi.org/10.1007/978-3-319-61391-8_10

the workplace is often a natural source of social connection and social support and may enhance self-actualization (Okada et al. 2015). Due to peak ages at the time of diagnosis, pediatric cancer affects primarily young, working families (Ward et al. 2014). In one investigation of newly diagnosed pediatric cancer patients at a major academic medical center, 96% of households had at least one working parent (Bona et al. 2016). Consequently, understanding the impact of a child's diagnosis and treatment on employment is an opportunity to broadly address a family's quality of life across the trajectory of care.

Work disruptions due to a child's cancer diagnosis and treatment are ubiquitous, begin early after diagnosis and persist throughout the course of care, ranging from decreased hours to formal leaves of absence or loss of employment (Bona et al. 2014; Dussel et al. 2011; Eiser and Upton 2007; Fluchel et al. 2014; Rosenberg-Yunger et al. 2013; Tsimicalis et al. 2012; Warner et al. 2014). In an investigation of pediatric acute lymphoblastic leukemia families (the most common childhood cancer diagnosis), 51% of families reported turning down work or educational opportunities in the first year after diagnosis (Lau et al. 2014). Parents of children with cancer are at significantly higher risk of extreme work disruption, namely, loss of employment, as compared to the general population, with over 40% reporting job loss in the settings of both up-front and advanced cancer treatment (Bona et al. 2014; Lau et al. 2014; Limburg et al. 2008). In one study of newly diagnosed pediatric cancer families in the USA only 53% of parents who took a leave of absence utilized the Family Medical Leave Act (FMLA) to protect their jobs, and a minority (34%) received pay during their leave (Bona et al. 2016). Whether early in the process of building careers or struggling to ensure secure long-term employment, young families are by definition in the midst of establishing financial savings—including cash savings for emergencies, retirement savings, and college savings. The implications of disrupted or terminated employment and financial needs of families of children throughout the cancer care trajectory can thus be daunting and include concrete loss of income, disruption to employer-associated insurance benefits, disrupted social networks, disrupted opportunities for career advancement, and disrupted financial planning (Dussel et al. 2011; Limburg et al. 2008; Pelletier and Bona 2015). Yet attention to this basic family experience is often limited in the medical setting, a reality which has been documented as a source of frustration for parents (Cadell et al. 2012). Parents have reported a perceived lack of sharing of financial and other resource information by healthcare providers and felt they discovered many resources through non-systematic approaches including other parent caregivers with whom they had contact and online blogs from organizations dedicated to the treatment of a child's particular disease (Cadell et al. 2012). The near universality of employment disruption and its wide-ranging impact on family well-being provide a significant opportunity for palliative care providers to intervene by addressing this topic as part of the care process.

Beyond the concrete work disruptions of diagnosis and emergent evaluations, life-threatening illness in a child often leads to a shift in parents' perspectives on many aspects of their lives, including employment. Many parents describe a reevaluation and restructuring of life and family priorities that occur following their child's life-threatening diagnosis such that employment becomes less of a priority and more of a necessity to maintain financial security (Wakefield et al. 2014; Okada et al. 2015; Syse et al. 2011; Schweitzer et al. 2012). Parents report feeling reluctant to commit to employment tasks when it requires embracing new skills or challenges as their emotional energy is depleted, both throughout the trajectory of illness and more acutely in end-of-life settings (Wakefield et al. 2014; Syse et al. 2011). This shift away from seeking career advancement and other employment-related opportunities, coupled with emotional exhaustion and fatigue associated with a child's care, is a reality for many parents caring for a child with cancer and may be a source of distress (Gibbins et al. 2012).

In addition to a renewed awareness of the importance of spending as much time as possible with their child, practical barriers to maintaining employment are abundant. In particular, a lack of reliable respite care and support makes continuing with employment all but impossible for some parents (Cadell et al. 2012). This may be particularly true in the context of single-parent households. In keeping with societal role expectations, mothers more often than fathers either leave work completely or reduce their hours significantly to care for their child throughout their illness (Lau et al. 2014; Alam et al. 2012). Fathers may spend more hours at work trying to meet the financial demands placed upon the family as a result of their child's illness but, also, as a strategy to cope with their emotional pain and as a refuge from crisis (Alam et al. 2012). Research on parental well-being during end-of-life care has identified an association between an inability to secure resources and achieve financial stability and negative paternal emotions (Bennett Murphy et al. 2008). Fathers have also reported a sense of conflict between their employment requirements and wanting to be with their ill child; lack of understanding from employers and feeling penalized in the workplace for performance-related issues contribute to reported distress in fathers (Nicholas et al. 2016).

Opportunities for providers to address employment-related distress are numerous. On a basic level, acknowledgment of this source of social distress and normalization of the experience within the context of childhood cancer are important. Liaison with employers to help navigate available benefits and preserve employment can be helpful. Further, assisting families in navigating burdensome paperwork—such as Family Medical Leave Act (FMLA) applications—may facilitate preservation of employment in at risk families.

Case Vignette

Jennifer is a 3-year-old girl who was diagnosed with metastatic osteosarcoma. Jennifer's mother, Susan, was pregnant at the time of Jennifer's diagnosis and delivered her baby in a hospital in the family's home city 300 miles from the Children's Hospital where her daughter was being treated. Susan had just begun a maternity leave of absence from her work at the time of the diagnosis. Susan returned to the Children's Hospital within 5 days of delivering her baby as she felt she could not be away from Jennifer any longer. Because Jennifer's husband, Frank, needed to continue to work in their home city, Susan cared for Jennifer and her new son, Toby, in the Children's Hospital. She had some extended family support which allowed her brief respite at the Ronald McDonald House. Although the separation of the family was stressful, they felt this was their only solution as they needed to have at least one parent employed to meet their financial obligations.

While on treatment, Jennifer's osteosarcoma recurred, and her parents were told they would need to consider changing treatment protocols to a more intensive regimen which would prolong their time away from their home city. Because Susan was so depleted emotionally and physically from trying to care for her ill daughter as well as her new baby, Frank felt he needed to explore taking a leave of absence from his employment to support his wife and children. Frank moved into the local Ronald McDonald House and invited a relative of the family to come and stay to assist with care of the baby so that Frank and Susan could spend more time together with Jennifer, who was not coping well with treatment and was not expected to survive her disease. Local and national financial support programs were explored with the family but, even with assistance, their financial needs were far from being met.

The stress of trying to meet their child's medical and emotional needs, high demands of caring for an infant, loss of income due to both parents being on extended leaves of absence from their employment, financial obligations being unmet, and lack of ongoing extended family respite support have the potential to lead to significant short- and long-term psychological concerns in these parents.

Employment Impact

- Nearly all pediatric cancer families will experience work disruption due to diagnosis and treatment.
- In 30–50% of pediatric cancer families, at least one parent will quit or lose a job due to their child's cancer.
- Life-limiting illness in their child may lead to a shift in priorities for parents away from previous career goals which may have long-term repercussions for career advancement.
- Loss of employment may result in the loss of social networks.
- Evidence supports gender differences in the meaning of employment in one's life when caring for an ill child.

Palliative Interventions

- Provide opportunities for parents to dialogue about the impact of lost or changed employment in their lives
- Serve as medical liaisons to employers to communicate expected impact of child's illness on availability and productivity
- Assist families in navigating practical supports for employment protection (such as completion of Family Medical Leave Act paperwork)
- Develop communication strategies to keep the parent who is employed and engaged in treatment decision-making
- Identify respite for the parents providing bedside caregiving

10.2 Financial Hardship as a Source of Social Distress

In addition to impact on parental identity and career trajectory, illness-related disruptions to parental employment result in financial hardship for many pediatric cancer families (Pelletier and Bona 2015). An awareness of family economic burden during the treatment of children with life-threatening illness is essential to ensuring the provision of high-quality palliative care. Pediatric providers increasingly recognize the importance of addressing social determinants of health, including financial hardship, as part of the care of children and their families. In 2016, the American Academy of Pediatrics issued a policy statement recommending that screening for social determinants, including financial hardship and concrete resource needs, be integrated into the routine care of all children based on overwhelming evidence that poverty negatively impacts child health outcomes and quality of life (American Academy of Pediatrics 2016). Concurrently, strong evidence of the ubiquity and relevance of financial burden in the pediatric cancer setting led to the recent recommendation to incorporate assessment of financial burden as a standard of care in pediatric psychosocial oncology (Pelletier and Bona 2015). Evidence supports the assertion that family financial hardship, *whether pre-existing or resulting from a child's treatment course*, is highly prevalent in the pediatric cancer setting and has significant impact on families. Data have identified financial burden while caring for a child with cancer as a source of distress for families with notable implications for parental emotional and mental health (Rosenberg-Yunger et al. 2013; Creswell et al. 2014; Heath et al. 2006; Rosenberg et al. 2013a; Williams et al. 2014). Financial hardship in the course of a child's cancer treatment results in increased burden on parental relationships (Heath et al. 2006; Fletcher 2010) and increased risk of serious parental psychological distress (Creswell et al. 2014; Rosenberg et al. 2013a). Despite this correlation with parental well-being, discussion of finances is frequently overlooked by the care team. Understanding the scope of financial hardship in pediatric cancer is essential to the provision of high-quality pediatric palliative care for three keys reasons. First, children living in low-income families may face disparities in accessing high-quality palliative care that must be addressed in a focused fashion by the medical care team. Second, the presence of concrete resource needs—food, heat, and housing—in the setting of pediatric cancer may have implications for the care recommendations provided. Third, understanding financial hardship as a correlate of parental suffering and actively addressing finances in the course of care can contribute significantly to improving communication and quality of life for families facing a child's life-threatening diagnosis.

10.2.1 Evidence: Financial Hardship in the Context of Childhood Cancer

One in five children in the USA lives in poverty (Macartney 2011). This basic epidemiology means that one in five children diagnosed with cancer comes from an impoverished family (Ward et al. 2014). Children in the USA who are socioeconomically disadvantaged and/or racial/ethnic minorities experience disparities in access to healthcare in general (American Academy of Pediatrics 2016; Linton and Feudtner 2008). Data on how these general pediatric disadvantages specifically translate to pediatric palliative care in the cancer setting are limited. However, existing data highlight potential poverty-related disparities to which providers should be attentive as they seek to serve families of children with cancer.

Specialty pediatric palliative care is a limited resource dependent on non-standard referral patterns, meaning that children from low-income families may be at a disadvantage in even accessing appropriate palliative care services depending on the hospital from which they receive care (Lewis et al. 2011). Pediatric palliative care seeks to provide care that maximizes goal-oriented quality of life, and relies heavily on robust communication with pediatric families. In the hospital setting, potential poverty-related barriers to achieving the family-clinician trust necessary for such care include historical precedents of institutionalized medical bias in disadvantaged populations (Linton and Feudtner 2008)and inadequate access to medical interpreters to facilitate the subtleties essential in discussion of sensitive topics of value-oriented care (Linton and Feudtner 2008). Beyond the establishment of family trust, poverty has the potential to concretely impact a family's ability to access recommended medical treatment and decision-making around locations of care. Integrating the social context—including poverty or financial hardship—into care recommendations will facilitate successful maximization of quality of life.

A family's ability to travel frequently to clinic or the hospital may be limited by access to reliable transportation or cash to pay for parking. Conversely, their ability to support a child at home may be limited by resources in the home or community. As providers provide care recommendations to maximize quality of life, it is valuable to consider the following data. Pharmacies in racial/ethnic minority neighborhoods (which are disproportionately low income in the USA) are significantly less likely to stock pain medications which may pose challenges for families seeking appropriate symptom management for their children (Morrison et al. 2000). Home care services and supports (adequate nursing, medication, medical equipment) necessary to enable a child with complex medical needs to be at home may not be available in low-income areas (Beaune et al. 2014). Finally, household material hardship—meaning an inability to meet basic resource needs of food, heat, electricity, and housing—is common in the pediatric cancer setting. Data from one large referral center demonstrate that nearly 30% of pediatric cancer families report either food, housing, or energy insecurity after the first 6 months of chemotherapy (Bona et al. 2016). The implications of such concrete deprivation for pediatric palliative care have not been studied; however, it is reasonable to hypothesize that concrete insecurity might affect a family's decisions about locations of care or ability to adhere to medical recommendations. Prior studies have demonstrated that children with complex chronic illness (including but not limited to cancer) who live in more affluent neighborhoods are more likely to die at home, though the causes of this differential outcome are not known (Feudtner et al. 2002). It is certainly plausible that insufficient home supports in low-income families may contribute to such decisions. Parents who are skipping meals to ensure adequate food at home for their children, or whose homes have had the heat or electricity shut off may have reasonable concerns about providing care at home to a medically fragile child.

Above and beyond the epidemiology of childhood poverty, childhood cancer treatment inflicts an enormous financial burden on families across the economic spectrum (Pelletier and Bona 2015). Income losses due to employment disruptions addressed in the initial portion of this chapter are significant. Additionally, families experience unavoidable out-of-pocket expenses from medical co-pays, travel to and from treating institutions, overnight accommodation near hospitals, childcare for other children at home, and food while in the hospital (Eiser and Upton 2007; Cohn et al. 2003; Dockerty et al. 2003; Tsimicalis et al. 2013). Additional out-of-pocket expenses include those aimed at maximizing quality of life for a child—gifts, recreational distraction, and favorite foods. Consistent data across studies demonstrate that, collectively, these income losses and out-of-pocket expenses account for over 30% of family income (Tsimicalis et al. 2012; Barr et al. 1996) and that low-income families are disproportionately impacted (Bona et al. 2014; Dussel et al. 2011). One in four pediatric cancer families report that their child's diagnosis and treatment were a great financial hardship (Bona et al. 2016, 2014; Dussel et al. 2011).

The often catastrophic financial impact of a child's cancer diagnosis speaks to the importance of providers being aware of the issue, systematically screening families for this source of anxiety and distress and mobilizing resources to support family financial burden. As noted above, while many families are able to cope with the significant financial impact of diagnosis and treatment, a significant proportion reports an inability to meet the basic daily needs of their families. Specifically, nearly 30% of pediatric cancer families may be facing an inability to put enough food on the table, keep the heat or electricity on in their home, or pay the monthly rent or mortgage (Bona et al. 2016). Screening for and addressing these immediate needs can serve as an essential first step in the provision of high-quality palliative care for many families, one not always recognized within the current paradigm of care. While the above fundamental realities of poverty and financial hardship are likely to impact a family's experience of palliative care, it is a topic not uniformly addressed in the exam room (Beaune et al. 2014). Providers may experience discomfort in addressing money with families, and families express concerns about stigma or differential care if they raise the issue (Beaune et al. 2014). Despite these challenges, overlooking poverty and financial hardship in the context of palliative care may limit the ability to successfully provide adequate care for a child. Ensuring that providers are cognizant of the high prevalence of poverty and financial hardship and potential barriers to care, it may pose an excellent first step in addressing this source of social distress for families. Screening for financial hardship or concrete resource needs using published tools (Hager et al. 2010; Garg et al. 2015; Beaune et al. 2014) can identify families in need of assistance meeting basic needs. Concurrent with this effort, identifying a team member to serve as a knowledgeable and up-to-date resource regarding community supports for families or partnering with others to serve this role is key to ensuring optimized care. Parents strive to maintain quality of life for their children no matter how high the cost. Interdisciplinary providers can play an essential role in supporting parents by ensuring that there is adequate food on the table, heat in the house, and a roof over their head as they navigate the journey of cancer therapy.

Poverty and Financial Hardship in Pediatric Cancer

- 1 in 5 children with cancer will come from an impoverished family in the United States.
- 1 in 3 children with cancer will live in a home that has food, energy or housing insecurity during chemotherapy.
- Low-income families may face challenges finding pharmacies to fill pain medications and accessing essential home care services.
- Family decisions regarding locations of care may be impacted by concrete financial resources.

Palliative Interventions

- Screening for financial hardship and concrete resource needs should be systematic.
- Multiple published screening tools can be integrated into clinical practice including a 2-item food security screen (Hager et al. 2010), the WeCare 6-item basic needs assessment (Garg et al. 2015), or the Child Poverty Tool and Resource Guide (Beaune et al. 2014). Additional resources are available through the American Academy of Pediatrics (AAP) website www.aap.org.
- Normalization of the experience of financial hardship in the pediatric cancer setting.
- Identifying a team member to serve as a "sign-post" for families with an up-to-date awareness of local and governmental financial supports and familiarity with facilitating applications to such programs.
- Establishment of dedicated institutional funds to provide for the concrete resource needs of families (may be done in conjunction with institutional development office).
- Raising staff awareness of how financial hardship may affect families (e.g., highlighting "impossible" parental choices in the context of poverty such as leaving a child's bedside to maintain employment necessary to feed and clothe the family) so that they can remain sensitive to the needs of these families.

10.3 Social Support

In addition to social distress posed by employment disruptions and financial hardship, social isolation and the disrupted relationships created by a child's life-threatening cancer diagnosis may serve as targets for social intervention (Hosoda 2014). In the setting of a child's cancer diagnosis, parents often desire to increase the amount of time spent attending to their child's well-being, providing comfort, and cherishing moments together—and this time may increase even further in settings of acute but reversible illness, advanced disease, and end-of-life. Parents of children at end-of-life describe the experience as intensely personal and all-consuming. (Lou et al. 2015; van der Geest et al. 2014; Whiting 2013; Kars et al. 2011) Parents report an obligation to remain at their child's side and make medically beneficial decisions (Hinds et al. 2009). Integral processes such as "piloting, providing, protecting, and preserving" all contribute to parents' sense of actively doing something for their child (Price et al. 2011). The consequences of such ubiquitous parental focus on a sick child include significant disruption to the social structure of family, home, and friendships—including relationships which served as prior sources of support (Gerhardt et al. 2016). This disruption may be amplified in the end-of-life setting (Ling et al. 2016). As much as parents recognize the importance of maintaining some normalcy in family life, and avoiding chaos for their other children, it is often difficult to accept relief in caregiving responsibilities. Helping parents to recognize these challenges and strategize approaches to strengthening relationships that provide family support or respite is an important role for the care team to play (Kazak and Noll 2015).

Barriers to maintaining strong social relationships during a child's cancer treatment are numerous and cumulative. Parents report being too fatigued to leave their child's side or worrying that in their absence others may engage in conversations with their child that cross boundaries (Kars et al. 2011; Knapp et al. 2010). Isolation from social supports may result in a decrease in parents' emotional ability and willingness to invest in and connect with family and friends which leads to a void in social engagement impacting coping, self-care, personal needs, and parental mental health (Cadell et al. 2012; Kars et al. 2011; Price et al. 2011; Knapp et al. 2010; Champagne and Mongeau 2012; Robert et al. 2012). Parental vulnerability to social isolation may be heightened in vulnerable groups—fathers, single parents, those from other countries or ethnic, and religious minority cultures—and in settings of advanced cancer or end-of-life. Fathers have reported feeling alienated from family and friends, misunderstood, and abandoned. Particularly in the setting of advanced cancer or end-of-life, fathers endorse feeling their world is less predictable and more uncertain with regard to their role and what is expected of them (Ware and Raval 2007). Whereas mothers may have more support networks within the healthcare setting, fathers perceive inadequacies in professionals acknowledging or understanding their distress (Nicholas et al. 2016; Ware and Raval 2007). Single parents may experience significant worsening of relationships with their other children as well as their friends (Wiener et al. 2015). They also report worsening of self-care, including diet and nutrition, less sleep, less time doing activities they previously enjoyed, and a decrease in physical activities (Wiener et al. 2015). Parents of children from non-Western cultures may experience limited understanding of their unique support needs by healthcare teams and other parents. The growing number of children who travel to other countries for therapy results in isolation and lack of emotional and social support from family and friends who may be extremely geographically distant. Despite these numerous practical and emotional barriers to maintaining healthy social supports and relationships, possibilities for intervention by the palliative care team are numerous.

Caregiver relief or respite care has been defined as "complementary care in the home or another setting with appropriate medical and nursing support, offering parents or caregivers relief…other venues may not provide direct medical or nursing care, instead providing relief of caregiver burden." (Carter and Mandrell 2013) Caregiver relief has been identified as crucial for parents of children to achieve rest, maintain social support networks, and support their other children (Whiting 2013; Champagne and Mongeau 2012; Robert et al. 2012; Vollenbroich et al. 2012). While applicable across the spectrum of childhood cancer care, particularly in the setting of advanced disease or end-of-life care, the benefits of respite for parents may be significant. All parents, regardless of cultural background, have a desire to fulfill their roles as caregivers, comforters, and protectors of their child (Wiener et al. 2013; Meyer et al. 2006). Helping families to prioritize the need for respite, and strategize how best to achieve it, is an important role for the interdisciplinary team. Few parents have the emotional energy to search for reliable, in-home respite care, and there is variability in what families may be able to negotiate with insurance companies around assistance at home and the cost of comfort measures for their child (Dussel et al. 2011; Neufeld et al. 2001). Further, parents from lower socioeconomic backgrounds as noted in the prior section may not have the practical or financial assistance necessary to access respite care even if available (Monterosso et al. 2009). Providers can offer guidance and education on the toll of caretaking, promoting resilience, and supporting the parental need for individual support (O'Donnell et al. 2013; Rosenberg et al. 2013b). Providers should be attentive to support needs that vary by language or culture, which may themselves augment social isolation. Parent-to-parent support for mentorship, relief of isolation, and sharing of practical resources have also been identified as important throughout the cancer treatment trajectory (Cadell et al. 2012; Konrad 2007).

Case Vignette

Sarah, a 9-year-old girl diagnosed with acute lymphoblastic leukemia, had disease recurrence shortly after completing her final course of chemotherapy. Emily, Sarah's mom, was separated from her husband prior to Sarah's diagnosis, and he was not involved with Sarah or her siblings aged 5, 7, and 12 years. Emily reported being financially dependent on social services as she had been unable to maintain regular employment given she was a single parent. As Sarah lived more than 3 h from the treatment center, she and Emily remained at the hospital during much of Sarah's up-front chemotherapy, and Emily's mother cared for Sarah's siblings in their home community. Although Sarah coped well with the demands of therapy up until the time of her recurrence, following relapse she became very fearful and was not comfortable with her mother leaving her alone. Emily was deeply shaken by the news of the relapse and responded to her daughter's need to have her mother close by; Emily only left Sarah's hospital room once or twice daily to get food from the hospital cafeteria and was gone for very short periods.

During Sarah's re-induction, Emily was sleeping infrequently and poorly, and nutrition was minimal and with very few visitors to provide relief for her. Emily became increasingly weepy with angry outbursts directed at the staff around care requirements. Emily and Sarah both became more agitated, and Emily found it difficult to encourage Sarah to cooperate with necessary procedures.

Recognizing that Emily was likely experiencing caregiver fatigue and burnout, the team arranged to have a meeting with her to explore her feelings and perceptions. Emily described feeling isolated and frustrated that she alone was carrying the responsibility for making treatment decisions, providing 24-hr daily care for Sarah, missing her other children, and beginning to resent Sarah's clingy behavior but feeling guilty for voicing those thoughts when she knew her child was critically ill and might not survive her relapsed disease. She reported feeling that she had given everything she had emotionally to get through the therapy and could not imagine going through all of it again with the recurrence.

The team addressed the normalcy of Emily's emotions and talked with her about the need for self-care and to reflect upon the road ahead and what she felt was important for herself and all of her children in light of Sarah's prognosis. A plan was established to engage a hospital volunteer to regularly schedule time with Sarah to provide respite time for Emily, recognizing Sarah may take some time to accept this. A plan was also made to reengage the child life therapist and psychologist who had been previously involved with Sarah to help her cope with the demands of therapy. Emily was encouraged to invite friends to come from home and bring her other children every other weekend so that both Emily and Sarah could benefit from their presence. Emily's financial status was also reassessed to look for areas where the burden of providing financial support to her mother for care of the siblings could ease Emily's stress. Finally, in addition to psychosocial support from the team, Emily was strongly encouraged to attend the weekly parent support group on the inpatient unit so she could begin to develop more support networks and dialogue with other parents.

Clinical Pearls: Social Distress in Pediatric Palliative Care

Employment

- Nearly all parents of children with cancer will experience work disruptions or loss of employment due to the demands of treatment. Palliative providers should provide opportunities for parents to dialogue about the personal and financial impact of reduced or lost employment. Providers can serve as liaisons with employers, and familiarity with employee legal protections within the state may be of benefit in advocating for parents.

Finances

- In the USA, one in three children with cancer will live in a home that has food, energy, or housing insecurity and one in five children will come from an impoverished family. Ongoing assessment of practical and financial needs using published screening tools throughout the cancer trajectory will identify at risk families. Ensuring a team member has up to date knowledge regarding available community resources to which families can be referred for concrete supports is essential.
- The capacity for parents to make decisions regarding location of care for their child with advanced disease may be impacted by financial and social resources. Understanding these practical barriers to achieving a family's goals of care is a crucial step in the provision of holistic care.

Social Supports and Respite

- Social isolation as a consequence of parental reluctance to leave a child's side as his/her emotional and physical care needs escalate is common and may impact parental mental health. Proactively addressing the issue, facilitating engagement opportunities (such as with parent groups), and facilitating respite care is a vital role for providers.
- Acknowledging and appreciating the important role of diversity, culture and health beliefs on treatment decisions, family coping, and family-team relationships will enhance a family's ability to care for their child in a way that is meaningful for them.

10.4 Summary

In summary, opportunities to address social distress throughout a child's cancer care are numerous and essential to high-quality care. Recognizing the impact of a child's diagnosis and treatment on employment, family finances, and social supports is essential to holistically addressing quality of life in the pediatric cancer setting. As ubiquitous as physical symptoms during chemotherapy, these domains are of particular import for pediatric providers in part due to the fact that they are not systematically addressed within the context of the medical system. Yet the numbers are striking. Nearly all pediatric cancer families will experience work disruptions (Pelletier and Bona 2015). One in five children with cancer will live in poverty. (Ward et al. 2014; Macartney 2011) One in three children with cancer will live in a home struggling to put food on the table, keep the heat and electricity on, or pay the rent or mortgage (Bona et al. 2016). All parents will face the struggle of fulfilling their caregiving duties while simultaneously maintaining marriages and friendships from which they derive support. Addressed or unaddressed, these social realities form the context within which a child receives care and create opportunities for disparities in care and child and family outcomes. Pediatric cancer families will benefit from systematic efforts to screen for and address these issues throughout the trajectory of their child's illness and care. As providers seek to maximize quality of life and facilitate the provision of goal-oriented care, an active awareness of these issues has the potential to improve both communication and outcomes.

References

Alam R, Barrera M, D'Agostino N, Nicholas DB, Schneiderman G (2012) Bereavement experiences of mothers and fathers over time after the death of a child due to cancer. Death Stud 36:1–22

American Cancer Society (2012) Cancer facts & figures 2012. American Cancer Society, Atlanta. Available at: http://www.cancer.org/acs/groups/content/@epidemiologysurveilance/documents/document/acspc-031941.pdf. Accessed 3 April 2012

American Academy of Pediatrics (2016) Poverty and Child Health in the United States. Pediatrics 137(4):e20160339

Barr R, Furlong W, Horsman J, Feeny D, Torrance G, Weitzman S (1996) The monetary costs of childhood cancer to the families of patients. Int J Oncol 8:933–940

Beaune L, Leavens A, Muskat B et al (2014) Poverty and pediatric palliative care: what can we do. J Soc Work End-of-Life Palliat Care 10:170–185

Bennett Murphy LM, Flowers S, McNamara KA, Young-Saleme T (2008) Fathers of children with cancer: involvement, coping, and adjustment. J Pediatr Health Care 22:182–189

Bona K, Dussel V, Orellana L et al (2014) Economic impact of advanced pediatric cancer on families. J Pain Symptom Manage 47:594–603

Bona K, London WB, Guo D, Frank DA, Wolfe J (2016) Trajectory of material hardship and income poverty in families of children undergoing chemotherapy: a prospective cohort study. Pediatr Blood Cancer 63:105–111

Cadell S, Kennedy K, Hemsworth D (2012) Informing social work practice through research with parent caregivers of a child with a life-limiting illness. J Soc Work End-of-Life Palliat Care 8:356–381

Carter KB, Mandrell BN (2013) Development of a respite care program for caregivers of pediatric oncology patients and their siblings. J Pediatr Oncol Nurs 30:109–114

Champagne M, Mongeau S (2012) Effects of respite care services in a children's hospice: the parents' point of view. J Palliat Care 28:245–251

Cohn RJ, Goodenough B, Foreman T, Suneson J (2003) Hidden financial costs in treatment for childhood cancer: an Australian study of lifestyle implications for families absorbing out-of-pocket expenses. J Pediatr Hematol Oncol 25:854–863

Creswell PD, Wisk LE, Litzelman K, Allchin A, Witt WP (2014) Parental depressive symptoms and childhood cancer: the importance of financial difficulties. Support Care Cancer 22:503–511

Dockerty JD, Skegg DC, Williams SM (2003) Economic effects of childhood cancer on families. J Paediatr Child Health 39:254–258

Dussel V, Bona K, Heath JA, Hilden JM, Weeks JC, Wolfe J (2011) Unmeasured costs of a child's death: perceived financial burden, work disruptions, and economic coping strategies used by American and Australian families who lost children to cancer. J Clin Oncol 29:1007–1013

Eiser C, Upton P (2007) Costs of caring for a child with cancer: a questionnaire survey. Child Care Health Dev 33:455–459

Feudtner C, Silveira MJ, Christakis DA (2002) Where do children with complex chronic conditions die? Patterns in Washington State, 1980–1998. Pediatrics 109:656–660

Fletcher PC (2010) My child has cancer: the costs of mothers' experiences of having a child with pediatric cancer. Issues Compr Pediatr Nurs 33:164–184

Fluchel MN, Kirchhoff AC, Bodson J et al (2014) Geography and the burden of care in pediatric cancers. Pediatric Blood Cancer 61:1918–1924

Garg A, Toy S, Tripodis Y, Silverstein M, Freeman E (2015) Addressing social determinants of health at well child care visits: a cluster RCT. Pediatrics 135:e296–e304

van der Geest IM, Darlington AS, Streng IC, Michiels EM, Pieters R, van den Heuvel-Eibrink MM. Parents' experiences of pediatric palliative care and the impact on long-term parental grief. J Pain Symptom Manage 2014;47:1043–1053.

Gerhardt CA, Salley CG, Lehmann V (2016) The impact of pediatric pancer on the family. In Pediatric Psychosocial Oncology: Textbook for Multidisciplinary Care. Abrams AA, Muriel AC, Wiener L (Eds). Springer International Publishing, Switzerland, 143–155

Gibbins J, Steinhardt K, Beinart H (2012) A systematic review of qualitative studies exploring the experience of parents whose child is diagnosed and treated for cancer. J Pediatr Oncol Nurs 29:253–271

Hager ER, Quigg AM, Black MM et al (2010) Development and validity of a 2-item screen to identify families at risk for food insecurity. Pediatrics 126:e26–e32

Heath JA, Lintuuran RM, Rigguto G, Tikotlian N, McCarthy M (2006) Childhood cancer: its impact and financial costs for Australian families. Pediatr Hematol Oncol 23:439–448

Hinds PS, Oakes LL, Hicks J et al (2009) "Trying to be a good parent" as defined by interviews with parents who made phase I, terminal care, and resuscitation decisions for their children. J Clin Oncol 27:5979–5985

Hosoda T (2014) The impact of childhood cancer on family functioning: a review. Grad Stud J Psychol 15:18–30

Howlader NN, Krapcho AM et al (2011) SEER cancer statistics review, 1975–2008. National Cancer Institute, Bethesda, MD

Kars MC, Grypdonck MH, van Delden JJ (2011) Being a parent of a child with cancer throughout the end-of-life course. Oncol Nurs Forum 38:E260–E271

Kazak AE, Noll RB (2015) The integration of psychology in pediatric oncology research and practice: collaboration to improve care and outcomes for children and families. Am Psychol 70:146–158

Knapp CA, Madden VL, Curtis CM, Sloyer P, Shenkman EA (2010) Family support in pediatric palliative care: how are families impacted by their children's illnesses. J Palliat Med 13:421–426

Konrad SC (2007) What parents of seriously ill children value: parent-to-parent connection and mentorship. Omega 55:117–130

Lau S, Lu X, Balsamo L et al (2014) Family life events in the first year of acute lymphoblastic leukemia therapy: a children's oncology group report. Pediatr Blood Cancer 61:2277–2284

Lewis JM, DiGiacomo M, Currow DC, Davidson PM (2011) Dying in the margins: understanding palliative care and socioeconomic deprivation in the developed world. J Pain Symptom Manage 42:105–118

Limburg H, Shaw AK, McBride ML (2008) Impact of childhood cancer on parental employment and sources of income: a Canadian pilot study. Pediatr Blood Cancer 51:93–98

Ling J, Payne S, Connaire K, McCarron M (2016) Parental decision-making on utilisation of out-of-home respite in children's palliative care: findings of qualitative case study research—a proposed new model. Child Care Health Dev 42:51–59

Linton JM, Feudtner C (2008) What accounts for differences or disparities in pediatric palliative and end-of-life care? A systematic review focusing on possible multilevel mechanisms. Pediatrics 122:574–582

Lou HL, Mu PF, Wong TT, Mao HC (2015) A retrospective study of mothers' perspectives of the lived experience of anticipatory loss of a child from a terminal brain tumor. Cancer Nurs 38:298–304

Macartney S (2011) Child poverty in the United States 2009 and 2010: selected race groups and Hispanic origin. American Community Survey Briefs. US Census Bureau. Available at http://www.census.gov/prod/2011pubs/acsbr10-05.pdf

Meyer EC, Ritholz MD, Burns JP, Truog RD (2006) Improving the quality of end-of-life care in the pediatric intensive care unit: parents' priorities and recommendations. Pediatrics 117:649–657

Monterosso L, Kristjanson LJ, Phillips MB (2009) The supportive and palliative care needs of Australian families of children who die from cancer. Palliat Med 23:526–536

Morrison RS, Wallenstein S, Natale DK, Senzel RS, Huang LL (2000) "We don't carry that"—failure of pharmacies in predominantly nonwhite neighborhoods to stock opioid analgesics. N Engl J Med 342:1023–1026

Neufeld SM, Query B, Drummond JE (2001) Respite care users who have children with chronic conditions: are they getting a break. J Pediatr Nurs 16:234–244

Nicholas DB, Beaune L, Barrera M, Blumberg J, Belletrutti M (2016) Examining the experiences of fathers of children with a life-limiting illness. J Soc Work End-of-Life Palliat Care 12:126–144

O'Donnell EH, Eddy KT, Rauch PK (2013) Parenting with chronic and life-threatening illness: a parent guidance model. In: Heru AM (ed) Working with families in medical settings: a multidisciplinary guide for psychiatrists and other health professionals. Routledge/Taylor & Francis Group, New York, NY, pp 130–147

Okada H, Maru M, Maeda R, Iwasaki F, Nagasawa M, Takahashi M (2015) Impact of childhood cancer on maternal employment in Japan. Cancer Nurs 38:23–30

Pelletier W, Bona K (2015) Assessment of financial burden as a standard of care in pediatric oncology. Pediatric Blood Cancer 62(Suppl 5):S619–S631

Price J, Jordan J, Prior L, Parkes J (2011) Living through the death of a child: a qualitative study of bereaved parents' experiences. Int J Nurs Stud 48:1384–1392

Pui CH, Pei D, Pappo AS et al (2012) Treatment outcomes in black and white children with cancer: results from the SEER database and St Jude Children's Research Hospital, 1992 through 2007. J Clin Oncol 30:2005–2012

Robert R, Zhukovsky DS, Mauricio R, Gilmore K, Morrison S, Palos GR (2012) Bereaved parents' perspectives on pediatric palliative care. J Soc Work End-of-Life Palliat Care 8:316–338

Rosenberg AR, Dussel V, Kang T et al (2013a) Psychological distress in parents of children with advanced cancer. JAMA Pediatr 167:537–543

Rosenberg AR, Baker KS, Syrjala KL, Back AL, Wolfe J (2013b) Promoting resilience among parents and caregivers of children with cancer. J Palliat Med 16:645–652

Rosenberg-Yunger ZR, Granek L, Sung L et al (2013) Single-parent caregivers of children with cancer: factors assisting with caregiving strains. J Pediatr Oncol Nurs 30:45–55

Schweitzer R, Griffiths M, Yates P (2012) Parental experience of childhood cancer using Interpretative phenomenological analysis. Psychol Health 27:704–720

Syse A, Larsen IK, Tretli S (2011) Does cancer in a child affect parents' employment and earnings? A population-based study. Cancer Epidemiol 35:298–305

Tsimicalis A, Stevens B, Ungar WJ et al (2012) A prospective study to determine the costs incurred by families of children newly diagnosed with cancer in Ontario. Psycho-Oncology 21:1113–1123

Tsimicalis A, Stevens B, Ungar WJ et al (2013) A mixed method approach to describe the out-of-pocket expenses incurred by families of children with cancer. Pediatr Blood Cancer 60:438–445

Vollenbroich R, Duroux A, Grasser M, Brandstatter M, Borasio GD, Fuhrer M (2012) Effectiveness of a pediatric palliative home care team as experienced by parents and health care professionals. J Palliat Med 15:294–300

Wakefield CE, McLoone JK, Evans NT, Ellis SJ, Cohn RJ (2014) It's more than dollars and cents: the impact of childhood cancer on parents' occupational and financial health. J Psychosoc Oncol 32:602–621

Ward E, DeSantis C, Robbins A, Kohler B, Jemal A (2014) Childhood and adolescent cancer statistics, 2014. CA Cancer J Clin 64:83–103

Ware J, Raval H (2007) A qualitative investigation of fathers' experiences of looking after a child with a

life-limiting illness, in process and in retrospect. Clin child Psychol Psychiatry 12:549–565
Warner EL, Kirchhoff AC, Nam GE, Fluchel M (2014) Financial burden of pediatric cancer for patients and their families. J Oncol Pract 11(1):12–18
Whiting M (2013) Impact, meaning and need for help and support: the experience of parents caring for children with disabilities, life-limiting/life-threatening illness or technology dependence. J Child Health Care 17:92–108
Wiener L, McConnell DG, Latella L, Ludi E (2013) Cultural and religious considerations in pediatric palliative care. Palliat Support Care 11:47–67
Wiener L, Viola A, Kearney J et al (2016) Impact of caregiving for a child with cancer on parental health behaviors, relationship quality, and spiritual faith: do lone parents fare worse. J Pediatr Oncol Nurs 33:378–386
Williams PD, Williams KA, Williams AR (2014) Parental caregiving of children with cancer and family impact, economic burden: nursing perspectives. Issues Compr Pediatr Nurs 37:39–60
Wolfe J, Klar N, Grier HE et al (2000a) Understanding of prognosis among parents of children who died of cancer: impact on treatment goals and integration of palliative care. JAMA 284:2469–2475
Wolfe J, Grier HE, Klar N et al (2000b) Symptoms and suffering at the end of life in children with cancer. N Engl J Med 342:326–333

11 Care at the End of Life for Children with Cancer

Eva Bergstraesser and Maria Flury

Long after parents ask "Will she die?," there will be a question about time: "When will my child die?" followed by several additional questions, such as "Will he suffer?"; "What will it be like?"; "What does she need?"; and "How can we be of help?" These are all questions about the end of life, which is what this chapter is about.

11.1 Definition of End of Life and End-of-Life Care

There is no standardized definition of end of life (EOL) (Wolfe et al. 2011), particularly concerning the length of this particular phase of palliative care and stage of disease, irrespective of whether we are thinking about an adult or a child[1] of any age between birth and adolescence. EOL refers to the closeness of death, when the prognosis of death is almost certain and close in time. For EOL care this means "preparing for an anticipated death (e.g., advanced discussion about using life-support technologies in case of cardiac arrest or any other crisis, arranging a last family trip, notifying relatives and friends) and managing the end stage of a fatal medical condition" (Institute of Medicine 2003). Sometimes terms such as terminal care or comfort care are used; however, these are even less clear and should therefore be avoided.

The UK charity organization "Together for Short Lives" (TfSL) describes "end of life" as follows (Together for short lives 2016):

> *The end of life phase begins when a judgment is made that death is imminent. It may be the judgment of the health/social care professional or team responsible for the care of the patient, but it is often the child/young person or family who first recognizes its beginning.*

In consequence "end-of-life care" is defined as (Together for short lives 2016):

> *... care that helps all those with advanced, progressive, incurable illness, to live as well as possible until they die. It focuses on preparing for an anticipated death and managing the end stage of a terminal medical condition. This includes care during and around the time of death, and immediately afterwards. It enables the supportive and palliative care needs of both child/young person and the family to be identified and met throughout the last phase of life and into bereavement. It includes management of pain and other symptoms and provision of psychological, social, spiritual and practical support and support for the family into bereavement.*

[1] "Child" is used for the whole age group from 0 to18 years if not specified otherwise.

E. Bergstraesser, M.D., M.Sc. (✉) • M. Flury
University-Children's Hospital Zurich—Eleonore Foundation, Steinwiesstrasse 75, CH-8032 Zurich, Switzerland
e-mail: eva.bergstraesser@kispi.uzh.ch

J. Wolfe et al. (eds.), *Palliative Care in Pediatric Oncology*, Pediatric Oncology,
https://doi.org/10.1007/978-3-319-61391-8_11

11.2 Particularity of End of Life in Children Dying from Cancer

Illness trajectories of children dying of cancer are in some ways typical and comparable and different to those of children dying from cardiac or neurological disorders (Hynson 2012). Murray et al. (2005) was probably the first to describe characteristics of illness trajectories in adults. Following the description of patterns for the patient himself, he started to envision a more complex perspective, including psychological, social, and spiritual aspects not only of the patient but also his or her family caregivers (Murray et al. 2010). Children dying from cancer are comparable to adults dying from cancer, with high quality of life or "function" prior to diagnosis, variable patterns during treatment, and a rather fast decline during the EOL phase (Murray et al. 2005). The EOL phase comprises a time frame which can vary from days to months as exemplified by the vignette and Fig. 11.1.

Vignette (Fig. 11.1)
Until his fourth birthday, Nick[2] was a healthy child. Shortly after his birthday, he was diagnosed with a metastatic rhabdomyosarcoma after presenting with back pain due to spinal cord involvement. Intensive chemotherapy was started, however, with poor tumor response. Even following further treatment intensification, the tumor remained unresponsive. Nick's parents were informed about the poor prognosis, and a less burdensome treatment was suggested. This happened 4 months after initial diagnosis. Surprisingly, Nick recovered well under this treatment, and the tumor remained stable for 8 months. However, 13 months following diagnosis, Nick experienced weakness in his left leg and was found to have progression of the spinal tumor; other tumors had remained stable. He responded well to local radiation. The whole family spent their summer holidays in the mountains, and Nick was able to accompany them on shorter hiking tours. In August further progression developed and Nick's general condition deteriorated. A network for his care at home was set up, and he died at home 6 weeks later, 16 months following diagnosis.

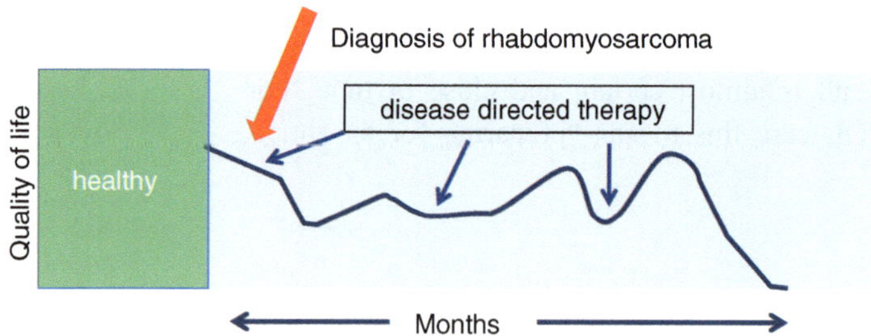

Fig. 11.1 Illness trajectory of a child with rhabdomyosarcoma

[2]All vignettes are based on real patients. Names have been changed to protect the families' identities.

11.3 Needs at the End of Life

When the burden of disease increases and poor quality of life outweighs the potential benefit of prolongation of life, the focus of care is shifted toward the individual needs of the patient. EOL care needs may be defined following the dimensions of palliative care: physical, psychological, social, and spiritual. This is depicted in the holistic model of adults' EOL care needs (NEST) developed by Emanuel et al. (2001): **n**eeds (social), **e**xistential matters, **s**ymptoms, and **t**herapeutic matters.

In children, particular needs at the EOL have to be considered. This imperatively includes the family and their needs. For the EOL care of a child, the parents' perspective is involved by discussing and evaluating the following themes with them (Hinds et al. 2009; Klick and Hauer 2010):

- Identifying communication preferences of the child and the family
- Discussing goals of treatment that may mitigate unnecessary suffering and facilitate comfort
- Balancing quality of life with duration of life
- Limiting interventions that cause unnecessary suffering
- Anticipating, assessing, and treating symptoms
- Deciding on discontinuation or pursuing life-sustaining therapies
- Discussing resuscitation
- Ensuring coordination and continuity of care
- Planning the location of death based on the preferences of the child and the family
- Anticipating and discussing the dying process
- Speaking about faith, spiritual, and cultural practices and needs

In adolescents, additional aspects become important, and their own preferences need to be clarified and integrated into the care plan. Several studies suggest that their preferences and needs may include (Jacobs et al. 2015; Rosenberg and Wolfe 2013; Rosenberg et al. 2014; Wein et al. 2010):

- Being physically comfortable
- Being free from pain
- Knowing what to expect
- Understanding treatment choices
- Completing an advance directive
- Being able to stay in their own home
- Being off machines at end of life
- Dying a natural death
- Being connected with others, having a sense of belonging
- Creating meaning and purpose
- Being at peace spiritually
- Choosing people who should be alongside them during the last hours and days

11.4 Care Setting

In the majority of children with advanced cancer, EOL care still takes place in the hospital, either in an oncology ward or an intensive care unit. This varies by country and strongly depends on palliative care service availability (Feudtner et al. 2007; Vickers and Chrastek 2012; Vickers et al. 2007). Children with hematological malignancies are more likely to be cared for in hospital compared with children with solid tumors. Additional factors of place of care include age, cause of disease deterioration and dying (treatment related versus disease progress), discussions with the healthcare team, and presence of a do-not-resuscitate order (Montgomery et al. 2016). Within these rational reflections, the needs and wishes of the individual child and his or her family should be weighted strongly. In general, many families wish to spend the last weeks of their child's life at home (Vickers et al. 2007; Friedrichsdorf et al. 2015; Siden et al. 2008), and death at home is more common for children with cancer than in other chronic conditions (Pousset et al. 2010).

However, planning and feeling prepared for the child's EOL seem to be even more important than the actual place of death (Dussel et al. 2009). In any case high flexibility is needed concerning uncomplicated and rapid transfers between care settings. When anticipated, the realization of rapid transfers should not be a problem. This also includes inviting families to openly communicate their wishes, doubts, or changing perspective as well as changes in perceived needs. It is helpful to let families know that changes are expected and that we as professionals regard them as normal events in an extraordinary life situation.

For a successful outcome, the care setting should suit the individual needs of the child and his or her family. There is no "best" setting. The best setting for child and family is the one that best answers needs and wishes and the specific situation and circumstances of the family. This also depends on the structure and extent of the local healthcare system (Vickers and Chrastek 2012). Irrespective of these individual factors, for each care setting, three cornerstones are central: communication, coordination, and continuity. Facilitators include clear responsibilities; a so-called key worker, who can serve as connector between settings and teams; and well-established relationships between the co-players.

Not every healthcare professional caring for an affected child and family will have specific or specialized palliative care training. Therefore, pediatric clinicians working with children with cancer at end of life and their families need basic training in palliative and EOL care (that is primary palliative care skills) (Blinderman and Billings 2015; Quill and Abernethy 2013). Primary care clinicians may also play a role at the EOL and therefore need to be involved and trained.

Importantly, recent literature suggests that the support and availability of a specialized pediatric palliative care team improve the outcomes of children with cancer at end of life (Hilden 2016; Kassam et al. 2015; Schmidt et al. 2013).

11.4.1 Hospital

Even when the condition of the child makes EOL care at home possible, some children and families will prefer the hospital as place of care. Reasons may be the need of reassurance by the hospital environment and the hospital staff to whom close and long-lasting relationships have developed during therapy. As a result, these families would rather stay at the hospital than have home care for their child (Cancer.Net 2015).

Vignette
Anna-Lia was 5 years old when diagnosed with neuroblastoma stage 4. She died 2 years later with relapsed disease, spending most of her time at home. The oncology team was surprised and somehow stunned by the wish of this extraordinary, self-confident girl to spend what turned out to be her last night on the oncology ward and to drive to the hospital by ambulance. Nobody could convince her to stay at home. No medical reasons could justify this step. Finally, her wish was granted. She arrived late in the evening and died peacefully at her preferred place of death, a place where she had spent a great deal of time during her cancer care.

More common reasons for children with cancer dying in the hospital setting are disease and symptom related. For example, children dying from treatment- or cancer-related complications commonly die in the hospital, several of them on intensive care units. In the case of relapse and disease progression, reasons for hospital admission may be difficult-to-control symptoms or the need to quickly change a treatment, such as rotating a pain medication, which may be done more rapidly in the hospital setting. Experience suggests that some of these crises may be foreseeable and even prevented with advance care planning and well-delineated symptom management recommendations.

Vignette

Nora was 10.5 years old when diagnosed with acute myelogenous leukemia (AML). Only 3 weeks later, she developed respiratory decompensation and was transferred to the intensive care unit, where noninvasive ventilation was initiated. Further deterioration occurred, and treatment was intensified including extracorporeal membrane oxygenation (ECMO), which was continued without improvement of her respiratory status. Therefore, 6 weeks after diagnosis of AML, ECMO was discontinued and she died shortly afterward. An autopsy concluded that respiratory decompensation was most probably caused by treatment-related acute respiratory distress syndrome with development of lung fibrosis. Regardless of her location of death, she and her family received intensive EOL supportive care.

11.4.2 Home

Many children, adolescents, and families prefer dying at home (Jacobs et al. 2015; Dussel et al. 2009; Kassam et al. 2014). Caring for a child at home allows the family greater choice and control over their environment. They experience more privacy and time together as a whole family, fewer attending health professionals and a clearly defined role in their child's care (Vickers and Chrastek 2012). The comfort of "normal" family life supports the child and reduces disruption to family life, particularly for siblings and parents.

To facilitate EOL care of children with cancer at home, different services providing home visits are involved. Community-based pediatric palliative care can be realized through pediatric community nursing supported by the family physician and/or the oncologist/palliative care physician from the tertiary hospital. The pediatric community nursing team provides home visits, has telephone contacts, or communicates electronically or by Skype—a potentially helpful tool to assess symptoms without being on site. This helps to ensure a safe environment for the child and the family. In some countries there are specialized outpatient palliative care teams supporting families in the care of a child with advanced cancer (Knapp et al. 2008; Bona et al. 2011). These services can also be hospital, medical practice, or hospice-based and bundle medical, emotional, social, and spiritual services. Caregivers from volunteer organizations may also be available to offer respite to the family (Meyers et al. 2014). In any case, availability of a physician is helpful to allow such an individualized means of care.

EOL care at home requests anticipatory planning. Potential needs of the child and the family have to be evaluated and existing supportive resources in the community clarified. To guarantee the family and the primary care team security while caring for a dying child, the 24/7 availability of a member of the dedicated palliative care team is very helpful; hospital-based pediatric oncology teams also serve this role. Anticipatory prescribing of medications for the most likely expected symptoms and having these medications in place are further requirements to allow safe and well-arranged care at home. The aim of anticipatory guidance is to empower and support the family in managing symptoms and problems as they arise (Foster et al. 2010). Poor symptom management, particularly concerning hemorrhage, seizures, pain, odor from wounds, or an unexpected course of the disease can be reasons for hospital admission during EOL care. Nevertheless, as noted previously, hospital admission may be very beneficial for a suddenly overburdened family system due to circumstances of the disease or events surrounding the family. The option of hospital admission should thus be consistently offered to the family; it may help in better controlling the symptoms and suffering of the child and may provide temporary relief for the parents and the broader family.

Vignettes

Marie was a 5-year-old girl, diagnosed with diffuse intrinsic pontine glioma. Due to the glioma, she lost her ability to talk, a symptom that caused her and her parents great suffering. During rapid tumor progression, she developed further cancer-related symptoms such as loss of mobility, spasticity causing pain, difficulties with swallowing, and uncontrollable nausea and vomiting, which was not improved with tube feeding. To enable an appropriate intake of fluids and calories, she was started on parenteral nutrition. The greatest wish of the parents, who were aware of the impending death of their only child, was to spend time in their beloved mountain resort. The community-based pediatric nursing team from the family's hometown offered to accompany the family. Supported by the oncologist and palliative care physician, the team worked out how to facilitate parenteral feeding and symptom management in this desired place. Marie died peacefully during the last week of the stay, only 5 months after diagnosis.

Jan was 7 years old when he developed a second relapse of his leukemia, limited to the central nervous system (CNS). He suffered from severe and debilitating headaches due to high intracranial pressure. Fortunately, he quickly responded to the CNS-directed treatment. As the general prognosis was poor, a decision was made—together with his parents—not to start systemic treatment. He spent 5 months in excellent condition, enjoyed his first day of school, and attended school for several weeks before his condition deteriorated, with obvious signs of bone marrow involvement. As previously with his leukemia, he developed severe nosebleeds and was begun on a strict transfusion program. He enjoyed being at home with a close network of support and some visits to the outpatient clinic. During his final days of life, the bleeding episodes worsened and often caused him to panic. These recurrent bleeds also led to an objectionable odor, which became unbearable for his brothers. During his last night, Jan asked his father to take him to the hospital, to the oncology ward, where he expected more effective help. The team also had the impression that he wanted to protect his beloved brothers from his suffering and the whole family from the odor of blood pervading the home.

11.4.3 Children's Hospices

Inpatient children's hospices, also known as "free-standing pediatric hospices" (FSPH), with long tradition in the United Kingdom (Burne et al. 1984), usually provide short break (respite) care and are more commonly used by families with children suffering from complex chronic diseases other than cancer. Due to the particular disease trajectories of children with cancer, hospices are less often chosen by this patient group (Vickers and Chrastek 2012). However, children with CNS tumors may constitute an exception (Fraser et al. 2011). Some hospices also provide hospice-to-home services including home visits. In selected cases, they may visit patients in hospital and thus can contribute importantly to continuity of care. Respite care has been recognized as an important supportive service in PPC, particularly in families of children with disabilities, where it enables parents to better cope with the burden of caring (Remedios et al. 2015).

On a more general level, the role of FSPHs within PPC services should be discussed frankly, allowing questioning aspects. Kassam and Wolfe (2013) discussed the high operating costs of FSPHs compared to home- and hospital-based PPC and emphasized the paucity of evidence concerning superiority of quality of EOL care in FSPHs.

11.5 Patient- and Family-Centered Care

Patient- and family-centered care has become the standard of care in pediatrics (Committee on Hospital Care and Institute for Patient and Family-Centered Care 2012; Kuo et al. 2012) and corresponds to the principles of PPC. It acknowledges the fact that illness and death affect the entire family.

Family interventions support the family, help to preserve and facilitate family integrity and processes, involve family members in the physical and emotional care of the child, enable patients and families to use their strengths, and reinforce them with information and practical help (Friedman 1998). Putting the family into the center of care implies treating all family members with respect, appreciating their expertise with their child, working together to reach the negotiated goals, and honoring their wishes, even if they are incomprehensible for some of the healthcare team (Wright and Bell 2009).

Wright and Bell (2009) describe: "A family is a group of individuals who are bound by strong emotional ties, a sense of belonging and a passion for being involved in one another's life." The family defines who is a member of their family. The management and the emotional pressure of an anticancer treatment for a child need the inclusion of all family members and quite often, new members, such as friends or neighbors annexed to the extended family system. All families have strengths and coping strategies developed during the illness trajectory. Assessing—if possible with the whole family—how the family is structured and functions will help to understand how the family reacts to the illness and suffering of the child. The assessment can disclose who has to be involved in communication and decisions. It helps to detect the illness beliefs of family members—often unspoken and unknown even to family members themselves (Wright and Leahey 2005). To support families during the EOL phase of their child, the following interventions can be helpful:

- Commending the strengths of family individuals and the complete family in a time when the family is struggling
- Empowering caregiver competencies
- Informing them about options for managing the situation and—if the family asks—offering opinions
- Confirming the normality of the family's emotional reactions to the extraordinary situation
- Supporting rituals
- Making further support and practical help accessible
- Encouraging respite for the primary caregivers

11.5.1 Parents

Hinds et al. (2009) identified four clinician behaviors that support parents during the EOL of their child: affirming that they are "good parents," doing their best for the child, providing ongoing support options, delivering coordinated EOL care, and not forgetting the child and the family after the death of the child.

Particularly in care at home, the empowerment of parents is important to ensure safe and appropriate care for the child. This includes ongoing training and support based on the individualized care plan and the parents' individual needs.

11.5.2 Siblings

Healthy siblings have to adjust to family changes through which parents are physically and emotionally less available for them due to caring for the ill child. They have been referred to as "shadow children," as they tend to become invisible. This puts them at risk for psychological problems (Sharpe and Rossiter 2002; Vermaes et al. 2012). It is therefore important to include healthy siblings in conversations, to inform them age appropriately about the ill child and the impending death of the sister or brother. Inviting them to take part in the care of the sick child, such as visits to the hospital, the hospice, or the sickroom at home or caring for the ill brother or sister, may help them to perceive themselves as an important member of the family and to better cope with the situation. Doing small things like reading a story, helping cook a meal, or picking clothes for the ill child can be encouraging for the sibling (Foster et al. 2010). In addition, siblings need to be encouraged to continue their life, by going to school and spending time with peers without a guilty conscience and negative feelings like anger. Feelings of guilt and jealousy should be acknowledged and, if possible, normalized.

11.5.3 Grandparents

Due to the rising life expectancy and health of older people, the EOL and death of a child often affect grandparents. The majority of grandparents perceive their grandparenting role as essential to their lives, and they deliver high social and emotional support to their grandchildren (Charlebois and Bouchard 2007; Youngblut et al. 2010). When a child is treated for cancer, grandparents are often involved in various tasks, such as providing emotional support for the parents, looking after healthy siblings, or doing household chores, but also in continuing to live their particular relationship to their beloved grandchild (Charlebois and Bouchard 2007). In this duty they experience a heavy burden and "double grief" by worrying about their own child and the grandchild (Charlebois and Bouchard 2007; Wakefield et al. 2014). However, treatment teams often assume that grandparents know by experience how to cope with severe illness and the risk of dying and, therefore, most commonly offer less support or do not even perceive their duty as supporting grandparents as well (Gilrane-McGarry and O'Grady 2011). A grandchild's death disrupts the expected natural order that children and grandchildren should outlive grandparents. In close consultation with the child's parents, grandparents may be provided with information about the condition of their grandchild, including a perspective on prognosis and possibilities for care during EOL, such as symptom management. Grandparents should feel welcome to be involved in the care of the grandchild. This attentiveness can help them to cope better with the overwhelming situation. In parallel to siblings, these members of an individual family need acknowledgement and appreciated for all their endeavors in supporting the dying child and the whole family.

11.6 Advance Care Planning

Advance care planning (ACP) is an extension of the normal treatment plan, documenting the process of discussing issues and planning ahead with parents and, if possible, the child in anticipation of a future change in condition (Horridge 2015; Spicer et al. 2015). ACP specifies how and to what extent symptoms that may occur during the child's EOL phase should be treated. When discussing treatment options, benefits and burdens are considered and potential outcomes anticipated. Decisions must be made within an ethical and legal framework, depending on local rules and reevaluated on a regular basis to respond to the changing medical condition of the child. The ACP also includes decisions, such as resuscitation status and wishes or expectations, about how to arrange the last days and desired location of death and decisions about what is to happen post-death from the perspective of the family and child when appropriate. The treatment team is responsible to initiate ACP. Discussing these issues with the child and the family secures the flow of communication and clarifies common goals. To ensure continuity of care, the ACP should be disseminated to all professionals and places involved in the patient's care (Tsai 2008; Baker et al. 2008). ACP may help families to communicate about aspects of care which otherwise may have remained unspoken. It may also alleviate the grieving process and move into a more realistic area with hopes and thus improve resilience (Horridge 2015).

Components to be included in pediatric advance care planning (Horridge 2015; Sanderson et al. 2016):

- Advance statements of wishes and preferences
- Statement about discussions with the child and family about appropriate level of intervention
- Statement about resuscitation
- Statement about wishes concerning place of care and death

11.7 Symptoms and Suffering at the End of Life

Symptoms and suffering not only have high impact on the child during EOL but also on the family after the death of the child (Kreicbergs et al. 2007). Symptoms have been well documented for children with cancer at EOL, as compared with children with other complex chronic conditions. Focusing on the last 4 weeks of life, several predominantly retrospective studies including parents' evaluation or chart reviews have been performed (Jalmsell et al. 2006; Wolfe et al. 2000, 2008). One of the first and most highly regarded studies is that of Wolfe et al. (2000). According to this first publication, 89% of all participating parents (whole sample 103 parents, response rate of 62%) reported a great deal of suffering from at least one of their child's symptoms. Pain is certainly ranked highest among the most stressful symptoms by parents and healthcare professionals (Goldman et al. 2006; Pritchard et al. 2010). Wolfe et al. (2000) also reported on the disappointing efficacy of treatment, with success in less than 30% of children (including treatment of pain). In later studies, further symptoms, such as anxiety and fatigue (Wolfe et al. 2008, 2015; Ullrich et al. 2010), have been documented. One prospective study in the UK, involving 20 centers, documented symptoms and symptom management in a total of 164 patients on a monthly basis over a period of 6 months until the death of the child (Goldman et al. 2006). This approach allowed comparing the development of symptoms toward the child's EOL and also how symptoms could be controlled. Particularly intractable symptoms occurred in CNS tumors. A recent prospective study by Wolfe and her team (Wolfe et al. 2015) included 104 children with progressive, recurrent, or nonresponsive cancer and analyzed child-reported symptoms during a 9-month period. In a subgroup of 25 children, the last 12 weeks of life were studied. This is the first larger prospective cohort study reporting on patient-related outcomes in children with advanced cancer.

11.7.1 Most Common Symptoms

According to the literature, fatigue, pain, dyspnea, poor appetite, nausea and vomiting, constipation and diarrhea, changes in motor function and reduced mobility, weakness, difficulty swallowing, anxiety, sadness and depression, weight loss and cachexia, and changes in behavior are the most common symptoms in children dying of cancer (Montgomery et al. 2016; Friedrichsdorf et al. 2015; Jalmsell et al. 2006; Wolfe et al. 2000, 2008, 2015; Goldman et al. 2006; Pritchard et al. 2008, 2010; Hechler et al. 2008; Jalmsell et al. 2010). Symptoms and suffering vary depending on diagnosis and the underlying deterioration, which determine whether the child will die of cancer progression or treatment-related complications (Wolfe et al. 2000; Klopfenstein et al. 2001). Treatment-related complications are associated with more severe symptoms (Wolfe et al. 2000), which may be less controllable. In children with progressive tumors or leukemia/lymphomas, tumor type significantly influences the prevalence of symptoms. Thus, children with progressive hematologic malignancies (e.g., leukemia) may develop bleeding, whereas children with solid tumors more often suffer from pain and children with CNS tumors from headaches and swallowing difficulties (Jalmsell et al. 2006; Goldman et al. 2006). In addition, the age of the child may have an influence on symptom intensity, with older children (> 9 years) suffering more intensely as compared with younger children (Jalmsell et al. 2006). Quality of life during the last month of life can be severely affected not only by physical symptoms but also by psychological issues such as sadness, anxiety, and mood swings. Physical symptoms influence the social life of the child, such as going to kindergarten or school and leisure activities or seeing friends. For

parents, the symptoms of most concern during the final week of life included changes in behavior and changes in breathing and pain (Pritchard et al. 2010).
Before discussing specific symptoms, some aspects of symptom assessment at EOL will be considered.

11.7.2 Symptom Assessment

Effective symptom assessment is pivotal to guiding appropriate treatment (Foster et al. 2010). The symptoms that cause the most concern to clinicians can differ from symptoms the child and the family rate as causing the most suffering. Therefore, the best assessment of symptoms should occur via the patient him- or herself. In addition to carefully asking the child and his or her caregiver about symptoms and suffering, appropriate assessment instruments according to age and condition are important in evaluating and understanding the symptoms from the perspective of the child. Training on how to use the different assessment tools should start before a symptom occurs for the first time. The condition and the often seen withdrawal of a dying child can add to the complexity of assessing symptoms. Involving parents in this process and using assessment tools for noncommunicating children can then be helpful. However, at the EOL, it is important to be aware that the existence of a symptom may not be as relevant as the distress resulting from a particular symptom (Pritchard et al. 2010). Additionally, assessment may result in added burden for the child. Thus, simply asking about symptoms can be most helpful. For example, Pritchard et al. (2010) suggested asking parents "What symptoms are of most concern to you or to your child now?" and also inquiring about reasons for these concerns. It may also be helpful to explain causative and contributing factors to symptom distress.

For pain various validated assessment tools for the different age groups are available (Hunt 2012) and discussed in Chap. 6. At EOL it may be helpful to assess physical, psychological, and contextual factors directly with the child or with family caregivers who know the behavior of their child best (World Health Organization 2012). This approach is particularly important when the pain has changed in character. In young children and in children with limited verbal skills, the observation of the child's behavior is a valid approach for pain assessment. Main indicators for pain are crying, facial expression, body movement, and inability to be consoled. However, these cues may be absent and "replaced" by fear of being moved, lack of interest in playing, quietness or increased irritability, sleep disturbance, and low appetite. Children at EOL may even deny having pain out of the fear of upsetting their parents.

There are very few validated assessment instruments for symptoms other than pain, such as nausea or dyspnea, for children in EOL care (Rajapakse and Comac 2012). Nevertheless, these symptoms should be assessed. For verbally communicating children, verbal assessment scales can be used. Even children less than 5 years of age can rank their symptoms with the three levels: "a little," "some," and "a lot." Face scales, known from pain assessment, may be used to ask children about their nausea, although they have only been validated for postoperative nausea (Baxter et al. 2011). A similar approach can be used to assess dyspnea. Caregivers can be a resource in validating these statements. Various scales are also available, e.g., the Bristol Stool Form Scale©, to rate the severity of constipation and diarrhea (Lewis and Heaton 1997). Older children can be encouraged to use a symptom diary to document their symptoms and the impact of the symptoms on their quality of life.

11.7.3 Diagnostic Measures and Laboratory Evaluation

With the exception of examinations needed to plan interventions for symptom management, such as drainage, diagnostic measures are not typically considered at EOL. The necessity of blood tests also has to be considered carefully. Questions about the rationale for any test and the consequences of abnormal test results should be answered before obtaining the information.

11.8 Pain

At EOL, pain is one of the most prevalent and burdensome symptoms, particularly in older children with solid tumors. Uncontrolled pain may be a reason for patients and families to remain in hospital. Sometimes extraordinarily high doses of opioids and highly individual approaches are needed. Among patient with solid tumors, radiotherapy may lead to rapid and effective pain relief. However, even if radiotherapy can be provided in a timely manner and over just a few days, the role of radiotherapy at EOL should be evaluated critically with respect to burden and benefit and with regard to life expectancy. In general, radiotherapy should be initiated early enough to allow for benefit. The following vignette underscores this concept.

Vignette
Sarah was 13 years old when she was diagnosed with adenocarcinoma of the colon, metastatic to local lymph nodes. Following hemicolectomy she received chemotherapy for 6 months. After only 2 months following the completion of chemotherapy, she developed peritoneal carcinomatosis. She underwent surgery and was treated with second-line chemotherapy. During this treatment, 17 months after diagnosis, a new tumor mass and liver metastases were found, and chemotherapy was changed in accordance with the patient and her parents. In parallel, she received patient-controlled analgesia (PCA) with morphine (40 μg/kg/h), which she also used at home. Due to further tumor progression, chemotherapy was discontinued 3 months later. She subsequently underwent drainage of ascites and received local, low-dose radiotherapy (2 × 2.5 Gy). Sadly, she died only 1 week later. Her pain treatment ultimately included PCA with fentanyl (100 μg/kg/h), continuous infusion of ketamine (0.2 mg/kg/h), clonidine (2 μg/kg/h), and midazolam (maximal 0.3 mg/kg/h). Under this highly intensive treatment, she was fairly comfortable until she died.

At EOL opioids play a central role in the treatment of pain, as mentioned, sometimes in extremely high doses. The most commonly used opioids are morphine, hydromorphone, and fentanyl (Anghelescu et al. 2015; Drake et al. 2003; Mherekumombe and Collins 2015). An analysis of morphine equivalent doses (MED) of 44 inpatients (median age at death 14.7 years, range 1.2–24) during the last 2 weeks of life illustrates this (Anghelescu et al. 2015). The mean MED (mg/kg/day) (SD) for the whole group were 10.7 (17.9) and 19 (25.8), 14 days prior to death. Interestingly, in younger patients (<13 years), MED was higher as compared to older patients (>13 years) at day 14 prior to death and on day of death with 12.8 and 27.4, respectively, and 9.5 and 14.5. Sarah had a MED of 240 mg/kg/day; massive doses as such have also been described in the literature (Hewitt et al. 2008; Zernikow et al. 2009). In home care settings, lower MED doses are usually prescribed, as shown in a comparable population with 33 children (Mherekumombe and Collins 2015). In this study the mean MED at home was 2.13 mg/kg/day; however, children with high-stage neuroblastoma needed much higher doses.

Particularly with very high doses of opioids and fast dose escalation, the risk of neurotoxicity and opioid-induced hyperalgesia has to be considered (Zernikow et al. 2009; Wilson and Weissman 2004). A leading symptom of neurotoxicity is myoclonus, an uncontrollable twitching and jerking of muscles or muscle groups, usually occurring in the extremities. In an advanced stage, further neuroexcitatory signs such as hyperalgesia, delirium, and eventually seizures may appear. Isolated hyperalgesia is also described with low or moderate opioid doses and is characterized by unexplainable increase of pain and change of pain character with more diffuse pain unresponsive to increasing opioid doses which may induce even more pain.

11.8.1 Methadone

In cases of severe pain at EOL, methadone may be of high value, particularly in children with neuropathic pain (Anghelescu et al. 2011). Dosing of methadone is challenging due to its high pharmacokinetic variability. Methadone can be given enterally or intravenously. The dosage depends on the dosage of the previous opioid, because it is seldom used as first-line opioid. However, the pediatric methadone equianalgesic dose is currently unknown (Fife et al. 2016). When conversion rules from adults—with lower resulting methadone doses for higher previous MED—are used in children, under-medication appears to be a relevant risk (Fife et al. 2016). The same is true for conversion from enteral to intravenous application, where children needed 80% of the enteral dose instead of 50% (Davies et al. 2008). Therefore, the initiation of methadone as well as conversion should take place with a highly experienced physician in an inpatient or intensively followed outpatient setting.

11.8.2 Adjuvant Medications

Low-dose ketamine as continuous intravenous or subcutaneous infusion is frequently used for neuropathic and in chronic pain as an adjuvant treatment (Bredlau et al. 2013). The dosage ranges from 0.05 to 0.5 mg/kg/h. Treatment should be started carefully with low doses to prevent neurotoxicity. On peripheral wards continuous infusion is preferred rather than bolus doses. In severe pain it may also have an opioid-sparing effect (Bredlau et al. 2013; Finkel et al. 2007), as shown in children with severe mucositis (James et al. 2010). Oral ketamine has also been used as an adjuvant medication among children cared for in the home setting.

In severe pain at the EOL, propofol may be used (Hooke et al. 2007). A retrospective chart review by Hooke et al. (2007) included nine patients with difficult-to-control pain. Propofol was chosen as co-medication and not primarily with the aim of sedation. All patients received propofol until death (median 5 days, range 1–30 days).

Children with pruritus or severe nausea receiving opioids may be managed with co-medication with continuous intravenous naloxone (0.25 μg/kg/h) (Zernikow et al., 2009).

11.9 Anemia and Bleeding

In children with leukemia or treatment-related complications, anemia and bleeding are relevant and potentially debilitating symptoms. In the context of EOL, the aim of treatment through the transfusion of erythrocytes or platelets should be carefully considered with symptoms rather than blood counts guiding intervention. In patients with a high risk of bleeding, a pragmatic approach concerning transfusion of platelets should be considered. Particularly when the child is at home, platelet transfusions should be planned irrespective of counts and administered on a fixed schedule (see vignette Jan).

Whereas minor bleeds can be dealt with using oral tranexamic acid, major bleeds due to bone marrow failure or vessel rupture may be lethal. Massive bleeding causes the child to lose consciousness rapidly and therefore avoids long suffering for the child (Amery, 2016). However, terminal hemorrhage is very frightening for the family and should be anticipated.

11.9.1 Transfusion of Blood Products in the Home Care Setting

There is variable availability of being able to provide transfusions in the home care setting. However if available, the provision of transfusion at home may reduce stress and discomfort from transport to the hospital for both the child and family.

Potential risks have to be considered carefully, as in case of an acute transfusion reaction, and the administering healthcare worker has no access to life support systems. The most important precondition for home transfusion is a history of well-tolerated transfusions without known adverse reactions. Secure venous access is needed and premedication if indicated. Additionally, medications to treat adverse reactions should be available in advance. When erythrocyte transfusion is planned, it may be necessary to organize transport of a pre-transfusion blood sample to the hospital laboratory as well as transport of the blood product from the hospital to the child's home. A family member can be trained to execute the pre-transfusion checking together with a healthcare worker. Ensuring that the child's well-being is observed during and after transfusion is vital. The documentation of the entire transfusion process should be carried out according to national transfusion standards (Wilson et al. 2014).

11.9.2 Practical Aspects in Epistaxis and Other Mucosal Bleeds

In order to reduce anxiety caused by acute bleeding, instruction of the family is essential. If the child has a nosebleed, he should be seated with his head down. The blood will then flow out of the nose and not to the back of the throat where it will be swallowed. Swallowed blood can cause nausea and vomiting. A cold pack positioned on the child's neck and pressure to the septal area of the nose can help stop the bleeding. Pads impregnated with tranexamic acid can also be useful to stop the bleeding. In addition, tranexamic acid mouthwashes may be used to treat bleeding gums (Jassal 2016). To reduce anxiety further, a dark cloth can be held under the child's nose. This intervention hides the amount of blood and helps to steady the child and the caregiver in the acute situation.

11.10 Dyspnea

Dyspnea is an unpleasant subjective experience of being unable to breathe adequately that may increase in prevalence and severity as the cancer disease progresses (Brook et al. 2012). Like pain, dyspnea is a multidimensional symptom that is influenced by affective and physical components (Dudgeon and Shadd 2016). It can be triggered by physical, psychosocial, and environmental factors and can lead to physical limitations and increased dependence. At EOL, dyspnea may be a leading symptom, eliciting fear not only in the patient but also among the whole family. Moreover, the respiratory distress of a loved one during the last days and hours can result in long-lasting adverse family memories. Therefore, management of dyspnea is of high importance, even at times requiring palliative sedation or noninvasive ventilation.

The management of breathlessness depends on the severity of the symptom and underlying causes. If the benefit of treatment of the underlying cause outweighs the burden, the source should be treated. For the patient and family, clear information about the reasons for dyspnea are important and may help to reduce anxiety, particularly anxiety about suffocation.

Dyspnea, as described in detail in Chap. 6, is most often treated with low-dose morphine or other opioids. Less than half the starting dose of opioids can be effective in relieving dyspnea in opioid naive patients.

Several non-pharmacological approaches can provide additional support. Treatment with oxygen is frequently prescribed or requested by patients and families, irrespective of the underlying cause and PaO_2 values. Several randomized controlled trials with adults revealed no additional benefit of oxygen for the relief of dyspnea compared with room air (Abernethy et al. 2010). However, when families were used to administer oxygen earlier in the disease, it may be difficult to convince them that oxygen will not effectively relieve dyspnea but prolong the dying process. A calm, well-ventilated, not overheated environment with windows opened is helpful, followed by reduction of physical activity, comfort positioning, and the use of a fan. Non-pharmacological approaches further include breathing techniques. In addition, caregivers should be instructed to watch their own breathing and comportment, which has an influence on reassuring and calming the child (Brook et al. 2012).

Anxiety can significantly exacerbate dyspnea. Thus, relaxation strategies can be very helpful. Adolescents often benefit from anticipatory guidance and explanation about reasons for dyspnea. Additionally, benzodiazepines are frequently used synergistically with opioids to ease dyspnea.

Some family members, including siblings, view changing breathing patterns and sounds in the last hours of life as dyspnea and distress for the child (Ethier 2010; Lovgren et al. 2016). Information about the cause of noisy breathing and that experience suggests that is it not distressing for the child may be helpful.

11.11 Urinary Retention

Reasons for urinary tract problems at EOL, particularly low urinary output, are commonly a natural process due to progressive organ failure prior to death and do not require intervention. In contrast, ureteral obstruction caused by a growing abdominal or pelvic tumor mass, spinal cord compression, bleeding with clotting, or urine retention due to opioids should be addressed in a timely manner (Benyamin et al. 2008; Kouba et al. 2008). Urinary tract obstructions can generate significant pain and suffering, if not managed properly. In the terminal phase, a full bladder can cause restlessness and agitation. Pronounced weakness can lead to incontinence, a symptom that can also be stressful for the child (Davies 2012). Depending on the underlying cause, catheterization or stenting of the ureter can effectively reduce discomfort. The use of a urinary catheter at EOL may also help to avoid the painful movement associated with bed linen changing. A catheter may also help to avoid bedsores caused by wet diapers or clothes (Kyle 2010).

Families should be prepared for potential urinary tract problems and for the fact that during the last days and hours of the child's life, kidney function will decrease (Davies 2012).

Vignette

The 7-year-old Sven, with the second recurrence of a nephroblastoma, was admitted to the hospital because of uncontrolled pain, nausea, and vomiting. The ultrasound showed pronounced hydronephrosis of the single kidney and a huge abdominal tumor mass. In agreement with his parents, the decision was made to implant a ureteral stent to facilitate the flow of urine. After the intervention, Sven's pain decreased significantly and could be controlled with transdermal fentanyl. He was able to eat and drink again and could be discharged to home care 48 h later. Following this intervention he spent 4 additional months with rather good quality of life before he died at home.

11.12 Ascites and Pleural Effusion

Malignant ascites may be associated with symptoms and may create a significant burden for the patient. If repeated paracentesis is needed, the use of a tunneled indwelling peritoneal catheter should be considered. A most recent fast fact (Burleigh et al. 2016) discussed this issue for adults. Several systems are used for both ascites and pleural effusion drainage and may also be applicable in children, particularly when care takes place in the home care setting.

11.13 Malignant Bowel Obstruction

Fortunately, bowel obstruction is a quite rare event in children with cancer. It may arise in children with abdominal tumors, such as neuroblastoma, nephroblastoma, or rhabdomyosarcoma (Davies 2012; Friedrichsdorf et al. 2011). Clinical signs are nausea and vomiting and cessation of bowel movements, accompanied by severe abdominal pain and cramps. Medical management includes aggressive analgesia, antiemetic and anti-secretory medication, and the placement of a nasogastric tube with suction. As in adults, octreotide is reported in pediatric case reports (Watanabe et al. 2007; Davies et al. 2012) to effectively relieve nausea and vomiting and to provide reasonable quality of life. The dose of octreotide for children is uncertain. In these reports and a summary of the Federal Drug Administration (Department of Health and Human Services 2008), a starting dose of 2 μg/kg/h is suggested which should then be titrated to effect with a maximum dose of 10 μg/kg/h.

11.14 Psychological Symptoms

At the EOL almost all patients experience psychological symptoms. Many of these symptoms can be seen in relation to the child's awareness of death and their concerns about themselves but also their loved ones on how they will cope (Himelstein et al. 2004; Nitschke et al. 2000;

Kreicbergs et al. 2004). Anxiety, fear, and depression play a central role. Adolescents have a significantly higher rate of anxiety and depression compared with younger children (Rosenberg and Wolfe 2013; Jalmsell et al. 2006; Bell et al. 2010; Theunissen et al. 2007; Cohen et al. 2008). It is of great importance to treat such symptoms as much as possible and not to underestimate them, as they also play a significant role in the bereavement of parents (Jalmsell et al. 2010). In cases where the child's well-being was severely affected, parents showed significantly more psychological morbidity 4–9 years after the child's death (Jalmsell et al. 2010).

11.14.1 Agitation and Delirium

Agitation and delirium at EOL have high impact on the patient, the family, and also the medical staff. Therefore, agitation and delirium need a straightforward management, including effective medication and sometimes even palliative sedation, non-pharmacological measures, and intensive support of the child's family. Agitation may occur isolated or as a symptom of delirium. Further features of delirium in children are disturbed consciousness, change in cognition with a tendency to fluctuate during the course of a day (Goldsmith et al. 2011). Pharmacological treatment of agitation as well as delirium consists of benzodiazepines or antipsychotics, such as haloperidol, which may also be given intravenously as continuous infusion (Goldsmith et al. 2011; Stoddard et al. 2006), risperidone (Goldsmith et al. 2011), levomepromazine (Hohl et al. 2013), or dexmedetomidine (Schieveld and Janssen 2014). Depending on experiences and local regulations, this treatment will be supported by the psychiatric service.

11.15 Palliative Sedation

The term "palliative sedation therapy" was recommended by Morita et al. (2002) to prevent association with euthanasia, which was strongly linked to the earlier term "terminal sedation." "Palliative sedation" and "palliative sedation therapy" are used interchangeably. The primary aim of palliative sedation is to relieve the patient from refractory symptoms associated with high distress by a reduction of consciousness. Not many children with end-stage cancer, particularly solid tumors, may need and benefit from palliative sedation. However, this estimate differs between countries, as a study from Belgium and Flanders shows, where more than 20% of children were continuously and deeply sedated at the EOL (Pousset et al. 2011). In this context, a clear definition of "refractory symptom or distress" is important. Morita et al. (2002) proposed the following definition of refractory distress: "All other possible treatments have failed, or it is estimated that no methods are available for palliation within the time frame and the risk-benefit ratio the patient can tolerate." In a child with the need for palliative sedation, a do-not-resuscitate order should be in place and can be regarded as an essential precondition.

Concepts for palliative sedation in children stem from those for adults. Naipaul and Ullrich wrote a comprehensive overview of palliative sedation that includes most important perspectives and aspects of this particular part of treatment at the EOL Naipaul and Ullrich 2011). The most common drugs used for sedation are benzodiazepines, and among those, midazolam is the most commonly prescribed. A safe starting dose would be 0.05 mg/kg/h intravenously or subcutaneously; an initial bolus may be applied if necessary. In adults, it was shown that palliative sedation is not associated with worse survival (Pousset et al. 2011; Maltoni et al. 2012). If benzodiazepines do not work sufficiently, propofol may be an option and has shown some promising effects in case studies (Anghelescu et al. 2012). According to Anghelescu, the starting dose of propofol is 30 μg/kg/min. Certainly, this treatment should remain in the hands of highly experienced healthcare professionals and if necessary with the support of anesthesiology.

The depth of sedation can be varied in accordance with the patient's needs. Palliative sedation may be delivered continuously or intermittently to determine the correct dose.

11.16 Nutrition and Fluid Management

Poor appetite is one of the symptoms parents reported in the indicatory study of Wolfe et al. (2000). Nurturing and feeding their child is one of the strongest instincts in parents. The wish to feed the child orally can go beyond what benefits the child. The preparation and serving of food are an act of caring, and intake of food is essential for survival. When the amount of ingested food decreases, the family may take it as a barometer of condition. For adolescents as well, nutrition may remain highly important until the last hour, also in its meaning as a sign of being alive. Clearly, good nutrition either orally, enterally, or parenterally can improve the child's quality of life (Thompson et al. 2012).

The decision to start or end enteral or parenteral feeding and hydration in the EOL phase can cause clinically relevant problems. Possible disadvantages of reduction or withdrawal of nutrition and hydration can be thirst, xerostomia, fever, constipation, nausea, tachycardia, and an increased risk of bedsores. At the same time, continuing intravenous hydration can be associated with edema and respiratory secretion. Continuing enteral feeding may depend on the insertion of a feeding tube, an intervention associated with potential suffering of the child. Intravenous nutrition requires a central line, and if not in place, the entire process—including the aims of nutrition—needs careful evaluation. The child, depending on her age, and the family should be closely involved in this discussion. When dehydration results from correctable causes, such as diuretics, vomiting, or diarrhea, artificial hydration can be considered. Once the child is close to death, the need to eat and drink decreases, and giving intravenous fluid will not influence the time of death. Thirst and a dry mouth should be treated with regularly applied mouth care or with ice cubes to suck.

11.17 Experimental Therapies (Phase I and II Studies)

Enrollment in phase I or II studies of pediatric cancer patients at the EOL rarely results in direct benefit for the child, as most children will die from their disease. In addition, children continuing to receive cancer-directed treatment at EOL may experience greater distress (Wolfe et al. 2000). The motivation to participate in an early phase study is often led by the optimism of disease stabilization, symptom relief, and maintenance of hope. Further on, the altruistic aspect of contributing to research and helping future patients may also be a motivation for the child or adolescent himself, as well as for the parents. If a parallel approach is chosen, where advance care planning and EOL care with effective symptom management are not impeded by participation in phase I or II studies, this approach may be valuable (Levine et al. 2015). It should be considered that according to a study by Mack et al. (2008), 28% of parents (39 of 140) whose child had received treatment for incurable cancer at EOL would recommend experimental chemotherapy to the family of a child without symptoms and 19% to the family of a symptomatic child.

11.18 Complementary and Alternative Treatments

Complementary and alternative medicine (CAM) is defined by the National Center for Complementary and Alternative Medicine (NCCAM) (2016) as "a group of diverse medical healthcare systems, practices, and products that are not presently considered to be part of conventional medicine. If a non-mainstream practice is used together with conventional medicine, it's considered 'complementary'. If a non-mainstream practice is used in place of conventional medicine, it's considered 'alternative'."

Up to 90% of parents administer CAM to their children during curative anticancer treatment (Bishop et al. 2010). At the EOL, 30% of families use CAM in children, mostly in the form of diets, vitamins and herbal treatments, homeopathy and phytotherapy (e.g., mistletoe), and spiritual healing. Most families apply complementary medicine together with conventional therapy in order to make their child feel more relaxed, to give it strength, and to ease side effects of conventional treatment (Heath et al. 2012). To prevent the secret administration of CAM to children and thereby potential interactions, for instance, with St. John's wort, it is important to discuss the issue on a regular basis with the family. Counseling and care from the treatment team serve to protect families against the false promises of miracles delivered by alternative therapies to heal the advanced cancer disease.

Using CAM may help families to cope better and enables them to stay active while facing the impending death of their child. The use of herbal tea, e.g., valerian, can help with sleeping (Bent et al. 2006). Aromatherapy with Melissa (lemon balm) may be helpful in reducing agitation (Ballard et al. 2002). Cool and warm wet packs can help in managing pain and are sometimes used complementarily to drug therapy. The application of massage techniques can also reduce pain (Kutner et al. 2008). Some children can even be trained in relaxation practices.

11.19 General Aspects of EOL Care

11.19.1 How to Change Treatment Plans and Standing Procedures

During active cancer treatment, most children's hospitals have standing operating procedures regarding hygienic and safety issues, such as how often to check vital signs or change dressings of central lines. These rules help to prevent infections and detect side effects of the therapy, before they become life-threatening. Quite a few of these procedures can cause discomfort and pain, disrupt sleep, and increase irritability and agitation (Bruera et al. 2014). At the EOL it is therefore important to assess the actual status of the child and the impact of specific interventions and consequences when they are skipped and to adapt procedures to individual needs and desires.

Need-adapted handling with the aim of maximizing comfort also applies to the prevention of pressure ulcers in children with increased weakness and impaired mobility. Regular repositioning may lead to significant pain and discomfort for the dying child. Therefore minimal handling may better meet the child's needs.

11.19.2 Monitoring in the Context of Family's Needs

Monitoring vital signs like heart rate, oxygen saturation, or blood pressure is commonly done with electronic equipment. Children and families are used to monitors, and during treatment they have learned to interpret figures and graphs and to rely on them. EOL is associated with significant changes in vital signs (Bruera et al. 2014). Therefore, the alarm of the monitor can induce unnecessary stress and fear in the patient and the family. Likewise, withdrawing electronic monitoring might also be (over-)interpreted as withholding support and, accordingly, should be discussed carefully with the family. Parents need the reassurance that intense suffering and the death of the child will be noticed without monitoring.

11.20 Mouth Care

A dry mouth and dry lips induced by mouth breathing, medications such as morphine, and decreased oral fluid intake can cause significant discomfort in the child. Cleaning the teeth with a soft brush and keeping the mouth moist with regular mouthwashes can help to prevent or improve an unpleasant sensation (Jassal 2016). Lips can be moisturized with cream. Older children may prefer to suck ice cubes made of their favorite beverage. To administer small amounts of beverage to younger children, swabs can be soaked with any kind of liquid. If the result of these interventions is insufficient, different artificial saliva products are available.

11.21 Wound Care

Wound problems, for instance, pressure ulcers, caused by decreased mobility of the child, or diaper dermatosis induced by illness-related incontinence or diarrhea can be seen in any kind of advanced cancer. During EOL care the primary goal of wound care, that is, wound healing, is often out of reach. The aim of intervention should be to stabilize the wound and to alleviate pain and suffering (Bower et al. 2011).

Malignant fungating wounds can be seen in pediatric oncology mainly in children with advanced sarcomas. They are caused by the invasion of the primary or metastatic tumor through the skin. The perfusion of the affected tissue is altered, and therefore, tumor necrosis can be found. Colonization of the necrotic tissue by anaerobic bacteria can lead to infection with pain and odor. Malignant wounds can affect the body image of the child and induce suffering for the child and the family (Bower et al. 2011). In the management of malignant wounds, antineoplastic interventions should be considered. Radiation therapy can reduce pain. An orthopedic intervention such as limb amputation can increase quality of life for the child and prevent the onset of a malignant wound (European Oncology Nursing Society 2015).

Vignette

Lina was 11 years old, when she was diagnosed with osteosarcoma of the left femur. At the time of diagnosis, bilateral lung metastases were also detected. She did not respond to neoadjuvant chemotherapy, which could already be assumed when she came to her regular treatments. Her leg still hurts and mobility was restricted. It was therefore decided not to force extremity-preserving surgery but to perform transfemoral amputation in the context of palliation. This somewhat radical procedure induced discussion in the oncology team as to whether the intervention was compatible with a palliative care approach. However, Lina and her parents—probably because of or at least influenced by their farming background—were quickly in favor of this procedure. She tolerated this aspect of treatment best compared to every other treatment. The benefit was a long period free of pain, which once again allowed her to enjoy horseback riding and mobility for the last few months of life.

Careful wound assessment is important in intervention planning. This also includes estimating the impact the wound will have on the child. Wound-related symptoms beside pain can be bleeding, odor, exudate, and sometimes pruritus. To prevent further colonization, the use of antiseptic agents to clean the wound as well as antimicrobial wound dressing (e.g., dressings with silver, honey) is recommended. The size and location of the wound may influence the dressing. A close-fitting dressing with absorbent materials helps to manage exudate, and the use of hemostatic agents can control potential bleeding. The most effective management of associated odor, the debridement of necrotic tissue, is an intervention that requires hospital admission. In home care, activated charcoal dressings can be used, and the odor can be managed with environmental procedures (aromatherapy candles or oils, cat litter) especially if the child is too fragile for dressing changes (European Oncology Nursing Society 2015). Effective treatment of pain due to malignant wounds has not yet been established. Systemic opioids are often used, and topical opioids (e.g., morphine) may produce local analgesia (Chuang et al. 2016).

11.22 Parenteral Administration of Medication in End of Life Care

Some children will have a central venous access device (e.g., Port-a-Cath® or a Hickman catheter) in place from their anticancer therapy, which can be used for the administration of medications (Ballantine and Daglish 2012). The use of central lines is associated with different risks, such as infections or clotting.

Safe and easy-to-manage alternatives are subcutaneous infusion devices. Various devices with different infusion capacities are available. The insertion of a subcutaneous device is only slightly invasive for the child, especially when local anesthetic cream is administered in advance. A trained nurse can do the insertion in the home setting as well. The subcutaneous line can be used to administer bolus injections as well as continuous medication and fluid infusions. The line can be inserted into the infraclavicular or abdominal subcutaneous tissue or into the upper side of the femur. Children may prefer the insertion in the thigh. Most devices can be in situ as long as 7 days. The subcutaneous administration of some drugs will possibly be off-label use. The mixture of different medications in the same syringe should be considered carefully with respect to stability and interaction. References for drug stability, interactions, and tissue compatibility can be found on www.palliativedrugs.com. Commonly used drugs in EOL care are morphine and midazolam, which can be administered without problem. The rate of infusion and absorption from the tissue will be limited, especially in young or cachectic children. A higher concentration can lead to more tissue irritation and pain. The insertion side has to be observed carefully for irritation and inflammation. Swelling of the surrounding tissue is normal, due to slow resorption of the fluid out of the tissue. Sometimes it is advisable to work with two subcutaneous lines to avoid drug interactions or to change between the lines to give the tissue time to regenerate. Any standard syringe driver can be used, but small syringe drivers are available for home care.

11.23 Nearing Death

Interventions prior to the child's death focus on management of distressing symptoms and should provide comfort care. Creating a comfortable environment with only selected people in the room, removing unnecessary equipment, and even reducing light can be helpful for the child and the family. Necessary interventions such as administration of pain medication should be carried out in an undisruptive manner. Whenever possible, a child lying in his parent's arms should not be moved. Healthcare staff should be available but never intrusive (Davies 2012). Sometimes families express the wish that only one or two members of the team carry out all necessary interventions; if possible this wish should be respected.

Anticipating with the family the physical changes that present near the time of the child's death may decrease distress. Physical signs particularly include a slowing down of the body with increased periods of sleep, reduced consciousness, mottled skin, cooling down of the body starting at the limbs, cyanosis, and changes in breathing. A change in breathing pattern and sounds can be worrying for family members, as they may associate them with distress for the child (Ethier 2010). Mouth care and comfort positioning with slightly elevated head can reduce potential discomfort. If oral suctioning is necessary, it should be done as carefully as possible (Eastern Metropolitan Region Palliative Care Consortium 2016). Feeling prepared for the child's dying process may help the family to handle the unbearable situation of losing their beloved child (Davies 2012).

11.24 Communication During EOL and Prior to Death

In this stage of a disease, communication still includes exchange of information as to the current medical status, out of which arise discussions about what to expect at EOL (e.g., anticipated symptoms), about goals and preferences of the patient and his or her family, and advance care planning, including the do-not-resuscitate order. Some families may appreciate having these discussions in a broader context, such as a family conference, involving all important professionals and possibly a relative or friend whom they trust most (Michelson et al. 2013). Even if cure is no longer a realistic goal, hope still plays an important role for patients and families (Kamihara et al. 2015). As Kamihara et al. (2015) point out, in this stage of the disease, hope may help families prepare for the death of the child and redefine goals, such as providing quality of life, love, or a good death.

Apart from providing hope for parents, the involvement of the child should also be considered. There is high variability in family perspectives regarding involving the child in EOL discussions. For example, in a study from the

Netherlands (Kars et al. 2015), it could be shown that parents were not prepared to actively include their child's voice in the decision-making process, even if they were of adolescent age. This was in discrepancy to the parents' self-perception of unselfish decisions and to the wish of older children and particularly adolescents. When they are asked directly about their preferences, they clearly formulate their wish to be involved and also want to be included when discussing their death (Jacobs et al. 2015; Jalmsell et al. 2016; Hinds et al. 2005; Nitschke et al. 1982).

In families with cultural backgrounds where discussions of dying and death are taboo, professionals who are in a trustful relationship with the family may initiate discussions about the family's choices concerning place of EOL care and death (Vickers and Chrastek 2012). On the other hand, there may be parents asking to hasten death due to unbearable pain or other uncontrolled symptoms. According to a study by Dussel et al. (2010) with 141 parents of children who died of cancer, more than 10% of parents had considered hastening death. The predominant reason for this wish was unrelieved pain. In this situation, open and honest information about options of treatment, including palliative sedation, may help to reduce the immense suffering of parents. But also talking open and honestly about death may decrease distress in the child as in the parents. Often, the initiative will be taken by the child, triggered by stories, movies, and music (Jalmsell et al. 2015).

11.24.1 Talking About Last Wishes

Advance care planning not only includes management plans for symptoms arising but also psychological, social, and spiritual needs of the child and its family. Children often have clear conceptions about who should be with them or where to die. Some of them have last wishes. This could involve meeting their favorite actor or singer, visiting a special place, or having a precious present. There are different organizations—some of them acting globally—that fulfill last wishes of children with a life-limiting disease, e.g., Make-A-Wish (www.worldwish.org). Enabling last wishes can generate invaluable memories for the whole family facing the impending death of their child.

Vignette

The last wish of the 9-year-old Laura, suffering from a highly aggressive brain tumor, was a visit to the zoo and have the chance to feed the Galapagos turtles and camels. Because of her increasing weakness and dyspnea, she was accompanied not only by her family but also by a nurse, who could administer morphine if necessary and manage the oxygen supply she needed due to breathlessness. She mobilized all her strength for this special event and enjoyed holding the baby turtle in her hands and the ice cream at the zoo restaurant. Back at the hospital she happily reported her wonderful experiences despite dyspnea. Two days after the zoo visit, she died peacefully. For her family this last adventure with their child was a precious gift.

11.24.2 Anticipation of Grief and Bereavement

Prior to the child's death, first considerations related to bereavement support and parental or siblings' risk factors for complicated bereavement should be made and actively discussed (see Chap. 11).

11.25 Interventions Shortly After the Death of the Child

Treatment of the body with respect and according to the cultural and religious practices of the family and in accordance with local law is of paramount importance.

After the child's death, the healthcare providers involved are informed. Legal confirmation of the child's death has to be given by a physician, who also signs the death certificate. If death was not caused by progression of the disease but, rather, was due to treatment complications, the physician will discuss a postmortem examination with the family of the child. If the family agrees with this procedure, tubes and lines stay inserted. Depending on region, postmortem examination will always be discussed with parents, irrespective of cause of death.

If the child died as a result of their disease, care of the body will take place in agreement with the family. Tubes and lines can be removed if culturally acceptable. Covering punctures with a tight dressing prevents leaking of body fluid. To avoid dirty clothes due to urine or stool, diapers or suitable incontinence material should be used.

The family should be informed about the physical processes starting after death. They should know that the body of the child will develop livor mortis. This process starts about 20–30 min after death, and the first signs can be seen on the lower-lying parts of the body, typically on the child's neck and back. To prevent livor mortis in the face, it is important to hold the child in a supine position. In children with hematological malignancies, livor mortis may start even earlier due to the blood disorder. After a preliminary muscle relaxation, rigor mortis develops about 1 hour after death due to changes in muscle proteins. If the child had a fever before death or in the context of high temperatures, this process may start earlier, even as soon as after 30 min.

The family members are encouraged to stay with their child as long as they wish, unless regional regulations prohibit this. Privacy should be respected if the family wishes to be alone with their child. Nevertheless it is important to check regularly whether the family has additional needs. Religious and cultural needs and wishes should be fulfilled whenever possible. Depending on religion and culture, some of the families desire to perform specific rituals with or without their spiritual leader. In some cultures, washing or bathing of the body is an act of spiritual cleaning and should therefore be done in agreement with the family.

11.25.1 Taking Home the Dead Child

Although very uncommon, some families may appreciate taking home their dead child from the hospital, particularly when the child and family had strongly wished to be at home during EOL. Transportation arrangements may vary from funeral home vehicle to private vehicle.

11.26 Spiritual and Cultural Needs

For many healthcare professionals, including those working in palliative care, it remains difficult to frame the concept of spirituality. Spirituality, in the context of palliative care, has been defined by the National Consensus Project for Quality Palliative care (USA) (Puchalski et al. 2009) as follows: "Spirituality is the aspect of humanity that refers to the way individuals seek and express meaning and purpose and the way they experience their connectedness to the moment, to self, to others, to nature, and to the significant or sacred." The European Association of Palliative Care used this definition as its foundation and adjusted it for the European context (Nolan et al. 2011): "Spirituality is the dynamic dimension of human life that relates to the way persons (individual and community) experience, express and/or seek meaning, purpose and transcendence, and the way they connect to the moment, to self, to others, to nature, to the significant and/or sacred."

For patients, families, and caregivers, spiritual aspects may become important during EOL, even without a religious affiliation (Hexem et al. 2011). For adolescents this may consist of a first critical analysis of the meaning of life and faith. This aspect is impressively shown by a case report of a 15-year-old boy diagnosed with osteosarcoma and dying 1 year later (Flavelle 2011). He keeps a journal and writes: "Sometimes I just wonder if it would be easier to give up. Then I think of everyone I would let down or all the things I would miss. I've been thinking a lot about who gets what if I were to die." Following a time of resistance against efforts of religious support, he starts to find a hold: "I pray every night for some strength and the strength to get through this." A little later, he writes: I know everyone here is doing everything they can and all my family are rooting for me and for the first time I feel safe and I do believe that there is a God and he is watching over me and protecting me." This speaks strongly for the positive psychological resources of adolescence, described under the concept of "resilience" among adolescents and young adults by Rosenberg et al. (2014).

For some parents, being "a good parent" includes spiritual care and guidance for their child (Hinds et al. 2009). For clinicians this means actively asking about spiritual and cultural needs. Some families may not wish to disclose their spiritual or religious values. However, many parents have also found religion helpful in their own coping (Hexem et al. 2011).

There is an array of literature which focuses on spiritual and religious practices surrounding death (Jones 2011; Dom 2011; Hasan 2012; Hedayat 2006; Lebens 2009). For example, Hedayat (2006) provides valuable insight into Muslim attitudes toward the death of a child.

11.27 Follow-Up Consultation After the Child's Death

Experience suggests that families should be invited by the oncologist to take part in a follow-up conversation several weeks following death. This allows reflecting on the child's disease as a whole, and questions around disease-directed treatment, and EOL care may be discussed. Families should have the opportunity to give feedback about care. If an autopsy was performed, results should also be discussed at this point. In addition, the physician may recommend support for the family, depending on suggestions of other team members or the current situation of the family related to their grief process.

It has been shown that parents appreciate this kind of contact, which may also be helpful in coping with their loss (Monterosso and Kristjanson 2008).

11.28 How Could Good Quality of EOL Care Be Measured?

In the future it will be even more important to justify additional resources in medicine, such as specialized pediatric palliative care (PPC). Therefore, we need to develop quality indicators for high-quality PPC, including EOL care. Besides cost and utilization outcomes, indicators should include the patient and family perspective, and with respect to a high quality of EOL care, and parental preparedness (Dussel et al. 2009; Mack et al. 2005). The development of instruments for the evaluation of care and health outcomes in these particular situations of severely ill and dying children could build on these indicators.

"Good death" has been defined by The Institute of Medicine, Washington DC (Institute of Medicine, 2003). "[A] decent or good death is one that is: free from avoidable distress and suffering for patients, families, and caregivers; in general accord with patients' and families' wishes; and reasonably consistent with clinical, cultural, and ethical standards." In contrast, a bad death has been characterized by: "needless suffering, dishonoring of patient or family wishes or values, and a sense among participants or observers that norms of decency have been offended." For children no such definition exists. However, some instruments have been developed which may support outcome research in the future (Wolfe et al. 2000; Kreicbergs et al. 2005; Widger et al. 2015; Zimmermann et al. 2015).

Summary of Key Take-Home Notes

- There is no standardized definition of EOL, either for adults or for children.
- The EOL phase of children dying from cancer often proceeds in a more predictable way as compared to children dying from cardiac or neurological disorders. This provides a chance for planning in advance with the child and family.
- At EOL, the focus of care is shifted toward the individual needs of the patient and family. Besides the four dimensions of palliative care (physical, psychological, social, and spiritual), particular needs of the child, adolescent, parents, and the whole family—including siblings—should actively be inquired about.
- The care setting at EOL highly depends on the cause of disease deterioration and dying. It also depends on communication between the family and the healthcare team and the presence of a do-not-resuscitate order. For each care setting, three cornerstones are central: communication, coordination, and continuity.
- Support and availability of a specialized pediatric palliative care team improve the outcome of children with advanced cancer, irrespective of the setting of care.
- Advance care planning documents the process of decision-making with parents and, if possible, the child in anticipation of the child's deteriorating health condition. Symptoms and suffering at EOL vary depending on diagnosis and the underlying situation of deterioration, whether the child will die of cancer progression or treatment-related complications. Treatment-related complications are associated with more severe symptoms, which may be harder to control. For parents, the symptoms of most concern during the last week of life include a change in behavior, a change in breathing, and pain.
- Pain is one of the most prevalent and burdensome symptoms at EOL, particularly in older children suffering from solid tumors. Uncontrolled pain may be a reason for patients and families to stay in the hospital.
- Dyspnea may be a leading symptom at EOL, eliciting fears not only in the patient but also in the whole family. Management of dyspnea has a major impact. In some children dyspnea may be a reason for palliative sedation.
- Concerning place of death, it has been shown that the opportunity to plan the child's EOL is as relevant a factor as the actual place of death.
- All families should be invited by the attending oncologist to take part in a follow-up conversation several weeks following death. This appointment allows reflecting on the disease of the child as a whole and questions connected with treatment, and EOL care may be discussed.

References

Abernethy AP, McDonald CF, Frith PA, Clark K, Herndon JE 2nd, Marcello J et al (2010) Effect of palliative oxygen versus room air in relief of breathlessness in patients with refractory dyspnoea: a double-blind, randomised controlled trial. Lancet 376(9743):784–793

Amery J (2016) A really practical handbook of children's palliative care. Lulu Publishing Services, United States

Anghelescu DL, Faughnan LG, Hankins GM, Ward DA, Oakes LL (2011) Methadone use in children and young adults at a cancer center: a retrospective study. J Opioid Manag 7(5):353–361

Anghelescu DL, Hamilton H, Faughnan LG, Johnson LM, Baker JN (2012) Pediatric palliative sedation therapy with propofol: recommendations based on experience in children with terminal cancer. J Palliat Med 15(10):1082–1090

Anghelescu DL, Snaman JM, Trujillo L, Sykes AD, Yuan Y, Baker JN (2015) Patient-controlled analgesia at the end of life at a pediatric oncology institution. Pediatr Blood Cancer 62(7):1237–1244

Baker JN, Hinds PS, Spunt SL, Barfield RC, Allen C, Powell BC et al (2008) Integration of palliative care practices into the ongoing care of children with cancer: individualized care planning and coordination. Pediatr Clin North Am 55(1):223–250. xii

Ballantine N, Daglish EB (2012) Using medications in children. In: Goldman A, Hain R, Liben S (eds) Oxford textbook of palliative care for children, 2nd edn. Oxford University Press, Oxford, pp 178–191

Ballard CG, O'Brien JT, Reichelt K, Perry EK (2002) Aromatherapy as a safe and effective treatment for the management of agitation in severe dementia: the results of a double-blind, placebo-controlled trial with Melissa. J Clin Psychiatry 63(7):553–558

Baxter AL, Watcha MF, Baxter WV, Leong T, Wyatt MM (2011) Development and validation of a pictorial nausea rating scale for children. Pediatrics 127(6):e1542–e1549

Bell CJ, Skiles J, Pradhan K, Champion VL (2010) End-of-life experiences in adolescents dying with cancer. Support Care Cancer 18(7):827–835

Bent S, Padula A, Moore D, Patterson M, Mehling W (2006) Valerian for sleep: a systematic review and meta-analysis. Am J Med 119(12):1005–1012

Benyamin R, Trescot AM, Datta S, Buenaventura R, Adlaka R, Sehgal N et al (2008) Opioid complications and side effects. Pain Physician 11(2 Suppl):S105–S120

Bishop FL, Prescott P, Chan YK, Saville J, von Elm E, Lewith GT (2010) Prevalence of complementary medicine use in pediatric cancer: a systematic review. Pediatrics 125(4):768–776

Blinderman CD, Billings JA (2015) Comfort care for patients dying in the hospital. N Engl J Med 373(26):2549–2561

Bona K, Bates J, Wolfe J (2011) Massachusetts' pediatric palliative care network: successful implementation of a novel state-funded pediatric palliative care program. J Palliat Med 14(11):1217–1223

Bower KA, Mulder GD, Reineke A, Guide SV (2011) Dermatologic conditions and symptom control. In: Wolfe J, Hinds PS, Sourkes BM (eds) Textbook of interdisciplinary pediatric palliative care. Elsevier Saunders, Philadelphia, pp 350–367

Bredlau AL, Thakur R, Korones DN, Dworkin RH (2013) Ketamine for pain in adults and children with cancer: a systematic review and synthesis of the literature. Pain Med 14(10):1505–1517

Brook L, Twigg E, Venables A, Shaw C (2012) Respiratory symptoms. In: Goldman A, Hain R, Liben S (eds) Oxford textbook of palliative care for children, 2nd edn. Oxford University Press, Oxford, pp 319–327

Bruera S, Chisholm G, Dos Santos R, Crovador C, Bruera E, Hui D (2014) Variations in vital signs in the last days of life in patients with advanced cancer. J Pain Symptom Manage 48(4):510–517

Burleigh J, Mehta Z, Ellison N (2016) Tunneled Indwelling Catheters for Malignant Ascites #308. J Palliat Med 19(6):671–672

Burne SR, Dominica F, Baum JD (1984) Helen House—a hospice for children: analysis of the first year. Br Med J (Clin Res Ed) 289(6459):1665–1668

Cancer.Net (2015) Caring for a terminally ill child: a guide for parents. American Society of Clinical Oncology. Available from http://www.cancer.net/navigating-cancer-care/advanced-cancer/caring-terminally-ill-child-guide-parents

Charlebois S, Bouchard L (2007) "The worst experience": the experience of grandparents who have a grandchild with cancer. Can Oncol Nurs J 17(1):26–36

Chuang C, Fonger E, Roth R, Campbell M (2016) Challenges with accruing a study of topical opioid for painful malignant wounds: lessons learned. J Palliat Med 19(6):586

Cohen LL, Lemanek K, Blount RL, Dahlquist LM, Lim CS, Palermo TM et al (2008) Evidence-based assessment of pediatric pain. J Pediatr Psychol 33(9):939–955. discussion 56-7

Committee On Hospital Care and Institute For Patient and Family-Centered Care (2012) Patient- and family-centered care and the pediatrician's role. Pediatrics 129(2):394–404

Davies D (2012) Care in the final hours and days. In: Goldman A, Hain R, Liben S (eds) Oxford textbook of palliative care for children, 2nd edn. Oxford University Press, Oxford, pp 368–374

Davies D, DeVlaming D, Haines C (2008) Methadone analgesia for children with advanced cancer. Pediatr Blood Cancer 51(3):393–397

Davies DE, Wren T, MacLachlan SM (2012) Octreotide infusion for malignant duodenal obstruction in a 12-year-old girl with metastatic peripheral nerve sheath tumor. J Pediatr Hematol Oncol 34(7):e292–e294

Department of Health and Human Services (2008) Update on pediatric postmarketing adverse events Sandostatin LAR (octreotide), NDA 021008. In: Food and Drug Administration (ed). Center of Drug Evaluation and Research

Dom HT (2011) The meaning of suffering and death in Hinduism. Eur J Palliat Care 18(4):179–181

Drake R, Frost J, Collins JJ (2003) The symptoms of dying children. J Pain Symptom Manage 26(1):594–603

Dudgeon D, Shadd J (2016) Assessment and management of dyspnea in palliative care [Internet]. UpToDate [cited 18.5.16]. Available from http://www.uptodate.com/contents/assessment-and-management-of-dyspnea-in-palliative-care—H89103965

Dussel V, Kreicbergs U, Hilden JM, Watterson J, Moore C, Turner BG et al (2009) Looking beyond where children die: determinants and effects of planning a child's location of death. J Pain Symptom Manage 37(1):33–43

Dussel V, Joffe S, Hilden JM, Watterson-Schaeffer J, Weeks JC, Wolfe J (2010) Considerations about hastening death among parents of children who die of cancer. Arch Pediatr Adolesc Med 164(3):231–237

Eastern Metropolitan Region Palliative Care Consortium (2016) Management of respiratory secretions in the terminal phase. Available from http://www.emrpcc.org.au

Emanuel LL, Alpert HR, Emanuel EE (2001) Concise screening questions for clinical assessments of terminal care: the needs near the end-of-life care screening tool. J Palliat Med 4(4):465–474

Ethier AM (2010) Care of the dying child and the family. In: Tomlinson D, Kline N (eds) Pediatric oncology nursing, 2nd edn. Springer, Berlin, Heidelberg, pp 565–578
European Oncology Nursing Society (2015) Recommendations for the care of patients with malignant fungating wounds [5.6.2016]. Available from http://www.cancernurse.eu/documents/EONSMalignantFungatingWounds.pdf
Feudtner C, Feinstein JA, Satchell M, Zhao H, Kang TI (2007) Shifting place of death among children with complex chronic conditions in the United States, 1989–2003. JAMA 297(24):2725–2732
Fife A, Postier A, Flood A, Friedrichsdorf SJ (2016) Methadone conversion in infants and children: retrospective cohort study of 199 pediatric inpatients. J Opioid Manag 12(2):123–130
Finkel JC, Pestieau SR, Quezado ZM (2007) Ketamine as an adjuvant for treatment of cancer pain in children and adolescents. J Pain 8(6):515–521
Flavelle SC (2011) Experience of an adolescent living with and dying of cancer. Arch Pediatr Adolesc Med 165(1):28–32
Foster TL, Lafond DA, Reggio C, Hinds PS (2010) Pediatric palliative care in childhood cancer nursing: from diagnosis to cure or end of life. Semin Oncol Nurs 26(4):205–221
Fraser LK, Miller M, McKinney PA, Parslow RC, Feltbower RG (2011) Referral to a specialist paediatric palliative care service in oncology patients. Pediatr Blood Cancer 56(4):677–680
Friedman MM (1998) Family nursing: theory, research and practice, 4th edn, Stamford, Appleton & Lange
Friedrichsdorf SJ, Drake R, Webster ML (2011) Gastrointestinal symptoms. In: Wolfe J, Hinds PS, Sourkes BM (eds) Textbook of interdisciplinary pediatric palliative care, 1st edn. Elsevier Saunders, Philadelphia, pp 311–334
Friedrichsdorf SJ, Postier A, Dreyfus J, Osenga K, Sencer S, Wolfe J (2015) Improved quality of life at end of life related to home-based palliative care in children with cancer. J Palliat Med 18(2):143–150
Gilrane-McGarry U, O'Grady T (2011) Forgotten grievers: an exploration of the grief experiences of bereaved grandparents. Int J Palliat Nurs 17(4):170–176
Goldman A, Hewitt M, Collins GS, Childs M, Hain R (2006) Symptoms in children/young people with progressive malignant disease: United Kingdom Children's Cancer Study Group/Paediatric Oncology Nurses Forum survey. Pediatrics 117(6):e1179–e1186
Goldsmith M, Ortiz-Rubio P, Staveski S, Chan M, Shaw RJ (2011) Delirium. In: Wolfe J, Hinds PS, Sourkes BM (eds) Textbook of interdisciplinary pediatric palliative care. Elsevier Saunders, Philadelphia, pp 251–265
Hasan U (2012) Health, sickness, medicine, life and death in Muslim belief and practice. Eur J Palliat Care 19(5):241–245
Heath JA, Oh LJ, Clarke NE, Wolfe J (2012) Complementary and alternative medicine use in children with cancer at the end of life. J Palliat Med 15(11):1218–1221
Hechler T, Blankenburg M, Friedrichsdorf SJ, Garske D, Hubner B, Menke A et al (2008) Parents' perspective on symptoms, quality of life, characteristics of death and end-of-life decisions for children dying from cancer. Klin Padiatr 220(3):166–174
Hedayat K (2006) When the spirit leaves: childhood death, grieving, and bereavement in Islam. J Palliat Med 9(6):1282–1291
Hewitt M, Goldman A, Collins GS, Childs M, Hain R (2008) Opioid use in palliative care of children and young people with cancer. J Pediatr 152(1):39–44
Hexem KR, Mollen CJ, Carroll K, Lanctot DA, Feudtner C (2011) How parents of children receiving pediatric palliative care use religion, spirituality, or life philosophy in tough times. J Palliat Med 14(1):39–44
Hilden J (2016) It is time to let in pediatric palliative care. Pediatr Blood Cancer 63(4):583–584
Himelstein BP, Hilden JM, Boldt AM, Weissman D (2004) Pediatric palliative care. N Engl J Med 350(17):1752–1762
Hinds PS, Drew D, Oakes LL, Fouladi M, Spunt SL, Church C et al (2005) End-of-life care preferences of pediatric patients with cancer. J Clin Oncol 23(36):9146–9154
Hinds PS, Oakes LL, Hicks J, Powell B, Srivastava DK, Spunt SL et al (2009) "Trying to be a good parent" as defined by interviews with parents who made phase I, terminal care, and resuscitation decisions for their children. J Clin Oncol 27(35):5979–5985
Hohl CM, Stenekes S, Harlos MS, Shepherd E, McClement S, Chochinov HM (2013) Methotrimeprazine for the management of end-of-life symptoms in infants and children. J Palliat Care 29(3):178–185
Hooke MC, Grund E, Quammen H, Miller B, McCormick P, Bostrom B (2007) Propofol use in pediatric patients with severe cancer pain at the end of life. J Pediatr Oncol Nurs 24(1):29–34
Horridge KA (2015) Advance care planning: practicalities, legalities, complexities and controversies. Arch Dis Child 100(4):380–385
Hunt A (2012) Pain assessment. In: Goldman A, Hain R, Liben S (eds) Oxford textbook of palliative care for children. Oxford University Press, Oxford, pp 204–217
Hynson JL (2012) The child's journey: transition from health to ill health. In: Goldman A, Hain R, Liben S (eds) Oxford Textbook of Palliative Care for Children, 2nd edn. Oxford University Press, Oxford, pp 13–22
Institute of Medicine (2003) Concepts and definitions. In: Field MJ, Behrman RE (eds) When children die improving palliative and end-of-life care for children and their families. The National Academies Press, Washington DC, pp 32–40
Jacobs S, Perez J, Cheng YI, Sill A, Wang J, Lyon ME (2015) Adolescent end of life preferences and congruence with their parents' preferences: results of a survey of adolescents with cancer. Pediatr Blood Cancer 62(4):710–714
Jalmsell L, Kreicbergs U, Onelov E, Steineck G, Henter JI (2006) Symptoms affecting children with malignancies during the last month of life: a nationwide follow-up. Pediatrics 117(4):1314–1320

Jalmsell L, Kreicbergs U, Onelov E, Steineck G, Henter JI (2010) Anxiety is contagious-symptoms of anxiety in the terminally ill child affect long-term psychological well-being in bereaved parents. Pediatr Blood Cancer 54(5):751–757
Jalmsell L, Kontio T, Stein M, Henter JI, Kreicbergs U (2015) On the child's own initiative: parents communicate with their dying child about death. Death Stud 39(1–5):111–117
Jalmsell L, Lovgren M, Kreicbergs U, Henter JI, Frost BM (2016) Children with cancer share their views: tell the truth but leave room for hope. Acta Paediatr 105(9):1094–1099
James PJ, Howard RF, Williams DG (2010) The addition of ketamine to a morphine nurse- or patient-controlled analgesia infusion (PCA/NCA) increases analgesic efficacy in children with mucositis pain. Paediatr Anaesth 20(9):805–811
Jassal SS (2016) Basic symptom control in paediatric palliative care Bristol 2016 [9.5]. Available from http://www.togetherforshortlives.org.uk
Jones R (2011) The meaning of suffering and death in Buddhism. Eur J Palliat Care 18(2):72–75
Kamihara J, Nyborn JA, Olcese ME, Nickerson T, Mack JW (2015) Parental hope for children with advanced cancer. Pediatrics 135(5):868–874
Kars MC, Grypdonck MH, de Bock LC, van Delden JJ (2015) The parents' ability to attend to the "voice of their child" with incurable cancer during the palliative phase. Health Psychol 34(4):446–452
Kassam A, Wolfe J (2013) The ambiguities of free-standing pediatric hospices. J Palliat Med 16(7):716–717
Kassam A, Skiadaresis J, Alexander S, Wolfe J (2014) Parent and clinician preferences for location of end-of-life care: home, hospital or freestanding hospice? Pediatr Blood Cancer 61(5):859–864
Kassam A, Skiadaresis J, Alexander S, Wolfe J (2015) Differences in end-of-life communication for children with advanced cancer who were referred to a palliative care team. Pediatr Blood Cancer 62(8):1409–1413
Klick JC, Hauer J (2010) Pediatric palliative care. Curr Probl Pediatr Adolesc Health Care 40(6):120–151
Klopfenstein KJ, Hutchison C, Clark C, Young D, Ruymann FB (2001) Variables influencing end-of-life care in children and adolescents with cancer. J Pediatr Hematol Oncol 23(8):481–486
Knapp CA, Madden VL, Curtis CM, Sloyer PJ, Huang IC, Thompson LA et al (2008) Partners in care: together for kids: Florida's model of pediatric palliative care. J Palliat Med 11(9):1212–1220
Kouba E, Wallen EM, Pruthi RS (2008) Management of ureteral obstruction due to advanced malignancy: optimizing therapeutic and palliative outcomes. J Urol 180(2):444–450
Kreicbergs U, Valdimarsdottir U, Onelov E, Henter JI, Steineck G (2004) Talking about death with children who have severe malignant disease. N Engl J Med 351(12):1175–1186
Kreicbergs U, Valdimarsdottir U, Onelov E, Bjork O, Steineck G, Henter JI (2005) Care-related distress: a nationwide study of parents who lost their child to cancer. J Clin Oncol 23(36):9162–9171
Kreicbergs UC, Lannen P, Onelov E, Wolfe J (2007) Parental grief after losing a child to cancer: impact of professional and social support on long-term outcomes. J Clin Oncol 25(22):3307–3312
Kuo DZ, Houtrow AJ, Arango P, Kuhlthau KA, Simmons JM, Neff JM (2012) Family-centered care: current applications and future directions in pediatric health care. Matern Child Health J 16(2):297–305
Kutner JS, Smith MC, Corbin L, Hemphill L, Benton K, Mellis BK et al (2008) Massage therapy versus simple touch to improve pain and mood in patients with advanced cancer: a randomized trial. Ann Intern Med 149(6):369–379
Kyle G (2010) Bowel and bladder care at the end of life. Br J Nurs 19(7):408. 10, 12–14
Lebens S (2009) The meaning of death and dying in Juadism. Eur J Palliat Care 16(5):220–223
Levine DR, Johnson LM, Mandrell BN, Yang J, West NK, Hinds PS et al (2015) Does phase 1 trial enrollment preclude quality end-of-life care? Phase 1 trial enrollment and end-of-life care characteristics in children with cancer. Cancer 121(9):1508–1512
Lewis SJ, Heaton KW (1997) Stool form scale as a useful guide to intestinal transit time. Scand J Gastroenterol 32(9):920–924
Lovgren M, Jalmsell L, Eilegard Wallin A, Steineck G, Kreicbergs U (2016) Siblings' experiences of their brother's or sister's cancer death: a nationwide follow-up 2–9 years later. Psychooncology 25(4):435–440
Mack JW, Hilden JM, Watterson J, Moore C, Turner B, Grier HE et al (2005) Parent and physician perspectives on quality of care at the end of life in children with cancer. J Clin Oncol 23(36):9155–9161
Mack JW, Joffe S, Hilden JM, Watterson J, Moore C, Weeks JC et al (2008) Parents' views of cancer-directed therapy for children with no realistic chance for cure. J Clin Oncol 26(29):4759–4764
Maltoni M, Scarpi E, Rosati M, Derni S, Fabbri L, Martini F et al (2012) Palliative sedation in end-of-life care and survival: a systematic review. J Clin Oncol 30(12):1378–1383
Meyers K, Kerr K, Cassel JBC (2014) Up close: a field guide to community based palliative care in California Sacramento, CA: California Health Care Foundation. Available from http://www.chcf.org/publications/2014/09/up-close-field-guide-palliative
Mherekumombe MF, Collins JJ (2015) Patient-controlled analgesia for children at home. J Pain Symptom Manage 49(5):923–927
Michelson KN, Clayman ML, Haber-Barker N, Ryan C, Rychlik K, Emanuel L et al (2013) The use of family conferences in the pediatric intensive care unit. J Palliat Med 16(12):1595–1601
Monterosso L, Kristjanson LJ (2008) Supportive and palliative care needs of families of children who die from cancer: an Australian study. Palliat Med 22(1):59–69
Montgomery K, Sawin KJ, Hendricks-Ferguson VL (2016) Experiences of pediatric oncology patients

and their parents at end of life: a systematic review. J Pediatr Oncol Nurs 33(2):85–104
Morita T, Tsuneto S, Shima Y (2002) Definition of sedation for symptom relief: a systematic literature review and a proposal of operational criteria. J Pain Symptom Manage 24(4):447–453
Murray SA, Kendall M, Boyd K, Sheikh A (2005) Illness trajectories and palliative care. BMJ 330(7498):1007–1011
Murray SA, Kendall M, Boyd K, Grant L, Highet G, Sheikh A (2010) Archetypal trajectories of social, psychological, and spiritual wellbeing and distress in family care givers of patients with lung cancer: secondary analysis of serial qualitative interviews. BMJ 340:c2581
Naipaul AD, Ullrich C (2011) Palliative sedation. In: Wolfe J, Hinds PS, Sourkes BM (eds) Textbook of interdisciplinary pediatric palliative care. Elsevier Saunders, Philadelphia, pp 204–214
National Center for Complementary and Alternative Medicine (NCCAM) (2016) Complementary, alternative, or integrative health: what's in a name? Maryland: U.S. Department of Health & Human Services, National Institutes of Helath, USA.gov; [updated March 2015]. Available from https://nccih.nih.gov/health/integrative-health
Nitschke R, Humphrey GB, Sexauer CL, Catron B, Wunder S, Jay S (1982) Therapeutic choices made by patients with end-stage cancer. J Pediatr 101(3):471–476
Nitschke R, Meyer WH, Sexauer CL, Parkhurst JB, Foster P, Huszti H (2000) Care of terminally ill children with cancer. Med Pediatr Oncol 34(4):268–270
Nolan S, Saltmarsh P, Leget C (2011) Spiritual care in palliative care: working towards an EAPC task force. Eur J Palliat Care 18(2):86–89
Pousset G, Bilsen J, Cohen J, Addington-Hall J, Miccinesi G, Onwuteaka-Philipsen B et al (2010) Deaths of children occurring at home in six European countries. Child Care Health Dev 36(3):375–384
Pousset G, Bilsen J, Cohen J, Mortier F, Deliens L (2011) Continuous deep sedation at the end of life of children in Flanders, Belgium. J Pain Symptom Manage 41(2):449–455
Pritchard M, Burghen E, Srivastava DK, Okuma J, Anderson L, Powell B et al (2008) Cancer-related symptoms most concerning to parents during the last week and last day of their child's life. Pediatrics 121(5):e1301–e1309
Pritchard M, Burghen EA, Gattuso JS, West NK, Gajjar P, Srivastava DK et al (2010) Factors that distinguish symptoms of most concern to parents from other symptoms of dying children. J Pain Symptom Manage 39(4):627–636
Puchalski C, Ferrell B, Virani R, Otis-Green S, Baird P, Bull J et al (2009) Improving the quality of spiritual care as a dimension of palliative care: the report of the Consensus Conference. J Palliat Med 12(10):885–904
Quill TE, Abernethy AP (2013) Generalist plus specialist palliative care—creating a more sustainable model. N Engl J Med 368(13):1173–1175
Rajapakse D, Comac M (2012) Symptoms in life-threatening illness: overview and assessment. In: Goldman A, Hain R, Liben S (eds) Oxford textbook of palliative care for children, 2nd edn. Oxford University Press, Oxford, pp 167–177
Remedios C, Willenberg L, Zordan R, Murphy A, Hessel G, Philip J (2015) A pre-test and post-test study of the physical and psychological effects of out-of-home respite care on caregivers of children with life-threatening conditions. Palliat Med 29(3):223–230
Rosenberg AR, Wolfe J (2013) Palliative care for adolescents and young adults with cancer. Clin Oncol Adolesc Young Adults 3:41–48
Rosenberg AR, Yi-Frazier JP, Wharton C, Gordon K, Jones B (2014) Contributors and inhibitors of resilience among adolescents and young adults with cancer. J Adolesc Young Adult Oncol 3(4):185–193
Sanderson A, Hall AM, Wolfe J (2016) Advance care discussions: pediatric clinician preparedness and practices. J Pain Symptom Manage 51(3):520–528
Schieveld JN, Janssen NJ (2014) Delirium in the pediatric patient: on the growing awareness of its clinical interdisciplinary importance. JAMA Pediatr 168(7):595–596
Schmidt P, Otto M, Hechler T, Metzing S, Wolfe J, Zernikow B (2013) Did increased availability of pediatric palliative care lead to improved palliative care outcomes in children with cancer? J Palliat Med 16(9):1034–1039
Sharpe D, Rossiter L (2002) Siblings of children with a chronic illness: a meta-analysis. J Pediatr Psychol 27(8):699–710
Siden H, Miller M, Straatman L, Omesi L, Tucker T, Collins JJ (2008) A report on location of death in paediatric palliative care between home, hospice and hospital. Palliat Med 22(7):831–834
Spicer S, Macdonald ME, Davies D, Vadeboncoeur C, Siden H (2015) Introducing a lexicon of terms for paediatric palliative care. Paediatr Child Health 20(3):155–156
Stoddard FJ, Usher CT, Abrams AN (2006) Psychopharmacology in pediatric critical care. Child Adolesc Psychiatr Clin N Am 15(3):611–655
Theunissen JM, Hoogerbrugge PM, van Achterberg T, Prins JB, Vernooij-Dassen MJ, van den Ende CH (2007) Symptoms in the palliative phase of children with cancer. Pediatr Blood Cancer 49(2):160–165
Thompson A, MacDonald A, Holden C (2012) Feeding in palliative care. In: Goldman A, Hain R, Liben S (eds) Oxford textbood of palliative care for children, 2nd edn. Oxford University Press, Oxford, pp 284–294
Together for short lives (2016) Introduction to children's palliative care. Definitions. Available from http://www.togetherforshortlives.org.uk
Tsai E (2008) Advance care planning for paediatric patients. Paediatr Child Health 13(9):791–805
Ullrich CK, Dussel V, Hilden JM, Sheaffer JW, Moore CL, Berde CB et al (2010) Fatigue in children with cancer at the end of life. J Pain Symptom Manage 40(4):483–494
Vermaes IP, van Susante AM, van Bakel HJ (2012) Psychological functioning of siblings in families of children with chronic health conditions: a meta-analysis. J Pediatr Psychol 37(2):166–184

Vickers J, Chrastek J (2012) Place of care. In: Goldman A, Hain R, Liben S (eds) Oxford textbook of palliative care for children, 2nd edn. Oxford University Press, Oxford, pp 391–401
Vickers J, Thompson A, Collins GS, Childs M, Hain R (2007) Place and provision of palliative care for children with progressive cancer: a study by the Paediatric Oncology Nurses' Forum/United Kingdom Children's Cancer Study Group Palliative Care Working Group. J Clin Oncol 25(28):4472–4476
Wakefield CE, Drew D, Ellis SJ, Doolan EL, McLoone JK, Cohn RJ (2014) 'What they're not telling you': a new scale to measure grandparents' information needs when their grandchild has cancer. Patient Educ Couns 94(3):351–355
Watanabe H, Inoue Y, Uchida K, Okugawa Y, Hiro J, Ojima E et al (2007) Octreotide improved the quality of life in a child with malignant bowel obstruction caused by peritoneal dissemination of colon cancer. J Pediatr Surg 42(1):259–260
Wein S, Pery S, Zer A (2010) Role of palliative care in adolescent and young adult oncology. J Clin Oncol 28(32):4819–4824
Widger K, Tourangeau AE, Steele R, Streiner DL (2015) Initial development and psychometric testing of an instrument to measure the quality of children's end-of-life care. BMC Palliat Care 14(1):1
Wilson RK, Weissman DE (2004) Neuroexcitatory effects of opioids: patient assessment #57. J Palliat Med 7(4):579
Wilson P, White A, d'Etremont S (2014) Guidelines for home transfusion: Nova Scotia Provincial Blood Coordinating Program. Available from http://novascotia.ca/dhw/nspbcp/docs/Home-Transfusion-Guideline.pdf
Wolfe J, Grier HE, Klar N, Levin SB, Ellenbogen JM, Salem-Schatz S et al (2000) Symptoms and suffering at the end of life in children with cancer. N Engl J Med 342(5):326–333
Wolfe J, Hammel JF, Edwards KE, Duncan J, Comeau M, Breyer J et al (2008) Easing of suffering in children with cancer at the end of life: is care changing? J Clin Oncol 26(10):1717–1723
Wolfe J, Hinds PS, Sourkes BM (2011) The language of pediatric interdisciplinary palliative care. In: Wolfe J, Hinds PS, Sourkes BM (eds) Textbook of Interdisciplinary Pediatric Palliative Care. Elsevier Saunders, Philadelphia, pp 3–6
Wolfe J, Orellana L, Ullrich C, Cook EF, Kang TI, Rosenberg A et al (2015) symptoms and distress in children with advanced cancer: prospective patient-reported outcomes from the PediQUEST study. J Clin Oncol 33(17):1928–1935
World Health Organization (2012) WHO guidelines on the pharmacological treatment of persisting pain in children with medical illness. Available from http://apps.who.int/iris/bitstream/10665/44540/1/9789241548120_Guidelines.pdf
Wright LM, Bell JM (2009) Beliefs and illness: a model for healing. 4th Floor Press Inc., Canada
Wright LM, Leahey M (2005) Nurses and families: a guide to family assessment and intervention, 4th edn. F.A. Davis Company, Philadelphia
Youngblut JM, Brooten D, Blais K, Hannan J, Niyonsenga T (2010) Grandparent's health and functioning after a grandchild's death. J Pediatr Nurs 25(5):352–359
Zernikow B, Michel E, Craig F, Anderson BJ (2009) Pediatric palliative care: use of opioids for the management of pain. Paediatr Drugs 11(2):129–151
Zimmermann K, Cignacco E, Eskola K, Engberg S, Ramelet AS, Von der Weid N et al (2015) Development and initial validation of the Parental PELICAN Questionnaire (PaPEQu)—an instrument to assess parental experiences and needs during their child's end-of-life care. J Adv Nurs 71(12):3006–3017

12 Family Bereavement Care in Pediatric Oncology

Malin Lövgren and Josefin Sveen

12.1 Introduction

The loss of a child is one of the most traumatic experiences a family can suffer. Intense and persistent grief reactions are common, such as depression and prolonged grief. As research shows that long-term psychological morbidity, including grief, among parents and siblings is affected by factors during illness, end of life, and after the loss, family bereavement care should start early during the palliative care of the child with advanced cancer and beyond the child's death. It is important that healthcare professionals are aware of the factors that can affect the grieving process and long-term mental health of family members. This chapter not only focuses on bereavement care after the death of a child to cancer but starts by describing what is known from existing research on parents and siblings with regard to aspects that have been found to have an impact on their grieving process and their long-term mental health. The chapter also includes bereavement care interventions for families after the loss. The views of healthcare professionals on bereavement care are also briefly described. We conclude by offering clinical implications, which can help to guide healthcare professionals and other individuals who care for these families from the child's illness to years after loss. Having knowledge about factors that are important for parents' and siblings' well-being, including the grieving process, gives healthcare professionals the opportunity to provide care that will positively affect the family for years after the loss.

M. Lövgren (✉) • J. Sveen
Department of Caring Sciences, Palliative Research Centre, Ersta Sköndal Bräcke University College, Stigbergsgatan 30, Box 11189, SE-100 61 Stockholm, Sweden
e-mail: malin.lovgren@esh.se; josefin.sveen@esh.se

12.2 The Death of One's Child in Cancer

"The grief comes in waves. In the beginning I could drive to the store but stayed in the car in the parking lot. The body wouldn't listen, I didn't have the strength to get out of the car" (cancer-bereaved parent, personal communication, April 2016).

Bereaved parents are at increased risk of developing mental and physical health problems (Stroebe et al. 2007), and bereavement is even associated with an increased risk of mortality in mothers (Li et al. 2003). Despite the traumatic experience of losing one's child, the majority of parents will adjust to the loss over time (Lichtenthal et al. 2015a).

J. Wolfe et al. (eds.), *Palliative Care in Pediatric Oncology*, Pediatric Oncology,
https://doi.org/10.1007/978-3-319-61391-8_12

12.2.1 "Normal" Grief

Grief is a normal reaction to loss and includes psychological, physical, spiritual, social, and cultural dimensions (Stroebe et al. 2008). However, psychological aspects of grief will be the main focus of this chapter. Typical grief reactions include a sense of disbelief, yearning, sadness, and overwhelming thoughts and memories of the deceased, as well as emotions of anxiety, guilt, and anger. Grief fluctuates over time, with fits and starts. The intensity and frequency of grief normally diminish with time and shift into a resolution of grief, which is accompanied by an increasing ability to have positive emotions when thinking of the deceased child, accepting and learning to live with the loss, as well as renewed appreciation for life (Stroebe et al. 2008; Bonanno and Kaltman 2001). The resolution of grief does not mean that the parent overcomes or forgets the loss but, rather, that they are able to have peaceful memories and thoughts of the child. This resolution may also include the ability to find new and meaningful ways of continuing the bond with the child (Stroebe et al. 2008). Nevertheless, episodes of grief may arise at certain occasions, such as around the anniversary of the child's death, the child's birthday, family holidays, and celebratory life events, as well as during stressful events.

Studies have shown that grief after the death of one's child is more intense and prolonged than after the loss of a spouse or a parent (Rando 1983; Middleton et al. 1998). There are few longitudinal studies that examine the duration of grief after the loss of a child to cancer. Cross-sectional studies assessing grief suggest that the grief continues for many years or is lifelong after the death of a child. One study reports that it takes at least 4–6 years to process the grief after the loss of a child to cancer (Kreicbergs et al. 2007).

Many parents express that they think of their child every day, remembering and missing the child. Parents do not get over the death: "You have to learn to live with it. But life will never be the same again" (cancer-bereaved parent, personal communication, April 2016).

It is well recognized that the grieving process differs among individuals and between cultures, and the grief reactions and their intensity and duration vary (Bonanno and Kaltman 2001). There is no "right way" to grieve and there is no absolute time frame for resolving the loss of one's child. Members within the family may be experiencing and expressing their grief differently, and thus clarifying these differences for the family may be important as not understanding these differences may cause misunderstanding, guilt, anger, and bitterness between parents and within the family, as well as feelings of loneliness.

Even though there is great strain on the family after losing a child, parents appear not to separate or divorce more than non-bereaved parents (Eilegard and Kreicbergs 2010; Syse et al. 2010). However, one study found that in average 18 years following the death, parents were more likely to have marital disruption than comparison parents (Rogers et al. 2008).

12.2.1.1 Maladaptive Responses to Bereavement

Although grief reactions as well as symptoms of depression and anxiety are common after the death of a child, most parents tend to adjust to the loss with time (Kreicbergs et al. 2004; Lannen et al. 2008). For a significant minority of parents (10–20%) (McCarthy et al. 2010; Lichtenthal et al. 2015b), the grief is unresolved, and they can be described as being "stuck" in their grief, which has been termed *prolonged grief* and *complicated grief*. The latest proposal to define complicated grief in WHO International Classification of Diseases' 11th revision (ICD-11) is prolonged grief disorder (PGD), characterized by an intense and persistent yearning for the deceased, a sense that life is meaningless, and difficulty accepting the loss and moving on with life. It is proposed that these reactions should be present at sufficiently high levels at least 6 months from the death and be associated with functional impairment (Maercker et al. 2013). The fifth edition of the Diagnostic and Statistical Manual of Mental Disorders (DSM-5) includes persistent complex bereavement disorder (PCBD) as a recommended condition for further study and not intended for clinical use. PCBD is similar but distinct from PGD, with a key difference being that PCBD holds that symptoms and functional impairment should persist beyond 1 year after bereavement (Lichtenthal et al. 2004; Prigerson et al. 2009).

Bereaved parents are a group who are at risk of developing complicated grief (Kersting et al. 2011), especially after the loss of younger children (Zetumer et al. 2015). A recent study (McCarthy et al 2010) reported that of those parents who lost a child to cancer, 10% met the criteria for PGD 4.5 years, on average, after the loss.

Proposed contributing factors for complicated grief in parents are the disruption of the natural life-order, feelings of guilt and failure, as well as the disruption of the family structure following the death of the child. Complicated grief is distinct from typical grief and other psychiatric disorders such as depression and posttraumatic stress disorder (PTSD). Furthermore, complicated grief is associated with increased rates of mental health disorders and sleep disturbance, suicidality, and physical health problems, such as cardiovascular disease and cancer (Shear 2015; Buckley et al. 2012). Thus, it is important to identify those individuals and offer them appropriate treatment.

A study (Kreicbergs et al. 2007) found that 26% of parents had unresolved grief 4–9 years after the loss of a child to cancer, and this was associated with symptoms of anxiety and depression. This association was higher for fathers than for mothers, and fathers with unresolved grief had higher rates of sleep difficulties, while mothers with unresolved grief had higher rates of physician visits and higher sick leave than parents reporting having resolved their grief. Research shows that parents of children who die from cancer have elevated rates of anxiety and depression, as compared to non-bereaved parents, and this was greatest at 4–6 years after the loss and approaching normative levels 7–9 years after the loss (Kreicbergs et al. 2004). Another study reported that 22% of parents had clinically significant levels of depression, which was strongly associated with symptoms of prolonged grief, and almost half had high levels of separation distress (McCarthy et al. 2010).

Posttraumatic stress symptoms have been less studied in cancer-bereaved parents; however, one longitudinal study measuring symptoms of posttraumatic stress, 1 year post-loss, found that 53% of mothers and 33% of fathers had symptoms of PTSD (Lindahl Norberg et al. 2011). It is important to be aware that these symptoms may co-occur together with other mental health problems.

Vignette: Andrew's Family (Part 1)

Andrew died of cancer at the age of 10. He, his parents, and younger sister Karen, 7, had lived with the uncertainty of the prognosis for several years. After Andrew's death, his mother tended to keep her feelings to herself and spent much time at Andrew's grave, and she did not go back to work during the first year. Andrew's father found it helpful to share his feelings with friends and returned to work within a month as he found working a relief and felt supported by his colleagues. The sister, Karen, was talkative and often tearful when talking with her aunt about her brother but did not show her sadness to her parents and avoided talking about Andrew other than in happy memories. She found it a help to be at school and to be with friends, as she found that she could take a break from the grief there.

Even though there is higher risk of complicated grief and other negative outcomes after the loss of a child, a search for meaning may follow, and there may be a changed self-perception, changes in interpersonal relationships, and a changed philosophy of life (Tedeschi and Calhoun 1995), characterized as posttraumatic growth.

12.2.2 Factors Impacting on Bereavement Outcomes in Parents

Research has identified several factors that might contribute to the psychological outcomes for parents after the bereavement of a child. These factors can be divided into either modifiable or avoidable factors within the healthcare and bereavement care settings or those factors that are not manageable.

12.2.2.1 Factors Healthcare Cannot Modify or Avoid

The child's age (Kreicbergs et al. 2004; van der Geest et al. 2014), the parent's gender (Li et al. 2003; Rostila et al. 2012a), previous loss (Rosenberg et al. 2012), and economic burden (Rosenberg et al. 2012) are all factors that healthcare cannot modify or avoid but that have been found to have an impact on parents' bereavement. For example, one study (Kreicbergs et al. 2004) found that bereaved fathers of older children (aged above 8 years) were more likely to have symptoms of anxiety and depression than fathers of younger children, but no difference was found among the mothers. A recent study reported that parents' long-term grief was associated with older age of the deceased minor child (van der Geest et al. 2014). In a study (Sirki et al. 2000) with bereaved parents of children who died of either cancer therapy-related complications or in terminal care, the mothers had a longer recovery time and returned to work later. Mothers have been shown to have a higher mortality rate after the loss of a child to cancer than is found for fathers (Li et al. 2003; Rostila et al. 2012a). The difference in bereavement outcomes between mothers and fathers could be because the mother is often the primary caregiver, and some research suggests that the attachment is often stronger between the mother and the child (Bowlby 1970). However, these differences may also be a reflection that mothers and fathers may grieve in different ways (Lannen et al. 2008). These factors are important for healthcare professionals to be aware of when supporting families.

12.2.2.2 Factors During the Child's Illness and End-of-Life Care Affecting Bereavement Outcome of the Parents

A growing body of evidence shows that factors during the care of the child with advanced cancer are important to parents' adjustment after the death of their child.

The child's suffering and medical care during the illness and at end of life can have an impact on the parents' psychological adjustment after death. It is thus important for healthcare professionals to provide adequate symptom management. Although adequate symptom management for a child may be challenging, it is important that clinicians are communicating with the family that they are doing their best. The child's psychological and physical symptoms, especially unrelieved anxiety and pain, have been associated with the psychological health of the parents after the child's death (van der Geest et al. 2014; Jalmsell et al. 2010). Research shows that bereaved parents of children receiving stem cell transplantation have worse long-term psychological health (Jalmsell et al. 2011; Drew et al. 2005) than parents of children who have not received transplantation. A reason for this may be that stem cell transplantation is associated with significant suffering and less opportunity to prepare for end-of-life care (Ullrich et al. 2010).

The location of the child's death is another factor that can have an impact on bereaved parents' adjustment after the death (Drew et al. 2005; Goodenough et al. 2004). Research has shown that parents whose child died at home had lower rates of complicated grief than those whose child died at the hospital. In addition, fathers appear to be more affected by in-hospital death, as they are reported to have more symptoms of anxiety and depression, as well as stress, than after child's death at home, but this was not found in mothers (Goodenough et al. 2004). The actual location of death may be less important than factors such as parental planning of location of death. Dussel et al. (2009) found that planning location of death was associated with more home deaths and being more prepared for the child's end of life.

Open and honest communication is essential in pediatric palliative care (Mack et al. 2005, 2006). A good relationship between the healthcare professionals and the parents with open and honest communication relating to diagnosis and prognosis improves the quality of palliative care of the child, and it allows the parents to emotionally prepare for the loss. Being emotionally prepared and having an awareness of the upcoming death allow the parents to say goodbye to their child and benefit other bereaved family members (McCarthy et al. 2010; Valdimarsdottir et al. 2007). Research shows that good communication with pediatric oncologists is associated with lower levels of long-term parental grief (van der Geest et al. 2014). Most parents and children want to be fully informed about the course and prognosis of the illness, even though many clinicians find it hard to talk about this with the family. Although these conversations may cause unease for the healthcare professionals, it is important to have honest communication as parents are more likely to be aware of the impending death if they are given such information (Valdimarsdottir et al. 2007). If parents are aware that the child will die, they are more likely to talk to their children about death, which provides an opportunity for them to talk about child's last wishes and place of death (Jalmsell et al. 2015). However, family preferences and cultural values may disagree with this view of open and honest communication. For example, in many cultures, family members include extended family and community members and may want information shared with community leaders to help them with decision making (Wiener et al. 2013) or that communication should be with the eldest member of the family. Another example of a cultural difference is that some cultures emphasize that once words are spoken out loud, they may become a reality, and thus families may be reluctant to talk about the impending death of the child as it may be self-fulfilling (Wiener et al. 2013).

Anticipatory grief can start at any time during the treatment trajectory including at diagnosis. It may be increasingly present as the family comes to realize the terminal prognosis of the cancer. Families may experience opportunities for family cohesion and communication as they approach the impending loss. Understanding the child's prognosis may also help families have information and preparation for the potential physical and emotional changes that can occur as death approaches. It is important that healthcare staff recognize anticipatory grief and that it can already begin at the time of diagnosis and identify strong or less helpful reactions that indicate that the family may need additional psychosocial support. Receiving psychosocial support from the healthcare staff during the last month of the child's life has the potential to facilitate the grieving process (Kreicbergs et al. 2007).

12.3 To Lose a Brother or Sister to Cancer

"I always came second. Sometimes couldn't bring friends home because of the risk of infection. Have difficulty talking with my parents today about things because I have taken care of myself and therefore I have drifted away from them when it comes to communication" (cancer-bereaved sibling in Lövgren et al. (2015)).

Siblings of children who die from cancer often stand outside the spotlight of attention and care. Until recently, research on siblings of childhood cancer has been limited, and the experiences of cancer-bereaved siblings are still relatively poorly studied. Siblings are often called "the forgotten grievers" based on the idea that they are not the focus of family, friends, and healthcare professionals, who often primarily focus on the ill child and the parents (Jenholt Nolbris et al. 2014; Warnick 2015).

The relation to a sibling is often the longest relation one has in life. Siblings play a special role in a child's growth and development. Siblings share family secrets and experiences. Siblings also have a special role to play in protecting each other in the wider environment of the school and playground. Cancer-bereaved siblings might not "only" lose their best and closest friend but also their parents' attention and care for long periods of time (Jenholt Nolbris et al. 2014): during the illness trajectory and after bereavement and during their childhood and youth, an important time for personal development and schooling, etc. Unfortunately, all distressing experiences of childhood cancer are ongoing and occur in parallel with the usual challenges of being a child, a teenager, and/or a young adult.

12.3.1 The Value of Being Involved and Supported During Illness

"I would have appreciated feeling involved and be able to help with the care of my brother. Trust and attention from care staff from the start I think is important. It don't need to take a lot of time. Just that everyone (children, parents, siblings, staff) are a team, where everyone can participate and help each other together. It is also important to remember that in many cases siblings are one's best and closest friends = difficult to lose" (cancer-bereaved sibling in Lövgren et al. (2015)).

Cancer-bereaved siblings describe that they are not included in the care of their brother or sister as much as they want (Nolbris 2009; Lövgren et al. 2016). Siblings of all ages benefit from inclusion in the care of their ill brother or sister during the illness trajectory, including the end-of-life phase of the disease (Lövgren et al. 2016; Giovanola 2005). Most siblings to pediatric palliative patients want to be involved in the brother's or sister's care; they have described the importance of helping the ill child with practical things, for example, transporting wheelchairs, fetching medications, and schoolwork. Siblings report that they help in order to worry less, provide comfort, keep things positive and normal, and feel the joy of helping (Gaab et al. 2014). On the other hand, cancer-bereaved siblings have also described that they grow up too fast and take too much responsibility for younger siblings and household chores at an early age. The pros and cons regarding sibling participation have been discussed in relation to their long-term well-being. Age, maturity, and type of participation might have an impact, but data from a nationwide survey in Sweden among cancer-bereaved siblings show that siblings' participation in the brother's or sister's care was not associated with long-term psychological morbidity. It has been highlighted by cancer-bereaved siblings that it is important to spend time on their own with their ill brother or sister when they visit him/her at the hospital as their time together creates valuable memories later on (Nolbris and Hellström 2005).

Cancer-bereaved siblings have been found to have a higher risk of anxiety 2–9 years post-loss if they perceived their need for social support as being unsatisfied during their brother's or sister's last month before death (Eilertsen et al. 2013). This is also true for siblings who are not satisfied with the amount of time they spent talking about their feelings with others during their brother's or sister's last month of life (Wallin et al. 2015). Those siblings who reported that their relationships with others were negatively impacted during the brother's or sister's illness did also report poorer social support years after the loss. This was also true for those siblings who were not satisfied with the amount of information given by parents and healthcare professionals during the illness trajectory. Siblings who described dissatisfaction with information during the illness also reported more psychological distress years after bereavement (Rosenberg et al., 2015).

When cancer-bereaved siblings gave their own advice to healthcare professionals, they described that the following areas were of significance during the illness trajectory:

- "See" and acknowledge the healthy siblings.
- Give psychosocial support to siblings during illness, e.g., talk about feelings and the situation but also talk about "normal" things.
- Give suitable information about the illness, the treatment, and the prognosis, together with the parents but also alone with healthcare professionals.
- Involve siblings in the care of the ill brother or sister.
- Give support to the parents as a way of supporting healthy siblings.
- Healthcare professionals should be honest, positive, cheerful, encouraging, strengthen hopes (but not false hopes), empathic, natural, patient, treat everyone warmly, don't butt in

but be nearby, and not do the same things as they have always done.

- Recognize the value of continuity in the care of the brother or sister but also in the contact with the healthy siblings (Lövgren et al. 2016; Steele et al. 2013).

12.3.2 Preparation for Death

"Hours before he died was agonizing. I had never seen anyone die, or a dead person and was afraid it would look scary when he died and afterwards. At the same time it was a relief as he suffered at the end and it was stressful to wait for death. You knew it was coming but not when, it was wearing me down. In hindsight it would have been good (nice) to talk to someone about how death can be and what would happen" (cancer-bereaved sibling in Lövgren et al. (2015)).

Siblings often notice that their brother or sister is getting sicker as their symptoms become worse, but many do not fully expect their brother or sister to die in the end. Lack of awareness about the impending death has been expressed by siblings, and this is often related to not realizing that death could come so suddenly. Many siblings report that it is important to discuss the impending death because it increases their understanding of the situation and also that knowledge gave them a greater appreciation of their sibling, which usually meant that they would spend more time with them. Siblings who have not understood that death was near expressed regret that they did not spend more time with their brother or sister during the illness period. Their reported explanations included that they were too busy with themselves or their own lives or that they did not understand that their brother/sister was going to die so soon (Lövgren et al. 2015; Gaab et al. 2014). Those siblings whose brother or sister died at home have reported that they were more aware of the impending death and felt more support from parents than siblings whose brother or sister died at the hospital (Giovanola 2005).

Some siblings reported how they felt left in the dark and described that they were confused and felt afraid of the brother's or sister's symptoms in the end of life without having them explained (Lövgren et al. 2015). Feeling misled at the end of their brother's or sister's life results in the sibling finding it harder to cope later (Gaab et al. 2014). Siblings described their brother's or sister's physical changes at the time of death: the slow breathing or the slow heart rate as signs that death was near. More dramatic bodily changes, such as rattle breath or seizure, were scary for the siblings as they did not understand what was happening or why nobody was helping their brother or sister. Some siblings also blamed others for the death, for example, the healthcare professionals or the parents, for taking the wrong decisions when they not have fully understood the situation/bodily changes that occur at the end of life, which influenced how they coped after the loss. Those siblings who reported that nobody talked to them about what to expect when their brother or sister was dying showed significantly higher levels of anxiety 2–9 years after the loss compared with those who did (Lövgren et al. 2015). Siblings who reported that they were not prepared for the circumstances at the time of their brother or sister's death perceived worse psychological distress and lower social support years after bereavement (Rosenberg et al. 2015).

Some siblings have described that their brother's or sister's death came so fast that they did not have the chance to be present or that they were on their way to their dying brother or sister but arrived too late. Research has shown that a vast majority of siblings who were not present at the time of death regretted it many years later after the loss, while siblings who were present expressed having positive feelings about it, for example, happiness and gratitude. Siblings who did not have the opportunity to say goodbye in a comfortable manner did report more psychological distress years after the loss (Rosenberg et al. 2015).

12.3.3 Grief Among Siblings and Youth

"I felt a bit in the way, didn't want to show how great my own grief was when I thought that my mother and my stepfather were busy with their own grief, and my little brother" (cancer-bereaved sibling in Lövgren et al. (2015)).

Grief after loss differs between children and adults because of children's developmental stages and cognitive abilities and lack of experience with death (Giovanola 2005; Nolbris and Hellström 2005). Siblings' psychosocial reactions to the death of a brother or sister differ among different age groups. For example, children between the ages of 3 and 5 years can express more hyperactivity and sleeping problems, and the 6–11-year-olds may express more depressive symptoms and daydreaming. Adolescence is likely to show a wide variety of symptoms, for example, impulsiveness, moodiness, worrying, and eating difficulties (Birenbaum 2000). It is common for younger children to either withdraw from family and friends or to act out in an aggressive manner. Children may also act as if nothing had happened and continue with their daily activities as though they were unaffected by the loss. Adolescents may exhibit exaggerated risk-taking behavior. Siblings have shown to use, e.g., drugs and alcohol the first year following the loss (Rosenberg et al. 2015). Self-destruction is also commonly seen in adolescents as a reaction to grief. Parents describe that siblings express their grief by having mixed emotions, such as sadness (crying) and anger at not having the dead child to play with. Some responses of children to the loss of a sibling can be misinterpreted by parents as callous. Because of this, the emotional response to a sibling's illness or death may be overlooked by family, friends, and healthcare professionals (Giovanola 2005; Barrera et al. 2013). As children's reactions to grief are so varied, it is hard to define what an abnormal grief response is. There is no timeline for the bereavement process. In fact, for most individuals, the pain of loss often continues for a lifetime, despite successful adaptation.

Research has found that 54% of siblings of children affected by childhood cancer still grieve 2–9 years post-loss (Sveen et al. 2014). It is also found that siblings' levels of depression and anxiety increased the first year following the loss (Rosenberg et al. 2015). Qualitative data describe how cancer-bereaved siblings go in and out of grieving randomly. They have also reported that they could not control their grieving and needed to have time-out periods from their grief (Nolbris and Hellström 2005), for example, take time to do something completely different, such as being with friends. These breaks usually last from a few hours to several days. Later, when more time has passed, cancer-bereaved siblings have described that they begin to think and to regain the courage to think, to reflect, and to accept what has happened. At that point, they also try to find words to express and communicate their grief (Jenholt Nolbris et al. 2014). Coping strategies for grief also involve using their spiritual beliefs and waiting for time to pass (Lövgren et al. in press). Parents report that the following strategies helped the surviving siblings to cope with their grief: getting back to their daily activities, talking about the child who died seeking social support from friends, and group support (Barrera et al. 2013). Some parents also describe that the siblings are aware of their parents' grief and distress and adjust their behavior so they do not add further to their parents' distress. About half of cancer-bereaved siblings report that they avoid talking to their parents about their deceased brother or sister out of respect for their parents' feelings following the loss. Their risk of anxiety increases as compared to those who talk with their parents (Wallin et al. 2015). Parents describe that they acknowledge their children's grief, but they feel that they are unable to always support them as much as they may need. Parents also report that the siblings want more parental attention and that they have concerns about the parents' well-being (deCinque et al. 2006). Unfortunately, large longitudinal studies on grief among cancer-bereaved siblings are lacking, which indicates that we lack knowledge about siblings' grief trajectories and their long-term concerns relating to grief in the family.

12.3.3.1 Factors Influencing Children's and Siblings' Grief

Grief among children and adolescents does not occur in isolation of those around them. Instead, the grief process can be influenced by the grief of the parent(s) (Warnick 2015; Morris et al. 2016), level of family cohesion, and their immediate caregiving environments (Warnick 2015). Unfortunately, there is limited research about factors that contribute to cancer-bereaved siblings' grief after bereavement with few exceptions (Sveen et al. 2014; Lövgren et al. 2017). Poor social support after the death and shorter time since the loss have been found to influence prolonged grief (Sveen et al. 2014). Other factors that have been found to predict prolonged grief among siblings are the siblings' perception that it was not a peaceful death, limited information being provided to siblings in the last month of life, information about the impending death on the last day before it occurred, siblings' avoidance of the doctors, and lack of communication with family and people outside the family about death (Lövgren et al. 2017). Cancer-bereaved siblings have also described other experiences that facilitated or complicated the grieving process. Facilitating factors included the knowledge that they had maintained contact with their brother or sister during the illness period and that their brother/sister looked peaceful shortly after death. Factors that complicated the grieving process included stressful situations at the time of death, for example, rapid deterioration or seizure, and that they did not show their own sadness within the family shortly after death because they thought others were too busy with their own grieving process (Lövgren et al. 2015).

When a child is dying, parents often conceal information from the surviving siblings to protect them from the death experience by, for example, leaving the siblings with a relative. When parents take this protective approach, the surviving siblings are left alone with no one to talk with about their emotions (Nolbris and Hellström 2005). Despite the best intentions of parents, a protective approach may create a lack of trust among the siblings and allows for misconceptions about events surrounding the illness and death, which can interfere with the grieving process. Allowing children to attend the funeral services may also beneficial to their bereavement (Giovanola 2005).

12.3.3.2 Memories: Important as Comfort and to Continue Having a Sibling Bond

Many siblings do not have the same need of visiting the grave as the parents. Siblings have reported multiple places for them to be able to feel close to their deceased brother or sister, for example, the sibling's room (Nolbris and Hellström 2005). A vast majority of the siblings choose reminders of the brother or sister who died, for example, visual representations, communication with the deceased brother or sister, activities honoring the dead, etc. The most common reminder is the deceased brother or sister's belongings, often toys or clothes. Having reminders stimulates positive memories about being with the deceased sibling and is perceived as comforting (Foster et al. 2011). Siblings have also reported that it is important to include the deceased sibling in the family, such as keeping a special place at the dinner table or making special arrangements during his/her birthday as a way of continuing having a sibling bond (Nolbris and Hellström 2005).

12.3.4 Changes and Consequences for Siblings After the Loss

"I was very much behind in school though one thing that can be improved is that the siblings of the ill should be able to some schoolwork, or at least do something to not get so much behind in school" (cancer-bereaved sibling, in Lövgren et al. (2015)).

Sibling loss may create several negative consequences and potential resilience for children, adolescents, and young adults. Parents have described that their children have problems concentrating at school, are fearful of dying, avoid revealing their feelings of sorrow to their parents, and engage in risk behaviors, such as drinking (Barrera et al. 2013). On the other hand, other studies have found no difference in alcohol and drug use between bereaved and non-bereaved siblings (Eilegård et al. 2013). They also perceive that the siblings change after the death in relation to their personality, life perspective, and interests. Many parents have also noted changes in siblings' relationships with family members and peers, either getting closer to each other or became more distant (Foster et al. 2012). Some siblings blame the parents for loving the decreased child more, which results in difficult relationships with their parents. Siblings must also adjust to a new role in the family, for example, being the only child, the oldest/youngest, etc., which can be challenging (Foster et al. 2012). Survivor guilt is also common among siblings if the relationship with the deceased child has been strained prior to the cancer diagnosis. It is common that older siblings take a parental role shortly after the loss when the parents are absorbed with their own grief, which can be negative in the long run (Wender and Committee on Psychosocial Aspects of Child and Family Health 2012). A higher risk of anxiety has been found for siblings if they do not perceive that their parents and neighbors cared for them after their brother or sister's death (Eilertsen et al. 2013). Moreover, siblings who reported that they shared none or less than half of their feelings about their deceased brother or sister with their family following the loss were at greater risk of reporting anxiety 2–9 years post-loss as compared to those who shared more of their feelings. The risk of long-term anxiety was increased in siblings who wanted to talk more with their family 2–9 year after the loss (Wallin et al. 2015).

On the other hand, siblings have expressed that they have learned to appreciate each day in life and live in the moment where daily problems became less important. They have pointed out that they tried to make the best of the situation, which they stated as being extreme, and learned that life was too short to throw away. The siblings also describe that losing a brother or sister can strengthen the bonds between family members. They emphasized that it was a positive experience that the family cared more for each other and became closer through their brother's or sister's illness and death (Bradley-Eilertsen et al. 2016).

Unfortunately, the experiences of sibling death during childhood have been found to have a negative effect on years of schooling and adult socioeconomic outcomes (Fletcher et al. 2013). It is also found that sibling loss is associated with a higher mortality rate in all age groups, but the association was stronger for those of a younger age (Rostila et al. 2012b). In addition, cancer-bereaved siblings are shown to have lower self-esteem, more sleeping problems, and lower levels of maturity 2–9 years post-loss in comparison with non-bereaved siblings (Eilegård et al. 2013). Teachers of cancer-bereaved siblings have reported that the siblings were more prosocial than comparable classmates. Peers perceived cancer-bereaved boys as being more sensitive-isolated and victimized than girls, while bereaved siblings in elementary grades were perceived by peers as being less prosocial, more sensitive-isolated, and less accepted and as having fewer friends. Peers and teachers viewed bereaved siblings in middle/high school grades as having higher leadership popularity (Gerhardt et al. 2012).

Vignette: Anna's Family (Part 1)

When Anna was 12 she died of leukemia. Even if her family knew she did have incurable cancer, death was experienced as coming suddenly. Both the parents and her little sister, Celia, aged 6 years, were present at the time of death. Anna died calmly at the hospital after a few days of deterioration. Paul, the older brother, aged 19 at the time of Anna's death, was studying in another town far from home. As the family experienced that Anna's death came suddenly, Paul was not present when Anna died. Anna, Celia, and Paul have grown up together, even though the sisters' father was not Paul's biological dad. Paul and Anna have always been close, and although

Paul spent the last year of her illness far from home, they did often talk on the phone. Anna loved her big brother's positive perspective on life and found strengths in their relationship. Paul knew that Anna's illness was incurable, but despite their good relationship, they never talked about death and dying with each other. When Anna died, Paul stopped going to class, slept a lot, and started to spend evenings and nights in clubs and with friends who his parents never had heard about before. The parents experienced that Celia, the little sister, seemed unaffected by the loss. She did not talk about Anna and lived her life as if nothing happened.

12.4 Family Bereavement Support

Family bereavement care should start before the child dies. The responsibilities and duties of the palliative care providers continue after the child has died, and ideally they would offer family bereavement support. With limited health resources, effective strategies for bereavement support are needed, and routine practice should be supported by the best evidence available. However, much of bereavement care is not evidence based or not even theoretically based, and evidence of family bereavement as being supportive in pediatric palliative care is scarce (Lichtenthal et al. 2015a).

12.4.1 Hospital-Based Bereavement Care

Families often develop close relationships with the healthcare team and want continued connection with the hospital after the loss (Darbyshire et al. 2013; Downar et al. 2014), and without such continuity, families may experience an additional loss (Darbyshire et al. 2013; D'Agostino et al. 2008; Prigerson and Jacobs 2001). Thus, hospital-based bereavement services that offer continuity of care are appreciated by parents (Darbyshire et al. 2013; Russo and Wong 2005) and should be offered to all bereaved families. It is widely recognized that the healthcare team becomes a significant part of the family support network during a child's illness and plays an important role in supporting the bereaved families. Mothers who have worked through their grief were more likely to have participated in post-death sessions involving a psychosocial clinician (psychologist or social worker) (Kreicbergs et al. 2007).

Bereavement follow-ups by healthcare services are frequently used in many countries, but universally accepted standards for bereavement follow-ups do not exist in palliative pediatric oncology. Without an existing standard of care, bereavement follow-ups are inconsistent and some families are never even contacted. Each site where deaths of children occur should have specific policies in place which provide guidance for healthcare professionals in addressing the needs of bereaved families and which describe the procedures that need to be followed when a child dies. This information should include details about asking for post-mortems; the need to provide for different religions, beliefs, and cultures; and the provision of mementos (e.g., photos, footprints, etc.) for the family. Practical guidance for what families will need is important, such as funeral arrangements. The standard of care should consist of at least one call, email, or letter from the team to the bereaved family after the death of a child to cancer. Follow-up should be provided to all those who accept it. Establishing contact between 1 and 2 months after the death provides opportunities to discuss the results of a post-mortem or other investigations which may shed more light on the precise cause of death. Healthcare professionals can support bereaved families by being empathic, by providing validation of feelings experienced by families, and by helping families have access to information about additional bereavement services. Contact from professionals may also help to identify families at risk or in need of professional bereavement support. Many families will find their own support in different ways, including social networks, and at different times. Families should be given access to information sources that enable them to make appropriate choices from the support and other services that are available (Larcher et al. 2015).

A systematic review (Donovan et al. 2015) found 19 different types of hospital-based bereavement services following the death of a child. The most common services were phone calls at key intervals, the provision of resource materials, and group programs. Remembrance programs were also identified as a well-utilized intervention in pediatric oncology. Post-bereavement meetings also exist, as well as interventions promoting linkage between the hospital and family, which included mailings at key intervals, sympathy cards, anniversary cards, newsletters, and home visits. Educational events and financial assistance (payment of utility expenses and funeral expenses) also existed. Staying in contact with the deceased child's healthcare professionals prevented secondary loss and feelings of abandonment with families feeling cared for, less isolated, and more supported. Parents, siblings, and grandparents described a reduction in their sense of isolation and the development of healing friendships with others whose situations were akin to their own. They also reported that the bereavement interventions improved coping and allowed for personal growth. Some also describe that they had fewer grief reactions. Worth noting is that all interventions described were primarily based on supporting parents—only a few were designed to support siblings (Donovan et al. 2015).

Healthcare professionals who are involved in treating the child at the end of life can help in the bereavement process by understanding that their contact with the family should not stop at the child's death (Knapp and Contro 2009). Parents and siblings have expressed a need for meeting healthcare professionals for various reasons, such as remembrance ceremonies, taking mementos, or asking questions about the child's care in the end of life (Lövgren et al. 2016; Knapp and Contro 2009).

The palliative care team must also be aware that there is not one intervention that works best for all family members and that a range of interventions, from brochures and support groups, should be offered and that referrals to professional support should be made when necessary. However, it is important to also be aware that providing bereavement care too soon after the loss may interfere with the natural grief process.

12.4.2 Support Groups for Parents

Many parents report that support groups are helpful and supportive. Support groups are often led by a professional and consist of a group of bereaved individuals, who provide each other with advice, information, and support. Support groups are often offered by church and other community organizations outside healthcare as well as being arranged by hospitals. Some parents experience that friends and relatives do not understand their situation, but by meeting other bereaved parents, they feel that they are being understood. Support groups can be suitable for most grieving parents but may not be suitable for everyone, especially when the grief reactions are prolonged or complicated.

A recent study (Lichtenthal et al. 2015b) found that 55% of bereaved parents were currently using or had previously attended support groups after the loss of a child. There were more parents attending support groups in the second year after their loss than in the first year, but the rate decreased in the third and fourth year post-loss, indicating that the parents' need of bereavement support changed over time. However, there is a lack of studies evaluating the effect of support groups on parents' psychological health.

12.4.3 Interventions for Complicated Grief for Parents

Interventions targeting those at risk of complicated grief or those with complicated grief have been shown to be more effective than interventions with less distressed individuals (Wittouck et al. 2011).

Interventions for complicated grief usually take place a much longer time after bereavement, primarily because it takes time to develop complicated grief.

The death of one's child is one of the highest risk factors for complicated grief (Kersting et al. 2011; Zetumer et al. 2015). It has been suggested that bereaved parents do not use mental health services as much as they may need despite the distress of losing a child (Institute of Medicine 2003; Thompson et al. 2011; Johnston et al. 2008). Suggested reasons for this are that those with complicated grief avoid psychosocial services as they may not want to accept the reality of their child's death or to avoid painful reminders of their loss. Other reasons may be that the families believe that the services will not help them in their grief or that the mental health providers lack specific training in bereavement and complicated grief.

Research on the treatment of complicated grief has received attention in recent years, which shows promising results. Unfortunately, there are few published trials that have evaluated treatments specifically for complicated grief and none for cancer-bereaved parents. There is a growing body of evidence that cognitive behavior therapy (CBT) is an effective treatment for complicated grief (Boelen et al. 2007; Shear et al. 2005; Bryant et al. 2014; Rosner et al. 2014). Elements of cognitive restructuring and exposure appear to be successful interventions in CBT for complicated grief (Boelen et al. 2007; Shear et al. 2005; Bryant et al. 2014). Internet-delivered cognitive behavior therapy (iCBT) is an increasingly employed modality, and it is reported to have several advantages over traditional treatments, such as anonymity, accessibility, and being less expensive (Andersson and Titov 2014). Only two trials of iCBT for bereaved individuals have been published to date, but these show promising results (Kersting et al. 2013; Wagner et al. 2006). One (Kersting et al. 2013) was a study among parents who had lost a child during pregnancy with positive treatment effect.

There is preliminary evidence that narrative-based treatment is effective in reducing complicated grief (Gillies et al. 2014; Gerrish et al. 2010), which is based on the constructivist approach (Neimeyer et al. 2010). Narrative-based treatment involves meaning-reconstruction and an assimilation of the loss memory into one's personal narrative. The treatment includes journal writing, retelling the story of the death, as well as other techniques based on the constructivist approach.

A challenge in helping bereaved parents is that many find it too painful to talk about their loss, and thus they do avoid support and many parents discontinue their therapy as they do not find it helpful. Nevertheless, many wish for support but they do not receive it (40%) (Lichtenthal et al. 2015b).

A systematic review (Endo et al. 2015) on interventions for bereaved parents concluded that there is "very limited evidence of sufficient quality to demonstrate the efficacy of intervention techniques used to assist bereaved families following a child's death," and they suggest that a CBT intervention for complicated grief for parents or siblings might be possible and useful, based on the literature.

Research on how to support bereaved individuals is mostly inconclusive (Currier et al. 2008; Kato and Mann 1999; Jordan and Neimeyer 2003). Some studies have shown that the effect of treatment for normal grief is small to moderate, whereas the effect is larger in individuals with more severe symptoms (Currier et al. 2008). This indicates that individuals with severe grief symptoms may benefit from psychotherapeutic interventions, while less distressed individuals will not. Hence, efforts should be made to identify those at risk and who are at a greater need of support. One psychometrically sound screening instrument for complicated grief is the prolonged grief disorder (PG-13) (Prigerson et al. 2009) which could be used at least 6 months to 1 year after the loss.

Vignette: Andrew's Family (Part 2)

One year after the loss, Andrew's father longed for more sharing with the mother in their grief, and the mother agreed to join a support group for bereaved parents together with the father. They both found it helpful to share their experiences with other bereaved parents, and the mother felt that her grief reactions were normal. Karen received support from the school psychologist, and with time, she was able to share more of her sadness and longing for her brother with her parents and used writing to express many of the feelings that she had kept to herself.

12.4.4 Bereavement Support for Siblings

The psychosocial needs of cancer-bereaved siblings are easily overlooked, both in clinical settings and in research. Few studies have evaluated bereavement support targeted on siblings. Although interventions designed for siblings are relatively rare, Prchal and Landolt (2009) found 11 different sibling interventions—most conducted during the illness trajectory. More recent intervention studies on siblings during illness have also been published (Nolbris et al. 2010; Gustafsson and Nolbris 2006; Salavati et al. 2014). Most of the studies used pre-/post-intervention design and consisted of programs using a group setting with 2–10 sessions with group sizes from 4 to 12 siblings. The objectives with the programs were enhancement of medical knowledge, coping, family communication, reduction of posttraumatic stress, and other negative thoughts and feelings and to provide peer support. Findings have been inconsistence with regard to anxiety, depression, behavioral problems, social adjustment, self-esteem, and posttraumatic stress symptoms, but satisfaction with the intervention was high in both siblings and parents. However, several methodological shortcomings exist and randomly controlled trial studies are needed. Unfortunately, few studies have examined the long-term psychological health of siblings. The evaluated bereavement support for siblings in pediatric oncology is primarily bereavement camps (Donovan et al. 2015), which are described below.

When the siblings themselves give advice to healthcare professionals who are working with children affected by cancer and their families, they ask for more bereavement support. They report that they need support many years after the loss because they were so young at the time of death/during the illness trajectory, which is the last time they were in contact with healthcare professionals who work in the pediatric oncology setting. Many described that they wanted to meet a counselor and other siblings who have lost a brother or sister. Some also described that they need more medical information in order to better understand the illness and the brother's or sister's death (Lövgren et al. 2016).

12.4.4.1 Bereavement Camps

The effectiveness of bereavement camps for children between the ages of 6 and 18 years has been examined. Unfortunately, there is only a small pool of existing studies that contribute to the examination of the effectiveness of bereavement camps. Even fewer have studied cancer-bereaved siblings. The few studies that have examined the effectiveness of such camps show that they are promising venues to help bereaved children, including siblings, to develop and build resilience in dealing with loss. Most camps involve children between the ages of 12 and 18 years. The main focus of the camps is related to promoting the psychological and behavioral well-being of the attendees through various activities, peer support, and support from professionals and volunteers. Three commonly shared objectives of the camps that are described in the literature include providing a safe place for children to share their feelings, providing psychological space where professionals guided and accompanied attendees in engaging their grief work, and facilitating the child's work on grief. The camps often involve play and recreation in an outdoor setting, which offers relief from grief in the form of play. The work of grief is woven into the camp's activities, offering healthy ways for children to deal with grief through activities such as arts and crafts, music, and group work. These camps have been found to contribute to several positive effects for children: decreased anxiety; decreased posttraumatic stress symptoms; increased knowledge about grief, death, and coping skills for grief; and the opportunity to express and share feelings. Many children appreciate these kinds of camps and reported that they realized that they were not alone and that they could talk about death more openly (Clute and Kobayashi 2013).

Vignette: Anna's Family (Part 2)

About a year after Anna's death, the parents went to a psychologist to discuss their surviving children. They have themselves found comfort in support groups for parents and have also found strengths in each other. Celia met a psychologist a couple of times together with her parents, which allowed Celia to make drawings about her experience of losing her sister at the meeting with the psychologist. The psychologist talked to the parents about different grief reactions and the parents could relax slightly with the new knowledge. Paul was also invited to the psychologist but never did show up. He had started to develop a destructive lifestyle and the parents were very worried but never did totally reach him. The first 2 years after Anna's death, Paul struggled with guilt and regret because of his absence during the end of life and the anxiety he experienced. He felt selfish that he had moved to another town to study during the last year of Anna's life. His loss occupied him for having a normal life for a long period and he found it hard to talk to his parents. He considered his little sister and his parents' well-being before talking about himself; they were, after all, full sisters and both the parents were biological parents to Anna. He started to go to therapy after a few years, but never felt that it helped him completely, but started to study again and started to enjoy some of the things he used to do before Anna's death.

12.4.5 Healthcare Professionals' Views on Bereavement Care

Healthcare professionals have reported that they find meaning and satisfaction in their role in bereavement care, but that they experience logistical barriers, lack of education, and lack of staff support, which has an impact on their own suffering. Hospital staff describe feeling overwhelmed, neglected, and ill-equipped to undertake bereavement care. Unfortunately, they also experience a lack of time to process the death of a child before having to move on to the next patient, which impacts negatively on healthcare professionals over time (Donovan et al. 2015). On the other hand, when staff engage in bereavement support, they have reported that they benefit from reaching out to the families (Lichtenthal et al. 2015a).

Support for pediatric oncology nurses is often informal and sporadic, and education relating to professional grief is often nonexistent or very limited in its content (Conte 2011). However, a few support programs have been evaluated. For example, bereavement debriefing sessions, which aim to provide emotional support and increase one's ability to manage grief, have been found to be helpful for healthcare professionals (Keene et al. 2010). Another supporting activity for pediatric oncology nurses is peer-supported storytelling. This consists of anecdotal reports of clinical practice and addresses nurses' experiences of caring for dying children. Participants have reported that this activity provided support, had an impact on grief, and had an impact on their meaning-making (Macpherson 2008). When nurses in the pediatric oncology setting gave recommendations for improving an organizational level of bereavement support, the following areas were mentioned: creating time and space for staff self-care, counseling or communicating with others who understand end-of-life issues and hospice or palliative care, spending quality time with patients and families, acknowledgement and reinforcement of nurses' special efforts, and work structures, work processes, and organization, for example, building a knowledge infrastructure through the Internet (Wenzel et al. 2011).

12.5 Clinical Implications

Based on today's knowledge about pediatric oncology bereavement care, as described above in this chapter, we have stipulated some recommendations for healthcare professionals and others who are in contact with these families:

- Important goals in pediatric palliative care to facilitate the families' bereavement outcome should include minimizing the ill child's suffering, especially pain and anxiety.
- Healthcare professionals play a key role in supporting the parents to talk to their children (the ill child and healthy siblings) about the impending death if parents want to, in order to prevent regrets later on.
- It is important for healthcare professionals to understand that the many varied grief reactions are normal and that there are no distinct stages of grief. For example, if a parent or sibling appears to lack grief reactions, it does not mean that this grief is abnormal or pathological. Professionals need to provide support for the family where they are and respect their cultural and familial values.
- It will help the family if healthcare professionals and others understand that individuals grieve in different ways, and thus each member within the family may be experiencing and expressing their grief differently.
- It is important to remember that most individuals will adjust to life without their child/brother/sister and without the need of therapeutic interventions. That does not mean that they have forgotten their loved one nor that they are not grieving just that they have learned to live after the death and with the grief.
- Having persistently high levels of distress that cause functional impairment may be indicative of prolonged grief disorder, depression, anxiety, or PTSD and may need professional support.
- If an individual has complicated grief, friends and relatives may feel frustrated that they cannot help or they believe it is time to move on; they may stop contacting the bereaved family, which may increase the isolation of the bereaved family.
- A death of a child to cancer is not always predictable, but in cases where death is unavoidable, it is important to prepare the whole family for the impending death.
- Lack of communication about what to expect when death occurs can result in anxiety many years after the loss among siblings. It is therefore important that healthcare professionals give appropriate and age-adapted information to the siblings in accordance with the parents' wishes and concerns.
- Create time and space for siblings to spend time with the ill child on their own in order to create important memories together.
- Help the family to identify an extended family member or friend who is in a position to help the siblings during the illness and after bereavement. For example, this allows for the young children to get the support they need during critical moments including funeral and rituals, as well as everyday events.
- As social support outside the family is of great importance for siblings' long-term mental health, and part of their need is outside the area of healthcare, information about other social services, e.g., support groups and other nonprofit organizations, should be given to the bereaved families.
- As much of the bereavement process is dependent on the child's understandings of death, all children need specific developmentally appropriate definitions, guidance, and support through the bereavement process.
- Adults must acknowledge the sibling's loss and give him/her permission to grieve. This allows him/her to grieve without feeling the need to protect parents from his/her sadness. This is another important time for extended family members to support the child.
- Open communication between surviving children and the family/people outside the family can be helpful for the sibling's grieving process.
- Communication, good relationships, and providing medical information during illness between healthcare professionals and siblings

can assist siblings' grief reactions many years after the loss.

- The existence of open communication and sharing of thoughts and feelings can be an important part of a positive relationship between parents and healthy siblings. Healthcare professionals should therefore encourage the family to talk openly and share feelings as fits their cultural and spiritual beliefs.
- Families should have access to the care team after the loss of the child. Parents and siblings have expressed a need for meeting professionals for different reasons, e.g., remembrance ceremonies, taking mementos, and obtaining more knowledge about the end-of-life care.
- Screening efforts need to be improved for families at risk of prolonged or complicated grief reactions. Thus, grief counselors or therapists should focus on those with complicated grief reactions. A newly developed assessment instrument is available for prolonged grief among children and adults (prolonged grief disorder, PG-13 (Prigerson et al. 2008, 2009)), which could be one alternative for identifying those parents and siblings with much distress. This psychometrically sound screening instrument could be used 6 months to 1 year after the loss.
- There is preliminary evidence that narrative-based treatment is effective in reducing complicated grief, but more research is needed.
- Parent support groups are much appreciated by the parents but lack evaluation of their effect.
- Sibling camps have shown to have positive effects, although more research is needed.
- Cognitive behavior therapy is the most promising of the psychotherapy interventions for parents with complicated grief but has yet to be evaluated in pediatric palliative oncology.
- The majority of the research that exists on cancer-bereaved sibling is based on children aged 12 and older. More knowledge is therefore needed about younger siblings' bereavement and their experiences of losing a brother or sister to cancer.
- Grief trajectories for both parents and siblings are lacking in the palliative pediatric oncology literature. There is therefore an urgent need for research in this area in order to better understand a typical grief response among these individuals.

References

Andersson G, Titov N (2014) Advantages and limitations of Internet-based interventions for common mental disorders. World Psychiatry 13(1):4–11

Barrera M et al (2013) Parental perceptions of siblings' grieving after a childhood cancer death: a longitudinal study. Death Studies 37(1):25–46

Birenbaum LK (2000) Assessing children's and teenagers' bereavement when a sibling dies from cancer: a secondary analysis. Child Care Health Dev 26(5):381–400

Boelen PA et al (2007) Treatment of complicated grief: a comparison between cognitive-behavioral therapy and supportive counseling. J Consult Clin Psychol 75(2):277–284

Bonanno GA, Kaltman S (2001) The varieties of grief experience. Clin Psychol Rev 21(5):705–734

Bowlby J (1970) Attachment and loss: separation, anxiety and anger, vol 1. Hogarth Press, London

Bradley-Eilertsen M-E et al (2016) Cancer-bereaved siblings' positive and negative memories and experiences of their brother's or sister's illness and death (unpublished manuscript). Karolinska Institutet, Stockholm

Bryant RA et al (2014) Treating prolonged grief disorder: a randomized clinical trial. JAMA Psychiatry 71(12):1332–1339

Buckley T et al (2012) Physiological correlates of bereavement and the impact of bereavement interventions. Dialogues Clin Neurosci 14(2):129–139

deCinque N et al (2006) Bereavement support for families following the death of a child from cancer: experience of bereaved parents. J Psychosoc Oncol 24(2):65–83

Clute MA, Kobayashi R (2013) Are children's grief camps effective? J Soc Work End Life Palliat Care 9(1):43–57

Conte TM (2011) Pediatric oncology nurse and grief education: a telephone survey. J Pediatr Oncol Nurs 28(2):93–99

Currier JM, Neimeyer RA, Berman JS (2008) The effectiveness of psychotherapeutic interventions for bereaved persons: a comprehensive quantitative review. Psychol Bull 134(5):648–661

D'Agostino NM et al (2008) Bereaved parents' perspectives on their needs. Palliat Support Care 6(1):33–41

Darbyshire P et al (2013) Supporting bereaved parents: a phenomenological study of a telephone intervention programme in a paediatric oncology unit. J Clin Nurs 22(3–4):540–549

Donovan LA et al (2015) Hospital-based bereavement services following the death of a child: a mixed study review. Palliat Med 29(3):193–210

Downar J, Barua R, Sinuff T (2014) The desirability of an intensive care unit (ICU) clinician-led bereavement

screening and support program for family members of ICU decedents (ICU bereave). J Crit Care 29(2):311e9–31116
Drew D et al (2005) Parental grieving after a child dies from cancer: is stress from stem cell transplant a factor? Int J Palliat Nurs 11(6):266–273
Dussel V et al (2009) Looking beyond where children die: determinants and effects of planning a child's location of death. J Pain Symptom Manage 37(1):33–43
Eilegard A, Kreicbergs U (2010) Risk of parental dissolution of partnership following the loss of a child to cancer: a population-based long-term follow-up. Arch Pediatr Adolesc Med 164(1):100–101
Eilegård A et al (2013) Psychological health in siblings who lost a brother or sister to cancer 2 to 9 years earlier. Psycho-oncology 22(3):683–691
Eilertsen ME et al (2013) Impact of social support on bereaved siblings' anxiety: a nationwide follow-up. J Pediatr Oncol Nurs 30(6):301–310
Endo K, Yonemoto N, Yamada M (2015) Interventions for bereaved parents following a child's death: a systematic review. Palliat Med 29(7):590–604
Fletcher J et al (2013) A sibling death in the family: common and consequential. Demography 50(3):803–826
Foster TL et al (2011) Comparison of continuing bonds reported by parents and siblings after a child's death from cancer. Death Stud 35(5):420–440
Foster TL et al (2012) Changes in siblings after the death of a child from cancer. Cancer Nurs 35(5):347–354
Gaab EM, Owens GR, MacLeod RD (2014) Siblings caring for and about pediatric palliative care patients. J Palliat Med 17(1):62–67
van der Geest IM et al (2014) Parents' experiences of pediatric palliative care and the impact on long-term parental grief. J Pain Symptom Manage 47(6):1043–1053
Gerhardt CA et al (2012) Peer relationships of bereaved siblings and comparison classmates after a child's death from cancer. J Pediatr Psychol 37(2):209–219
Gerrish NJ, Steed LG, Neimeyer RA (2010) Meaning reconstruction in bereaved mothers: a pilot study using the biographical grid method. J Constr Psychol 23(2):118.142
Gillies J, Neimeyer RA, Milman E (2014) The meaning of loss codebook: construction of a system for analyzing meanings made in bereavement. Death Stud 38(1–5):207–216
Giovanola J (2005) Sibling involvement at the end of life. J Pediatr Oncol Nurs 22(4):222–226
Goodenough B et al (2004) Bereavement outcomes for parents who lose a child to cancer: are place of death and sex of parent associated with differences in psychological functioning? Psychooncology 13(11):779–791
Gustafsson K, Nolbris M (2006) See-hear-do pictures. Teaching about children's cancer with cartoon tools. MediaCuben AB, The Swedish Childhood Foundation (Barncancerfonden), Stockholm
Institute of Medicine (2003) When children die: improving palliative and end-of-life care for children and their families. The National Academies Press, Washington, DC
Jalmsell L et al (2010) Anxiety is contagious-symptoms of anxiety in the terminally ill child affect long-term psychological well-being in bereaved parents. Pediatr Blood Cancer 54(5):751–757
Jalmsell L et al (2011) Hematopoietic stem cell transplantation in children with cancer and the risk of long-term psychological morbidity in the bereaved parents. Bone Marrow Transplant 46(8):1063–1070
Jalmsell L et al (2015) On the child's own initiative: parents communicate with their dying child about death. Death Stud 39(2):111–117
Jenholt Nolbris M, Enskär K, Hellström AL (2014) Grief related to the experience of being the sibling of a child with cancer. Cancer Nurs 37(5):E1–E7
Johnston DL et al (2008) Availability and use of palliative care and end-of-life services for pediatric oncology patients. J Clin Oncol 26(28):4646–4650
Jordan JR, Neimeyer RA (2003) Does grief counseling work? Death Stud 27(9):765–786
Kato PM, Mann T (1999) A synthesis of psychological interventions for the bereaved. Clin Psychol Rev 19(3):275–296
Keene EA et al (2010) Bereavement debriefing sessions: an intervention to support health care professionals in managing their grief after the death of a patient. Pediatr Nurs 36(4):185–189. quiz 190
Kersting A et al (2011) Prevalence of complicated grief in a representative population-based sample. J Affect Disord 131(1–3):339–343
Kersting A et al (2013) Brief internet-based intervention reduces posttraumatic stress and prolonged grief in parents after the loss of a child during pregnancy: a randomized controlled trial. Psychother Psychosom 82(6):372–381
Knapp CA, Contro N (2009) Family support services in pediatric palliative care. Am J Hosp Palliat Care 26(6):476–482
Kreicbergs U et al (2004) Anxiety and depression in parents 4–9 years after the loss of a child owing to a malignancy: a population-based follow-up. Psychol Med 34(8):1431–1441
Kreicbergs UC et al (2007) Parental grief after losing a child to cancer: impact of professional and social support on long-term outcomes. J Clin Oncol 25(22):3307–3312
Lannen PK et al (2008) Unresolved grief in a national sample of bereaved parents: impaired mental and physical health 4 to 9 years later. J Clin Oncol 26(36):5870–5876
Larcher V et al (2015) Making decisions to limit treatment in life-limiting and life-threatening conditions in children: a framework for practice. Arch Dis Child 100(Suppl 2):s3–23
Li J et al (2003) Mortality in parents after death of a child in Denmark: a nationwide follow-up study. Lancet 361(9355):363–367

Lichtenthal WG, Cruess DG, Prigerson HG (2004) A case for establishing complicated grief as a distinct mental disorder in DSM-V. Clin Psychol Rev 24(6):637–662
Lichtenthal WG et al (2015a) Bereavement follow-up after the death of a child as a standard of care in pediatric oncology. Pediatr Blood Cancer 62(Suppl 5):S834–S869
Lichtenthal WG et al (2015b) Mental health services for parents who lost a child to cancer: if we build them, will they come? J Clin Oncol 33(20):2246–2253
Lindahl Norberg A, Poder U, von Essen L (2011) Early avoidance of disease- and treatment-related distress predicts post-traumatic stress in parents of children with cancer. Eur J Oncol Nurs 15(1):80–84
Lövgren M et al (2015) Siblings' experiences of their brother's or sister's cancer death: a nationwide follow-up 2–9 years later. Psycho-oncology 25(4):435–440
Lövgren M et al (2016) Bereaved siblings' advice to health care professionals working with children with cancer and their families. J Pediatr Oncol Nurs 33(4):297–305
Lövgren M, Sveen J, Steineck G, Eilegård Wallin A, Eilertsen ME, Kreicbergs U (in press) Spirituality and religious coping are related to cancer-bereaved siblings' long-term grief. Palliat Support Care
Lövgren M, Sveen J, Nyberg T, Eilegård Wallin A, Prigerson Holly G, Steineck G, Kreicbergs U (2017) Care at End of Life Influences Grief: A nationwide long-term follow-up among young adults who lost a brother or sister to childhood cancer. J Palliat Med. Ahead of print. https://doi.org/10.1089/jpm.2017.0029
Mack JW et al (2005) Parent and physician perspectives on quality of care at the end of life in children with cancer. J Clin Oncol 23(36):9155–9161
Mack JW et al (2006) Communication about prognosis between parents and physicians of children with cancer: parent preferences and the impact of prognostic information. J Clin Oncol 24(33):5265–5270
Macpherson CF (2008) Peer-supported storytelling for grieving pediatric oncology nurses. J Pediatr Oncol Nurs 25(3):148–163
Maercker A et al (2013) Proposals for mental disorders specifically associated with stress in the International Classification of Diseases-11. Lancet 381(9878):1683–1685
McCarthy MC et al (2010) Prevalence and predictors of parental grief and depression after the death of a child from cancer. J Palliat Med 13(11):1321–1326
Middleton W et al (1998) A longitudinal study comparing bereavement phenomena in recently bereaved spouses, adult children and parents. Aust N Z J Psychiatry 32(2):235–241
Morris AT et al (2016) The indirect effect of positive parenting on the relationship between parent and sibling bereavement outcomes after the death of a child. J Pain Symptom Manage 51(1):60–70
Neimeyer RA et al (2010) Grief therapy and the reconstruction of meaning: from principles to practice. J Contemp Psychother 40(2):73–83
Nolbris M (2009) Att vara syskon till ett barn eller ungdom med cancersjukdom- Tankar, behov, problem och stöd (To be a sibling to a child or adolescence with cancer: thoughts, needs, problems and support). University of Gothenburg, Gothenburg, Sweden, p 53
Nolbris M, Hellström AL (2005) Siblings' needs and issues when a brother or sister dies of cancer. J Pediatr Oncol Nurs 22(4):227–233
Nolbris M et al (2010) The experience of therapeutic support groups by siblings of children with cancer. Pediatr Nurs 36(6):298–304. quiz 305
Prchal A, Landolt MA (2009) Psychological interventions with siblings of pediatric cancer patients: a systematic review. Psychooncology 18(12):1241–1251
Prigerson HG, Jacobs SC (2001) Perspectives on care at the close of life. Caring for bereaved patients: "all the doctors just suddenly go". JAMA 286(11):1369–1376
Prigerson HG, Vanderwerker LC, Maciejewski PK (2008) A case for the inclusion of prolonged grief disorder in DSM-V. In: Stroebe M et al (eds) Handbook of bereavement research and practice: 21st century perspectives. APA, Washington DC, pp 165–186
Prigerson HG et al (2009) Prolonged grief disorder: psychometric validation of criteria proposed for DSM-V and ICD-11. PLoS Med 6(8):e1000121
Rando TA (1983) An investigation of grief and adaptation in parents whose children have died from cancer. J Pediatr Psychol 8(1):3–20
Rogers CH et al (2008) Long-term effects of the death of a child on parents' adjustment in midlife. J Fam Psychol 22(2):203–211
Rosenberg AR et al (2012) Systematic review of psychosocial morbidities among bereaved parents of children with cancer. Pediatr Blood Cancer 58(4):503–512
Rosenberg AR et al (2015) Long-term psychosocial outcomes among bereaved siblings of children with cancer. J Pain Symptom Manage 49(1):55–65
Rosner R et al (2014) Efficacy of an outpatient treatment for prolonged grief disorder: a randomized controlled clinical trial. J Affect Disord 167:56–63
Rostila M, Saarela J, Kawachi I (2012a) Mortality in parents following the death of a child: a nationwide follow-up study from Sweden. J Epidemiol Community Health 66(10):927–933
Rostila M, Saarela J, Kawachi I (2012b) The forgotten griever: a nationwide follow-up study of mortality subsequent to the death of a sibling. Am J Epidemiol 176(4):338–346
Russo C, Wong AF (2005) The bereaved parent. J Clin Oncol 23(31):8109–8111
Salavati B et al (2014) Which siblings of children with cancer benefit most from support groups? Children's Health Care 43:221–233
Shear MK (2015) Clinical practice. Complicated grief. N Engl J Med 372(2):153–160
Shear K et al (2005) Treatment of complicated grief: a randomized controlled trial. JAMA 293(21):2601–2608

Sirki K, Saarinen-Pihkala U, Hovi L (2000) Coping of parents and siblings with the death of a child with cancer: death after terminal care compared with death during active anticancer therapy. Acta Paediatrica 89(6):717–721
Steele AC et al (2013) Bereaved parents and siblings offer advice to health care providers and researchers. J Pediatr Hematol/Oncol 35(4):253–259
Stroebe M, Schut H, Stroebe W (2007) Health outcomes of bereavement. Lancet 370(9603):1960–1973
Stroebe M et al (2008) Handbook of bereavement research and practice: advances in theory and intervention. American Psychological Association, Washington DC
Sveen J et al (2014) They still grieve-a nationwide follow-up of young adults 2–9 years after losing a sibling to cancer. Psycho-oncology 23(6):658–664
Syse A, Loge JH, Lyngstad TH (2010) Does childhood cancer affect parental divorce rates? A population-based study. J Clin Oncol 28(5):872–877
Tedeschi RG, Calhoun LG (1995) Trauma & transformation: growing in the aftermath of suffering. Sage Publications, Thousand Oaks, CA
Thompson AL et al (2011) A qualitative study of advice from bereaved parents and siblings. J Soc Work End Life Palliat Care 7(2–3):153–172
Ullrich CK et al (2010) End-of-life experience of children undergoing stem cell transplantation for malignancy: parent and provider perspectives and patterns of care. Blood 115(19):3879–3885
Valdimarsdottir U et al (2007) Parents' intellectual and emotional awareness of their child's impending death to cancer: a population-based long-term follow-up study. Lancet Oncol 8(8):706–714
Wagner B, Knaevelsrud C, Maercker A (2006) Internet-based cognitive-behavioral therapy for complicated grief: a randomized controlled trial. Death Studies 30(5):429–453
Wallin AE et al (2015) Insufficient communication and anxiety in cancer-bereaved siblings: a nationwide long-term follow-up. Palliat Support Care:1–7
Warnick AL (2015) Supporting youth grieving the dying or death of a sibling or parent: considerations for parents, professionals, and communities. Curr Opin Support Palliat Care 9(1):58–63
Wender E, Committee on Psychosocial Aspects of Child and Family Health (2012) Supporting the family after the death of a child. Pediatrics 130(6):1164–1169
Wenzel J et al (2011) Working through grief and loss: oncology nurses' perspectives on professional bereavement. Oncol Nurs Forum 38(4):E272–E282
Wiener L et al (2013) Cultural and religious considerations in pediatric palliative care. Palliat Support Care 11(1):47–67
Wittouck C et al (2011) The prevention and treatment of complicated grief: a meta-analysis. Clin Psychol Rev 31(1):69–78
Zetumer S et al (2015) The impact of losing a child on the clinical presentation of complicated grief. J Affect Disord 170:15–21

13 Easing Clinician Distress in Pediatric Cancer Care

Karen Moody, Deborah Kramer, Caitlin Scanlon, Lucia Wocial, Beth Newton Watson, and Adam Hill

13.1 Introduction

The rewarding field of pediatric oncology is one that must be entered into with determination and full awareness of oneself on account of the physical and emotional demands. A dear friend and colleague summed it up this way, "I tell residents that if they are considering a career in pediatric oncology, then they should ask themselves, 'Can I be happy and fulfilled doing anything else?'. If the answer is 'yes' then look elsewhere. Pediatric oncology has to be a calling like the drive to be an artist. No one wants to be a struggling artist, but if that is your passion then do you really have a choice?" (Levy, personal communication, 2017). There is a sacredness in caring for children with cancer likely due to the witnessing of profound bravery, honesty, self-awareness, and a warrior-like spirit at times in children living with cancer. In addition, the field of oncology draws in those who value scientific inquiry, discovery, and the potential to make a profound impact on humanity. However, these same aspects that draw a clinician into pediatric oncology can also lead to that clinician's downfall. Turned around, caring gives way to exhaustion, dedication and commitment can become workaholism and isolation, and searching for the cure can lead to feelings of defeat and failure. All across medical specialties, burnout rates are rising, and pediatric oncology is no exception (Shanafelt et al. 2015a).

This chapter will focus on four distinct (but often coexisting) types of distress described below:

- *Burnout*: a work-related, predominantly psychological syndrome of emotional exhaustion, depersonalization, and reduced feelings of personal accomplishment (Maslach et al. 2001).
- *Compassion Fatigue*: also known as secondary traumatic stress, is a state of emotional strain in a worker that occurs as a result of empathic engagement with those suffering from the consequences of traumatic events (Figley 1995).
- *Moral Distress*: the experience of believing one knows the ethical thing to do, but institutional

K. Moody, M.D., M.S. (✉) • C. Scanlon, M.S.W.
A. Hill, M.D.
Pediatric Palliative Care, Riley Hospital for Children at Indiana University Health, 705 Riley Hospital Drive, Room 3039, Indianapolis, IN 46202, USA
e-mail: kmoody1@IUHealth.org

D. Kramer, R.N., Ed.D., C.P.N.P., F.N.P.
Undergraduate Nursing Program, College of Mount Saint Vincent, Bronx, NY 10471, USA

L. Wocial, Ph.D., R.N., F.A.A.N.
Fairbanks Center for Medical Ethics and Indiana University School of Nursing, Indiana University Health, Indianapolis, IN 46202, USA

B.N. Watson, M.Div., B.C.C.
Spiritual Care and Chaplaincy, Indiana University Health, Academic Health Center, Indianapolis, IN 46202, USA

J. Wolfe et al. (eds.), *Palliative Care in Pediatric Oncology*, Pediatric Oncology,
https://doi.org/10.1007/978-3-319-61391-8_13

barriers prevent the individual from acting accordingly (Repenshek 2009).

- *Spiritual Distress*: a pervasive disruption in a person's belief system that prevents finding meaning and purpose in life through connection (Caldeira et al. 2014).

All of these types of distress can have profound results on the practitioner and manifest as physical and psychological symptoms that can drastically affect well-being, professional performance, the care of patients, and ultimately the healthcare system (Najjar et al. 2009).

While literature in the field of clinician distress for pediatric oncology physicians and psychosocial professionals is relatively scant, the pediatric oncology nursing literature is replete with descriptions of and interventions for distress (Simon et al. 2005).

13.2 Burnout

Maslach first described burnout in 1981 as a syndrome that occurs in response to chronic work-related stress manifesting as emotional exhaustion, depersonalization (treating people as objects), and decreased feelings of personal accomplishment. It has been measured in epidemiological studies primarily with The Maslach Burnout Inventory (Maslach and Jackson 1981). The International Society of Pediatric Oncology Working Committee on Psychosocial Issues described burnout as occurring through a series of stages (Spinetta et al. 2000). In the first stage, one experiences depleted energy reserves, emotional emptiness, finds work depressing, develops minor physiological disturbances (insomnia, hypertension, headache, bruxism, etc.), and experiences distress that spills over into their personal lives (Moody et al. 2013). The next stage is described as feeling indifferent or cynical, irritable, uncaring, and disinterested. One may start to withdraw from work and colleagues in this stage manifesting as absenteeism, procrastination, and isolation. In the third stage, clinicians fall into despair as they view themselves as professional failures; they may focus on the personal losses they witness at work and have little time to think about the successes (Potter et al. 2010).

In the fourth stage, they develop a feeling of personal failure. In this stage the clinician often withdraws from personal activities and family in addition to withdrawing from work. Clinicians may find themselves dreading coming into work and calling out frequently. Finally in the fifth stage, the clinician reports feeling "dead inside," leaves the profession, or suffers a major crisis such as turning to substance abuse and even suicide (Spinetta et al. 2000).

The prevalence of burnout as measured in one study of pediatric oncologists ranged from 38% (moderate burnout) to 72% (moderate and severe burnout combined) (Roth et al. 2011). Of particular concern in this study was the finding that 60% of pediatric oncologists that did not perceive themselves as having symptoms of burnout were found to have at least moderate levels of burnout. A study at a major cancer hospital estimated a nurse burnout rate of 44% in inpatient nursing staff (Roth et al. 2011; Emanuel et al. 2011). In psychosocial oncology professionals, the estimated prevalence of burnout was 26% (Turnell et al. 2016). In a meta-analysis of cancer professionals across disciplines, the prevalence of depersonalization was 34%, emotional exhaustion was 36%, and low personal accomplishment was 25% (Trufelli et al. 2008).

Although the effects of burnout are often most profound at the individual level, there are significant implications for patients and for healthcare in general. Burnout is associated with poorer patient satisfaction, less adherence to medical recommendations (Nedrow et al. 2013), and suboptimal care (Shanafelt and Dyrbye 2012). It is also associated with increased medical errors, absenteeism, and staff turnover as a result of job dissatisfaction and could lead to work force shortages in some specialties (Bowden et al. 2015; Hayes et al. 2005).

13.3 Compassion Fatigue

While burnout and compassion fatigue lead to similar outcomes, they represent different phenomena. Compassion fatigue, referred to interchangeably as secondary traumatic stress, is suggested to have a quicker onset of symptoms and occurs as a result of being directly exposed to traumatic material, whereas burnout seems to be more gradual and cumulative (Ross 1995; Figley 2002). To clarify, compassion fatigue is not a result of job dissatisfaction, frustrations with institutional policies, work hassles, or volume of patients, but rather a stress response including feelings of helplessness, isolation, and confusion that results from bearing witness to the suffering of a traumatized patient and internalizing it as "secondary trauma" (Figley 1995; Najjar et al. 2009; Orlovsky 2006; Sabo 2006). Additionally, while burnout is now commonly applied to all professions, compassion fatigue is still thought to be specific to the helping professions where compassion is practiced and applied each day (Slocum-Gori et al. 2013).

Compassion fatigue can result in poor judgment, clinical errors, avoidance of work, abandonment of patients, increased cynicism, detachment from patients, and becoming easily irritated with others (Figley 1995; Rourke 2007; Rossi et al. 2012; Bush 2009). Since compassion fatigue and burnout share the same risk factors and lead to similar outcomes in professionals and patients, the remainder of this chapter will refer to the two terms collectively as clinician distress.

While the patient population remains the same, professionals from distinct disciplines within pediatric oncology may experience clinician distress differently based on their different roles on the care team.

13.4 Nurses' Perspective

The nurse is the healthcare worker that spends the most time with the pediatric patient and his/her family. The nurse often stays with the child and family for 8–12 h a day providing care. This intensity of time and patient care leads to a very close relationship between the nurse and the family, and sometimes the nurse can be viewed by the family as part of the extended family. The nurse is with the patient while they are undergoing painful procedures and treatments and with the family throughout the hardship of watching their child going through the cancer trajectory, which sometimes ends in death (Spinetta et al. 2000; Moody et al. 2013; Mukherjee et al. 2009). Oncology nurses must follow protocols of care specific to each diagnosis. These protocols may include chemotherapy that can result in significant side effects, surgery that can result in disfigurement or reductions in function, and multiple invasive procedures that can result in fear and pain in the child. Furthermore, despite the best efforts of medical care, some children will die. The close relationships, provision of burdensome treatments, and experiencing the suffering and death of children often put oncology nurses at great risk for experiencing extreme stress, compassion fatigue, post-traumatic stress symptoms, emotional overload, and burnout (Moody et al. 2013; Hecktman 2012). In an international study of nurses, it was found that the United States and Canada had the highest levels of burnout in oncology nurses (Poghosyan et al. 2009). A survey of members of the Oncology Society of Nurses revealed that 72% of nurse executives were unable to retain their experienced oncology nurses (Hayes et al. 2005), and shockingly, in a study of interdisciplinary pediatric oncology staff (the majority of which were nurses) across two institutions, in two countries, the burnout level was 100% (Moody et al. 2013).

Nurse Vignette 1: Emotionally Challenging Family

Nurses coming into work have no idea what mood this patient and the family will be in. Nurse Sue described coming in one day, and the family was welcoming and warm; the next day or even later the same day, the family became angry and hostile, blaming her for the treatment not working and/or the child's pain. As a result, Nurse Sue wants to care for the child but has difficulty walking into the room and is not as physically present with this child and family as she normally would be. Sue felt undervalued by the family as they complained when she did her hourly physical assessments as required. The family complains that "no other nurse comes in as often to do these assessments." Nurse Sue feels that the nurses on the other shifts are providing poor quality of care. Having four other patients, it is easy for Sue to try to avoid this room and the hostile attacks from the family members. Nurse Sue feels anguished over not doing the job as competently as she would like to. She called in sick the next day knowing she would leave the staff short handed.

Nurse Vignette 2: Lack of Pain Relief and Staff Support

Nurse Daniel was working the night shift caring for a child in pain. The parents asked him for pain medication for which Nurse Daniel had no order. He contacted the covering physician, who did not get back to him with an order for one and a half hours. During this time the family was angry and hostile toward Nurse Daniel, thinking that he did not care about the child's welfare or was not sufficiently competent to get the medicine the child needed to be relieved of her pain. Nurse Daniel himself was in despair about watching this child in pain but had to suppress his own emotions. He was also distressed by being unable to get the child's pain relieved quickly. To compound nurse Daniel's feelings of distress, this child was not doing well in treatment, and the nurse felt a hopelessness that the treatment was not working despite the pain it was causing. Nurse Daniel's supervisor admonished him for not caring for this child's pain in a timely manner and Daniel feels undervalued. Not only did the family not value his efforts, but his supervisor was not giving him the support he deserved.

Nurse Vignette 3: Generally Positive Experience but No Boundaries Between Home and Work

Mary is a nurse who sees her work in pediatric oncology as a privilege and feels fulfilled working with the families. She maintains long-time relationships with some of the children she has cared for and their families and is considered by them as a cherished member of the family. She feels she is a good nurse and is there for the children. She is appreciated by the parents for helping them during these difficult times. At home, Nurse Mary worries about her patients instead of focusing on her own children's issues, which may seem minor in comparison. When her children talk to her about issues they are having, they tell her: "You think our issues are not important because they are not about cancer." Mary finds herself checking for lab values on her patients on her blackberry while she is home with her family. She is uncomfortable in social situations and impatient with petty talk about people and things in the community. Folks will say to her "we can never do what you do, working with such ill children and their families; I don't know how you do it." She senses that her friends feel uncomfortable with her because of the work she does. Nurse Mary has a list that she carries about in her mind of those children she cared for but whose treatment was not successful. She often reflects back on some of the very meaningful conversations they shared.

13.5 Psychosocial Professionals' Perspective

Psychosocial professionals (social workers, child life specialists, psychologists, etc.) are often in a unique position on an oncology team. While there are typically many nurses and physicians on any given team, there are likely far fewer psychosocial professionals. Psychosocial professionals are entrusted with the role of managing psychological distress of patients and families, in addition to assisting them in accessing resources, and acting as patient advocates (Simon et al. 2005; Gwyther et al. 2005). Furthermore, psychosocial professionals are expected to assist other team members in coping with caring for their patients (Gwyther et al. 2005). Social workers, because of the very role in which they function, are in a particularly vulnerable position. This vulnerability is due to an emphasis on the use of empathy and the fostering of a supportive relationship with the patient and family (Joubert et al. 2013). Since professionals from other disciplines, nurses in particular, also provide emotional support to families, social workers may find that their unique skills in empathic support, assessment, intervention, and coordination are not recognized. In fact, in one study, social workers reported that recognition for providing emotional support was more often given to professionals who seemingly held more power, thereby leading to higher stress and lower morale for the social workers (Dane and Chachkes 2001).

13.6 Physician Lens

The prevalence of burnout identified in the survey of US physicians across specialties is alarmingly high (46%) and on the rise (Shanafelt et al. 2012). Physician's long work hours are a significant contributor, which is hardly surprising with 61% of physicians reporting work hours of > 50 h per week and 36% reporting working > 60 h per week (Shanafelt et al. 2012). Whereas in other fields, higher levels of education and professional degrees correlate to reduced risk of burnout, in medicine an advanced degree actually increases risk (Shanafelt et al. 2012). Another personal factor that increases physician burnout risk is the perception of loss of control, which can occur when patients are dying or when staff is short handed. The complex, ever-changing healthcare system also contributes to physician burnout with its increasing administrative paperwork, increasing patient volumes, and complex payer mechanisms. More emphasis on documentation, and bottom line, rather than quality of the patient encounter has led to shorter face time between patients and doctors, which is what 73% of doctors identify as what they find most rewarding in medicine (Gundersen 2001). Physicians may learn to deny their own needs and emotions as a survival mechanism that eventually becomes not only counterproductive, but actually self-destructive (Gundersen 2001).

A Physician's Road to Recovery (Hill, Personal Communication, 2017)

Nothing could have prepared me for the emotional tsunami that rolled through my life in my first year of my pediatric oncology fellowship training. A few sick days turned into weeks without energy or motivation and eventually leading to a true loss of hope. Reeling, I started to self-medicate and before long I was drinking a pint of vodka every night just to fall asleep. In only a few short months, I found myself alone, sitting in my car, in the woods, with a fifth of vodka and a plan. Ending up in the woods involved a lot of denial, personal neglect, self-pity, chemical depression, and self-medication. Reflecting back now, I see how many factors collided into a perfect storm. At the time, I was newly married, moved halfway across the country, left my family/friends, and started a new challenging career in pediatric oncology. I started to feel isolated, alone, and developed signs/symptoms of depression. I was faced with a complicated and heavy patient load, long hours, and grueling academic demands in the context of a totally unsupportive work environment that left me feeling exhausted, burned out, and hopeless. I didn't really feel that I had anyone that I could trust and/or that understood what I was going through, so the easiest thing to do was to drink and forget all of my problems. I could delve further into spiteful specifics, but I feel there is a better part of the story to tell; the story of surviving to write this self-reflection at all. This is not a beautifully neat story of redemption; it's sometimes messy and angry: a story of unforeseen obstacles, humiliating judgment, and unexplainable societal stigma that I simply never understood before.

Growing up, I was never naïve to the powers of mental illness and substance abuse. My grandfather died of alcoholism in his 50s, and his son, my father, became a mental health and substance abuse counselor. By the time I was in my early 20s, five of my high school classmates had committed suicide, and in just the first 4 years of my career in medicine, two physician colleagues took their own lives. That all being said, I could not believe, I was wading in the dark waters of depression and alcohol addiction.

One thing that became instantly clear was that seeking help for mental illness and substance abuse carries massive stigma in our culture and, ironically, even more so among medical professionals. The first meeting I scheduled was with a physician at the academic hospital health center office. He asked me "Do you really know what you are getting into?" I did not know at the time, but he was not referring to the prospect of a happy life or a life in sobriety; instead he was referring to the years of hypocritical bureaucracy that would follow the rest of my career. At that moment, he was questioning my intentions of going down that road and actually offering a way out—a let's just forget this conversation happened moment. Call it what you will, but I call this my true moment of grace, a moment of blissful ignorant salvation and the catalyst from which I'm allowed to write this reflection. In my depressed state of alcohol-induced denial, personal hatred, and self-neglect, I would have never willingly signed into a recovery system of lawyers, medical board hearings, randomized drug testing, monitoring contracts, and physician health programs. Yet I did, willingly, and for that sole reason, I am still alive today.

I decided to go a 6-week treatment program, quit drinking, signed into a physician health program, started my random drug screening and compliance contracts, and hated every minute of my life. I resented everyone, the system, the people that loved me, and the idea that other people had power over me. I was not drinking, I was medicated, and I was learning skills to cope with my depression and substance abuse, and I was still miserable. My marriage was crumbling, my friends were distant, and my whole universe was turned upside down. The greatest fallacy in recovery is that you stop drinking and automatically your whole life is fixed and this simply isn't true. It takes a lot of work and time. After a few months, I was cleared to go back to work; however, then the medical board meetings started, my license was put on probation, and I had to further document my compliance with sobriety. A few months after that, I was turned down for an incredible job opportunity. I walked out of the chairmen's office in tears, after he told me that I wouldn't be hired, and those tears quickly turned into anger. I resented the hospital, the system, my sobriety, and I could not reconcile the fact that I deserved this opportunity, with not getting it. It simply isn't fair, I got sober, I changed my life around, and I deserved this.

I look back at that day as one of the greatest days of my life now. If I had gotten that job then, I would have failed. At the time, I wasn't drinking any longer, but I wasn't living a sober life quite yet either. There truly is a reason for everything. In recovery, there is often a saying "just do the next right thing," and then suddenly, without even knowing at the time, everything changes. That time came around 6 months of sobriety; it took nearly 6 months of living "one day at a time", not drinking, and practicing new life skills like yoga, meditation, mindfulness, and hemi-sync. During this time, I learned to keep a gratitude list that I kept in my wallet and read every night before I went to sleep. I didn't mind getting drug tested any longer, and I looked at the compliance meetings as an opportunity and not a punishment. In hindsight,

I truly don't know when the switch flipped, but I learned to reframe life experiences and to view the happenings of the past in a whole new way, and because of that I learned humility, gratitude, and grace.

I write this now having been sober for several years, working in a job that I love, with people that I love, in a marriage that was saved, and with a toddler filling our home with giggles of joy. There can be a light at the end of the tunnel. I fully acknowledge that the system is broken and the stigma of depression and substance abuse is real, it is dangerous, and good people die because of it. The system still treats anyone with substance abuse and/or mental illness as a delinquent and not as an individual with a medical problem that simply needs help. I don't know why I didn't take the "way out" offered in that physician's office, but I know for a fact that if I had I wouldn't be alive to tell my story. And the fact that it was offered still disturbs the part of me that mourns for those forever lost in this goliath struggle. I hope people know that I am as perfectly imperfect as any man can be, but I am alive, I am a survivor, and I am free. I truly hope that we can turn this scarlet letter system of public shaming addiction/mental illness into an empathic network of connecting loved individuals to the resources they need. I realize now that I have a breath and a voice. A voice solidified in hope, humility, gratitude, and grace, because every single day I choose to love myself and take care of myself first—the rest will simply fall into place, if you let it.

13.7 Risk Factors for Clinician Distress

Literature suggests that the single largest risk factor for clinician distress is human service work (Newell and MacNeil 2010). Pediatric oncology with its high-stakes decisions, chronic exposure to child and family suffering, and long hours can be a fertile ground for cultivating distress among healthcare professionals. Furthermore, the medical training model teaches young professionals to sacrifice themselves in order to meet the pressing service and educational demands. This model can create a culture of martyrdom and delayed gratification whereby the learner develops a philosophy of biding time until things get easier (e.g., after graduation, after licensing exams, after residency). Unfortunately, however, the demands do not lessen after training is completed, and yet an unrealistic philosophy of biding time may persist (Drummond 2015). Recent changes in technology (electronic medical record keeping), productivity pressures that leave little room for "face time" with patients, and challenges with insurance company reimbursements have compounded the problem (Shanafelt et al. 2015a).

Risk factors for clinician distress can be organized into personal (e.g., female, younger age), interpersonal (e.g., angry patients/families, poor team communication), professional (e.g., moral distress, chronic exposure to death), and institutional (e.g., understaffing, lack of flexibility (Spinetta et al. 2000; Khamisa et al. 2013)) (Table 13.1).

13.8 Interventions for Clinician Distress

It is now accepted that preventing and remedying clinician distress is not solely up to individuals, but must also be addressed by healthcare institutions (Shanafelt et al. 2012). Furthermore, promoting clinician well-being may inherently lead to improved patient satisfaction and outcomes, improved team morale, and a hardier (and larger) work force which is better equipped to handle the ever-changing demands of the healthcare system (Shanafelt et al. 2014). There have been few empirically based studies to examine burnout and compassion fatigue in clinicians, and the majority of published studies are in the nursing literature (Ruotsalainen et al. 2015). Interventions for

Table 13.1 Risk factors for clinician distress (Spinetta et al. 2000; Roth et al. 2011; Khamisa et al. 2013; Shanafelt et al. 2014)

Personal	
• Younger age • Female gender • Idealistic perspective • Over involvement/inappropriate boundaries with patients • Too high expectations of self • Inability to say "No" • Difficulty discussing feelings	• Low self-esteem • Lack of a spiritual practice • Cumulative losses • History of psychiatric disorder • Difficulty asking for help or using social support • Unsatisfactory work-life balance • History of own traumatic experiences
Interpersonal	
• Conflict with colleagues • Unsupportive managers • Low team morale	• Depressed, angry, or psychotic patient/family members • Poor communication among staff • Lack of recognition
Professional	
• < 5 years' experience • Exposure to death and dying (especially of children) • Insufficient training in palliative care and bereavement support	• Patients with uncontrolled symptoms • Moral and ethical dilemmas • Oncology practice • Insufficient time to grieve losses
Institutional	
• Increased clinical workload • Understaffing • Increased paperwork/EMR • Chaotic environment • Perceived inadequacy of resources • High rates of exposure to child and family trauma	• Lack of control or input on work policies and procedures • Working at an institution that does *not* have services available to address burnout • Culture of "martyrdom" • Long hours

clinician distress can be classified as personal, professional, and institutional.

13.8.1 Personal Interventions

Changes on a personal level are the most studied and may be the easiest to implement rapidly (Ruotsalainen et al. 2015). Recharging one's physical, spiritual, and emotional energy may require different approaches from person to person; however, one thing is certain: it requires paying attention to one's energy level in these areas and, if low, taking some action to improve it (Drummond 2015). Personal interventions can include physical changes (sleep, exercise, diet, massage), psychological changes (meaning making when facing death and relaxation), emotional expression (through supportive relationships at work or at home and support groups, writing narratives and poetry, engaging in art and music), developing a spiritual practice (protecting some personal time for self-reflection and discovery and cultivating mindfulness), and discipline-specific interventions (gaining expertise in pain management and goals of care conversations, connecting with the mission that attracted you to the field, reinventing role as a caregiver) (Shanafelt and Dyrbye 2012; Drummond 2015; Quill and Williamson 1990; Fanos 2007; Shanafelt et al. 2006). Interestingly, Susan Bauer-Wu, a nurse researcher and oncology nurse, describes a relationship between the attributes of extraordinary cancer survivors she met through her cancer healing programs and exceptional oncology nurses she worked with. In looking at the stories of remarkable cancer survivors, she identified nine characteristics that were present in each of them and realized that they were also present in the nurses. She coined the term "nurse thrivers" and prescribes the following traits to cultivate in order to be one: be self-sufficient and have a can-do attitude; do fulfilling and enjoyable activities; have at least one supportive and trusted relationship; express a full range of emotions; find meaning in the work every day; partner with patients and colleagues; engage often in stress-reducing activities; have a sense of spiritual connection, including connection with nature; and be flexible and willing to try new things and to think "out of the box" (Bauer-Wu 2005).

13.8.2 Professional Interventions

Professional level changes encourage clinicians to honestly appraise one's values and priorities and to set short- and long-term goals in personal and professional areas. Careful review of goals and values may reveal inherent conflicts (e.g., spend more time with family versus gain more professional visibility through public speaking and publication). Creating a work-life balance that is in line with values and goals, and sticking with it, can assist in achievement of professional and personal goals. A successful medicine-pediatric colleague was asked what she would change when looking back on her career. If she could do it over again, she said she would work a little less and be home and present with her children more, even as they aged through high school. When her children were teens, she had made the decision to move from part time to full time. Quickly, it became too easy for the workload to exceed a full time schedule. Therefore, when making choices about opportunities at work, she tried to use a mantra "I am the only mother of my children" while remembering that there were many other doctors to help care for patients. Nonetheless, it was still difficult to maintain a sense of balance between doctoring and mothering (Ciccarelli, personal communication, 2017). Some clinicians will intentionally carve out time with their families after a period of traveling, time on service, or grant writing. One author suggested that oncologists discover what they love most about their career (clinical time, leadership, healthcare administration, teaching, research, etc.) and ensure that at least 20% time is spent engaged in this activity (Shanafelt et al. 2006). Mostly, authors on clinician burnout highlight the need for clinicians to refocus on finding the joyful aspects of practicing medicine and cultivate them (Shanafelt et al. 2006).

13.8.3 Institutional Level Interventions

Healthcare institutions have an obligation to promote clinician wellness, and ultimately the institution will benefit from a healthier workforce (Shanafelt and Dyrbye 2012). Maslach and Leiter suggest institutions (and individuals) first take an inventory of the following factors to assess burnout (Maslach and Leiter 2005): workload (too much, lack of resources), control (micromanagement, accountability without power), reward (compensation, acknowledgment), community (isolation, conflict, disrespect), fairness (discrimination, favoritism), and values (ethical conflicts, meaningless tasks). Maslach and Leiter and others who are applying their work (Henry 2014) discuss identifying any mismatches between people and their work raised on the inventory and then developing interventions to support staff on an individual level as well as the institutional level to deal with the conflicts and reduce burnout. Not all risk factors can be addressed at once, but it is important for the well-being of the staff that the process begins and that social and organizational processes be addressed.

The nursing literature is the most plentiful regarding institutional level interventions to mitigate clinician distress. Mukherjee and colleagues developed a specific tool, Work Stressor Scale – Paediatric Oncology (WSS-PO), for nurses to help identify and ameliorate clinician distress. This tool assesses stressors and rewards experienced on the job and can be used to measure intensity and frequency of factors associated with burnout as well as assist in the development of staff interventions (Mukherjee et al. 2014). Various interventions have been investigated in oncology clinicians that fall primarily into four discrete categories: community support in the workplace, continuing education opportunities, reflective and supportive supervision, and bereavement debriefing.

13.8.3.1 Creating Community in the Workplace

Staff support groups are an important vehicle to address work-related stressors. Regularly scheduled support groups enable individuals to analyze their own personal feelings, gain new perspectives, share in finding solutions together, spread the responsibility for a positive work environment, and increase staff morale (Le Blanc et al. 2007). When clinicians feel they are part of a caring community, it helps them to better deal with the constant changes that take place on the oncology unit and prevent burnout (Dane and Chachkes 2001; Parker and Gadbois 2000; Medland et al. 2004). Schwartz Rounds offer healthcare providers a forum to discuss emotional and social impacts of caring for patients and families (Lee et al. 2015). Caregivers share their thoughts and feelings on provocative topics taken from real patient cases in order to connect to others and experience some level of catharsis (Thompson 2013). Notably only 36% of pediatric oncologists report the availability of a formal debriefing session to discuss their personal psychosocial concerns at their institutions (Roth et al. 2011).

Several programs described in the nursing literature were designed and implemented to foster community support in the workplace and reduce burnout. A few of these programs are outlined in Table 13.2.

13.8.3.2 Empowering and Educating Clinicians

A systematic educational framework can help empower clinicians to stay in the profession through skills development and promotion of

Table 13.2 Nursing programs designed to promote community in the workplace

Name of intervention	Population	Exposure	Intervention	**Outcome**
Circle of care retreat Medland et al. (2004)	Interdisciplinary oncology team members (> 150 staff members)	One-day retreat later followed up ongoing support/ planning groups that make decisions on how to improve systems of care	Assess how the staff copes with the high level of death and dying patients, as well as what can be done to create a psychosocial sense of caring in the workplace and a meaningful environment	Protocol on units changed for when patients die—body is prepared with a partner, patient care assignments reshuffled to allow for attending to needs of patient and family, direct staff encouraged to go to “safe space” for processing loss, symbol of another life passing displayed on door of room
Take careLe Blanc et al. (2007)	Direct care providers for oncology patients	Six monthly sessions, 3 h each	Meetings were designed to gather information on the policies and structures in the institution which were perceived to be the greatest contributors to job stress and burnout. They consisted of one part education on varying topics and one part action planning	Evaluators found reductions in depersonalization, emotional exhaustion, and burnout scores
Care for the professional caregiver Edmonds et al. (2012)	Three groups of oncology nurses (pediatric, surgical, and general oncology), and one group of nurse managers	Day-long retreat followed by a booster session 6 months later	Includes didactic learning with group discussion exploring coping strategies, vicarious trauma, consequences of burnout and self-care strategies, including mindfulness, to lessen the effects of workplace stressors. The booster session was designed to reinforce previously reviewed material	Compared to a control group, the program reduced emotional exhaustion significantly, feeling less overextended both physically. Additionally, improvements were demonstrated on the general health of the nurses

self-confidence. Through the development of new skills, clinicians are afforded improved self-efficacy to assist patients and lessen feelings of helplessness pertaining to the patient's condition (Cohen and Gagin 2005). One nursing graduate development program revealed that through the utilization of professional development, educational opportunities, mentorship, exposure to advanced practice, and continued reflection, the majority of new oncology nurses remained on the unit (Hayes et al. 2005). In addition, communication training of clinicians regarding end-of-life discussions is associated with improved job satisfaction (Puntillo and McAdam 2006).

13.8.3.3 Reflective Supervision

Reflective supervision enables staff to identify and understand their own feelings, thoughts, and reactions to the trauma they see in their daily work with their patients and families (Van Berckelaer 2011). It is not therapy but rather a dialog between a clinician and his/her supervisor and is characterized by active listening and thoughtful questioning by both to help guide the clinician to identify his/her feelings and prevent compassion fatigue. It can also be useful for helping to make decisions and as a source of empathetic, nonjudgmental discussion to process complex emotions and manage job stress (Parlakian 2001). It serves as a good model for the relationship the clinician will want to have with patients and their families and can be done on a regular basis (Parlakian 2001).

Similar to the nursing literature, social work literature suggests that supervision programs which focus on improving the intervention skills of the clinician have been shown to reduce the experience of burnout, as well as a decline in emotional exhaustion. This has been shown through both formal supervision with a supervisor, as well as informally with peer supervision (Cohen and Gagin 2005; Ben-Zur and Michael 2007). The benefits of supervision for social workers can be identified as being highly valuable in two ways: (1) linking work with individual patients and families to theoretical framework and (2) managing the emotional impact of the work on the social worker, as well as managing the challenges within the greater system and the multidisciplinary team (Joubert et al. 2013).

In the physician model, similar to the concept of supervision described above, it is suggested that institutions cultivate and promote leaders that exhibit attributes shown to be associated with decreased distress. Specific leadership attributes include leaders that mentor by facilitating young doctors to make values-based career decisions and create realistic goals. They treat others with dignity and respect, ask their opinion on work-related policies and issues, and keep staff updated on institutional changes, as well as provide helpful feedback and guidance. They empower, inspire, praise accomplishments (both personal and professional), and encourage the development of skills and talents that are valued to the physician and will help build their career (Shanafelt et al. 2015b).

Finally, all supervisors and managers could ensure that they are supporting their personnel to take care of themselves. For example, when clinicians are experiencing an overly difficult workload, managers could encourage staff to take frequent breaks such as a walk, coffee break, or alternating clinical care with administrative tasks (Maslach and Leiter 2005; Henry 2014).

13.8.3.4 Inclusion of Bereavement Debriefing in the Workplace

As with much of the published data on these topics, the majority of the literature on bereavement debriefing for clinicians is found nursing; however, the principles can be applied across all clinical disciplines.

Bereavement support groups and group debriefing help clinicians to share their feelings around a patient's death and reduce isolation (Saunders and Valente 1994). These groups allow clinicians to recognize that their feelings are part of normal grief and that sharing these feelings with colleagues can help facilitate collegial collaboration and assist with getting through the grieving (Saunders and Valente 1994). A study found that both nurses that have only been in the field for a year and those who are seasoned nurses find that diversional activities like exercising, shopping, and venting to others about work are not necessarily sufficient in handling their grief when a patient dies (Hinds et al. 1994). Every time a patient dies, the clinician is presented with his or her own mortality (Saunders and Valente 1994). Offering staff time with individual psychosocial personnel may provide additional help for those who are not helped by group psychological support and diversional activities (Saunders and Valente 1994).

One study identified four phenomenological themes of the nurses' lived experience following the death of a patient:

(1) Reciprocal relationship transcends professional relationship—the nurse reflects on the connection with the patient they make while caring for them. The nurse gains from the relationship to the patient and the family (and vice versa) something of value that is not tangible. When the patient dies, the nurse feels a loss for the relationship and needs to grieve.
(2) Initial patient death events are formative—when the first time of experiencing death of a patient is not well supported, the nurse will carry a negative perception with them into the future. If the supports were positive the first time, such as a positive role model, the nurse is more likely to be able to grieve and feel positive emotions and cope well in the future.
(3) Incorporating spiritual world views and caring rituals—the nurse's beliefs can help her cope, and the beliefs can change over time due to experiences with dying patients. Often the nurses' world beliefs in an afterlife deepen or transform because of his/her repeated exposure to death. Some nurses stated they felt as if they were being guided by a spiritual entity through the situation. They may gain control by having a set of caring rituals such as offering tissues and drinks to the family or attending the funeral of the patient.
(4) Compartmentalizing the experience to maintain professionalism—they need to separate the pain they experience due to the loss of the relationship they had with the patient from the questions they may have about hastening the death through their medical treatment of the patient. They may have to maintain a clear boundary between their emotional responses and the need to be present to continue with their day-to-day care of patients and then make time to grieve later (Gerow et al. 2010).

A bereavement debriefing session focuses on the emotional feelings of staff members, looking at the relationship with the patient and not just talking about the death. This session should be held within a week of the patient's death so that all clinicians and other staff can reflect and discuss how they are experiencing the death. Enabling these focus groups to happen by providing funding and release of time has been shown to reduce burnout and enhance staff retention (Keene et al. 2010). Each of these sessions should include a welcome and introductions of each participant which include how they were involved with the care of this patient and family, a factual review of the circumstances of the death, a case review describing what it was like taking care of the patient, what the most distressing and satisfying aspects were of the case, the individual grief responses experienced by each staff member (physical, emotional, behavioral, cognitive, or spiritual), what staff will each remember most about this patient and family (emotional component), staff strategies for coping with grief, available resources and strategy review, and lessons learned. The session should conclude with an acknowledgment of the care given and summarize bereavement support available for families and staff (Keene et al. 2010).

A comprehensive list of strategies for improving personal, professional, and institutional wellness and decreasing clinical distress can be found in Table 13.3.

13.9 Moral Distress

Although the term moral distress has been in the literature since 1984 (Jameton 1984), it is a complex construct with considerable debate over an exact definition (Fourie 2015;

Table 13.3 Interventions for clinical distress (Spinetta et al. 2000; Roth et al. 2011; Bowden et al. 2015; Quill and Williamson 1990; Shanafelt et al. 2006; Bauer-Wu 2005; Mougalian et al. 2013)

Personal interventions	
Psychological	*Physical*
• Positive reframing • Mindfulness • Relaxation • Self-awareness • Assertiveness training • Laughter/cultivating happiness	• Exercise (e.g., weight training, cardiovascular, yoga) • Massage • Breathing exercises • Sleep • Whirlpool • Diet
Emotional/social	*Spiritual*
• Boundaries • Support systems • Positive relationships with colleagues • Pursing hobbies/interests • Expression via writing, art, music, etc.	• Meditation • Religion • Prayer • Reiki • Retreats
Professional interventions	
• Work-life balance • Time management • Redefine role when child is dying • Develop philosophy on death • Identify professional values	• CE's in palliative care topics: pain management and goals of care conversations • Prioritizing and learning to say "No"
Institutional-level interventions	
• Schwartz Rounds • Town hall meetings • Flexible scheduling • Policies for nursing breaks/relief after a patient dies • Facilitated debriefing forums • Strengthen interprofessional community	• Calm and supportive environments • Team decision-making • Staff retreats • Education days • Supportive leadership • Bereavement support • Reflective supervision

Musto et al. 2015). In simple terms, moral distress is the experience of believing one knows the ethical thing to do; however internal or external barriers prevent the individual from acting (Wocial and Weaver 2013). There is no doubt that emotion, empathy, and compassion play a role in moral distress (Rushton and Kurtz 2015). Manifestation of moral distress may be indistinguishable from other forms of emotional stress such as burnout and compassion fatigue. However, what does distinguish moral distress from other forms of emotional stress is the perception that a person's professional integrity is violated and that person is constrained from taking ethically appropriate action (Epstein and Hamric 2009). It is also directly related to the well-being of a patient (Dudzinski 2016). Moral distress has been most widely discussed in nursing; however, a growing body of research confirms that it is experienced by individuals across disciplines in healthcare (Allen et al. 2013; Bruce et al. 2015; Ulrich et al. 2010), and it has negative consequences for clinicians and patients (Elpern et al. 2005; Houston et al. 2013; Whitehead et al. 2015).

The exponential growth in the number of publications on moral distress in recent years underscores the rise in recognition that moral distress is an issue not to be ignored (Lamiani et al. 2017). The presence of moral distress is not a personal weakness or an indication of emotional instability of a clinician, nor does it suggest that someone cannot practice in ethically complex situations. Moral disagreements should be expected in a complex specialty such as pediatric oncology. Disagreement does not have to result in conflict or distress. When moral distress is present, clinicians should view it as evidence that conscientious persons are practicing in challenging contexts (Garros et al. 2015). Furthermore, it must be addressed as failing to address moral distress may have negative consequences (Halpern 2011).

13.9.1 Risk Factors for Moral Distress

Constant exposure to suffering children that occurs in pediatric oncology puts clinicians at risk for developing moral distress (Rushton and Kurtz 2015), and there are many specific situations that may trigger moral distress. Examples of these include the use of experimental treatments, management of severe side effects of chemotherapy, and limb removal in the context of extremely poor overall prognosis. When one is legally obligated to administer or bear witness to treatment in accordance with family wishes that feels unethical, moral distress can occur. Moral distress is often associated with what clinicians perceive as futile or inappropriate treatment (Mobley et al. 2007; Piers et al. 2011; Trotochaud et al. 2015; Wilson et al. 2013) and poor physician-nurse collaboration (Hamric and Blackhall 2007; Kalvemark et al. 2004; McAndrew et al. 2011; Papathanassoglou et al. 2012). In pediatric oncology, physicians and parents are the central decision-makers even though it is the children who must undergo tremendously burdensome treatment and the nurses who are primarily responsible for administering those treatments. Nurses and social workers often voice that their perspectives are not included in decision-making nor respected (Bush 2009; Dane and Chachkes 2001; Mukherjee et al. 2014; Morgan 2009). This can lead to a moral hazard, a situation that often leads to moral distress. A moral hazard exists in a situation in which one party controls decisions about resources, but another party bears most of the benefits or burdens of the decision (Brumnquell and Michaelson 2016). In addition, moral distress can occur in clinicians caring for children at end of life when critical medical decisions must be made. The decision to pursue, continue, or withhold life-sustaining treatments at the end of life continues to be among the most emotionally charged issues that can contribute to moral distress (Keeler 2010). Because pediatric oncologists experience close longitudinal relationships with patients and develop a strong sense of fiduciary responsibility toward their patients, they may be less likely than other subspecialists to identify care as overly burdensome and tend toward a "try everything" approach (Johnson et al. 2015). When treating children who face life-threatening illness such as cancer, doing anything less than "everything" can be difficult (Clark and Dudzinski 2013). This in turn might hinder an oncologists' ability to recognize conflicting ethical principles concerning goals of care (Johnson et al. 2015). Furthermore, physicians may view death as a professional failure instead of an unavoidable part of the work (Buxton 2010) This is further complicated by the emerging autonomy of children and raises questions regarding how much information to provide to them and how much influence they should have over these critical end-of-life decisions (Kushnick 2010; Friebert 2010; Shepard 2010).

13.9.2 Interventions for Moral Distress

It is not enough for clinicians to state they are experiencing moral distress. They must be able to name the emotion they are experiencing, identify the source of the distress, name the forces preventing them from acting, identify the conflicting obligations and responsibilities, name an action that would alleviate the distress by addressing patient need, and, finally, name the action that could be taken to set a forward course (Dudzinski 2016). Beyond naming emotions, Rushton and Kurtz suggest that teaching clinicians to modulate their responses to morally troubling situations by developing self-awareness may help modify the effects of moral distress (Rushton and Kurtz 2015). Others see moral distress as a form of relational trauma and suggest there is a need to understand how nurses as moral agents are influenced by and influence the environments in which they work (Musto et al. 2015). Moral distress is a relational experience that is shaped by multiple contexts (Varcoe et al. 2012). If we can focus on the relational aspects of our practice, we may be able to overcome vexing ethical challenges (Browning 2010).

Nurses identify debriefing and ethics consultations as important strategies to address moral distress (Wilson et al. 2013). Promoting effective communication along with bioethics education must be part of strategies to address moral distress (Garros et al. 2015; Wocial 2008). This requires a supportive and nonjudgmental culture in the practice environment where open dialog about moral differences is honored and individual differences are respected and where we intentionally listen to typically silenced voices of those who must act on decisions made by others (Browning 2010; Pavlish et al. 2014; Wocial 2016). A space where feelings can be shared openly and honestly can influence the personal experience of clinicians and expose the perceived professional conflicts which is necessary to address moral distress (Austin et al. 2009). Seeking help from an ethics consultation service or ethics committee often will support the creation of such an environment (Johnson et al. 2015; Mekechuk 2006; Carter and Wocial 2012). Promoting open discussion about ethically challenging situations can lessen moral distress (Bruce et al. 2015; Karanikola et al. 2014; Wocial et al. 2010). These discussions can be led by psychosocial clinicians, such as social workers, who are competent in facilitating groups, supporting team members, and promoting conversations of ethical issues that emerge during the course of an illness through the end of life (Gwyther et al. 2005).

Much is unknown about moral distress in the ethically complex context of pediatric oncology. The impact of moral distress on clinicians is physical, emotional, and professional. Tools that may be helpful in managing, measuring, and tracking moral distress and interventions to address it include the 4 A's model (Rushton and Kurtz 2015), the moral distress thermometer (Wocial and Weaver 2013), the revised Moral Distress Scale (Hamric et al. 2012), and the moral distress map (Dudzinski 2016). Managing the impact of moral distress requires interventions on several levels, including the individual, team, facility, and policy level (Epstein and Hamric 2009; Shepard 2010; Nurses AAoCC 2008; Pauly et al. 2012). Eliminating moral distress is an unrealistic goal. Managing it, however, is not only possible; it must be a priority.

13.10 Clinician Spiritual Distress

The concept of spirituality can be viewed as ambiguous, due to it being personal, subjective, and distinctive from religion, while also being manifested through religious or symbolic practices and rituals (Tanyi 2002; Tanyi et al. 2009). Because of this variability in defining spirituality, clinicians likely experience spirituality profoundly different from one another, affecting each practice in a different way. Spirituality has been described also as the aspect of humanity regarding the way individuals seek and express meaning and purpose and the way they experience their connectedness to the moment, to themselves, to others, to nature, and to sacred and significant events (Puchalski et al. 2009). It can be expressed as a coping mechanism, a way of being, and relates to hope, faith, and one's relationship to God (Burke and Neimeyer 2014). Pellebon and Anderson put forth the notion that spirituality has the "most notable impact on an individual's attitudes, behaviors, and decision-making process" (Pellebon and Anderson 1999). Research suggests that clinicians that view spiritual care as important, as well as endorse a high spiritual well-being, have more positive attitudes toward spiritual care and are more likely to incorporate spiritual care in their care plans (Musgrave and McFarlane 2003). It seems that if providers place value on spiritual care, they are more likely to recognize the spiritual needs of others (Musgrave and McFarlane 2003; Piles 1990). In one study of nurses, researchers found that nurses in the oncology unit were least likely to talk with patients about and asses their spiritual needs than nurses on any other unit (Musgrave and McFarlane 2003; Bath 1992). This is concerning since 40–94% of cancer patients report that they would like their clinicians to address their spiritual needs (Ramondetta et al. 2013; Kang et al. 2012; Balboni et al. 2013). Unfortunately there are few data regarding the experience of spiritual distress in the clinician; however, surely we can learn from the research on spiritual distress of patients.

Exploration of a patients' spirituality including their hopes, fears, and wishes as well as the assessment of spiritual distress (often expressed as abandonment, guilt, and viewing illness as a punishment from God) can be critical in helping to manage patients' suffering and to guide patients through the medical decisions they are presented with when facing death (Ramondetta et al. 2013). Healthcare teams can engage spiritual providers on their team or in the community to support families and providers.

Providing such care is challenging to the spirit of the physician who has not explored their own spiritual distress (see Table 13.4, asking the "why" and "how" questions). Clinicians have not been traditionally trained to do this, yet we know that strong spiritual well-being correlates to better spiritual care of patients (Musgrave and McFarlane 2003; Piles 1990; Kaur et al. 2013). This spiritual care manifests as increased compassion and providing solace; helping to feel healed when cure is not possible through life review, forgiveness, and legacy making; and helping patients to make meaning and find connection and realistic hope in the midst of suffering, chaos, and pain (National Consensus Project 2013). For the provider, cultivation of spirituality and spiritual practice can provide respite during times of emotional distress by creating a sense of harmony and providing focus (Collins 2005). A clinician's spiritual well-being is protective against burnout and compassion fatigue and may reduce psychosocial and existential distress in patients (Ramondetta et al. 2013; Kaur et al. 2013; Desbiens and Fillion 2007; MacDonald and Friedman 2002). In patients, four domains of spiritual need have been identified: connectedness, peace, meaning/purpose, and transcendence (Burke and Neimeyer 2014). Perhaps these can be applied to clinicians to promote spiritual well-being as well. Specific to clinicians, however, is the original sense of mission and purpose that led to their choice of vocation and this can provide the bedrock of their daily work (Pfifferling and Gilley 1999). Daily work without connection to values may feel like work that is empty, meaningless, and sometimes brutalizing. Recapturing the joy and renewing the essence of why one was drawn to this work may also require acknowledgment of the pain experienced so that it can be processed and healed. Having clear values, strong support, a sense of humor, self-awareness of one's own needs, and a receptivity to receiving gratitude, love, and respect from patients can bolster clinicians' spiritual well-being (Pfifferling and Gilley 1999).

Table 13.4 For clinicians to consider asking the "why" and "how" questions (Myss 1996; Kjeldmand and Holmstroem 2008; Tillich 2000; Frankl 2014)

The "why" and "how" questions
How do I find hope when the prognosis is dismal?
What restores my soul in the face of the following? • When the suffering is not apparently meaningful • When the pain is not relieved • When the parents are demanding and delinquent
What shall I do with my search for meaning and my fear of meaninglessness?
Am I leaving my soul behind, safe from harm, when the magnitude of suffering is great?
Where can I find the strength to be with the suffering of others?
What do I require of the parents I admire? Can they falter? Have rage? Have despair?
Can I care enough for myself spiritually to receive a parents suffering with acceptance and grace?
Is it okay if I don't have answers to the "why" questions?
Connecting to one's mission and purpose
Why did I want to be a healer? Was I willing to give of myself to save the life of another? Was I committed to ending needless suffering?
Do I find sanctity in professionalism of the highest standards?
Am I willing to learn from my mistakes and improve from yesterday to today?
Can I encourage you in this agonizing journey and loan you hope when you have none?
Can I face the fact that I am not God and still continue to balance head and heart and body's strength in my care for you?

13.11 Employee Assistance Programs

When clinician distress is severe, individuals can seek help through employee assistance programs (EAPs). EAPs are free and confidential counseling services offered at institutions for employees. Typically, they provide assessments, information, referrals, and short-term counseling to assist with professional and/or personal difficulties interfering with a provider's success and job satisfaction. The number of sessions provided, associated fees, and availability of services varies among institutions. In a survey of 410 pediatric oncology physicians, only 40% of the providers were aware of services for burnout at their institution (Roth et al. 2011). Despite having access to a staff counselor or psychologist, they are not always able to be utilized by employees. In one survey of oncology nurses, an identified barrier to this assistance was lag time between request and a scheduled appointment. Instead, nurses reported turning to their social work colleagues and case managers for support during times of need (Aycock and Boyle 2009). While it seems these services may be underutilized for varying reasons, a multicenter study reported that between 40 and 58% of nurses and physicians who have attended EAP services rated them as moderately or very helpful. Still, less than 10% of survey respondents reported occasional or frequent usage of the resource (Lee et al. 2015). These studies highlight a need for more availability and flexibility of the programs, in addition to education to staff regarding availability and scope of services offered by these programs.

Physician assistance programs (PAPs) or physician health programs (PHPs) are specifically designed to assist physicians with mental health and/or drug-/alcohol-related conditions. Most PHPs have a multidisciplinary team of nurses, advanced practice nurses, social workers, case managers, and physicians. Individual states vary in the services they offer and the overall structure of their programs. National success rates for PHP enrolled physicians are > 75%, with some states reporting over 90% success (Knight et al. 2007, 2002; Morse et al. 1984; Shore 1987; Alpern et al. 1992) in sustained abstinence and return to active work. In most state programs, the structure is designed so that physicians can confidentially enroll, seek treatment, and formulate a long-term treatment plan without involvement of the state medical licensing boards. Referral to a PHP can be from the individual physician (self-referral), a colleague, family member, or any concerned individual. Ultimately, unless formal complaints have been issued to the medical licensing board or state government office, the decision to enroll in a physician health program is voluntary (Hill, personal communication, 2017).

Recommendations are case specific but can vary from continued follow-up with a local PHP to outpatient treatment programs, inpatient rehabilitation services, or partial hospitalization programs (± inpatient detoxification for patients with unstable medical conditions such as severe alcohol withdrawal). The decision to follow the treatment recommendations is voluntary—if no pre-existing claims exist—however, to participate and enroll in the PHP, most states will require compliance. In most states, as long as an individual physician remains compliant with their treatment program, the medical license board will not be made aware of the physician's recovery, and no punitive repercussions will be incurred. Physicians should be aware that most states have disclosure questions that must be answered upon renewal of a state license and/or at the time of applying for another out-of-state license. The handling of diagnoses and treatment disclosure is completely subject to the local medical board judgment, and physicians may have their license put on probation for a subjective amount of time. If more serious concerns arise, such as criminal arrests, patient safety concerns, and/or noncompliance with PHP, then additional sanctions may be imposed. After completion of a monitoring contract, physicians are encouraged to continue their recovery program but will no longer be subject to a monitoring program. The overall design of a PHP is to provide treatment resources, help safely return physicians to work, and advocate for physicians during their recovery process (Hill, personal communication, 2017).

Conclusion

Distress, regardless of type—burnout, compassion fatigue, moral distress, and spiritual distress—is a reality that professionals working in pediatric oncology will likely face at one time or another, either personally or in a colleague. The consequences of such distress can be severe for the individuals and their patients, as well as for the healthcare system as a whole. Many risk factors for distress in clinicians have emerged that can be addressed through personal, professional, and institutional interventions. Most of the intervention research in pediatric oncology has been studied in nurses. Much more needs to be learned regarding effective interventions for all healthcare providers including how to implement effective interventions in healthcare systems. Those working in this field need to become mindful of how they are being affected by this work in order to identify and address their distress. Clinicians working in pediatric oncology would benefit from education regarding strategies to reduce distress at personal, professional, and institutional levels. Providers already suffering from extreme distress can get help through institutional and state programs. The act of the clinician exploring their own beliefs, values, and emotions must be as important as knowing those of their patients and families because the caregiver must replenish himself if he is to continue to effectively care for others.

Key Take-Home Points

- Distress in a clinician can manifest as distinct but overlapping types of distress including burnout, compassion fatigue, moral distress, and spiritual distress; it is highly prevalent and rates are on the rise.
- Consequences of distress in clinicians can affect individuals personally (e.g., depression, suicide, substance abuse) and professionally (e.g., medical errors, procrastination), patients (e.g., depersonalized care), and healthcare systems as a whole (e.g., morale, staff attrition).
- Risk factors occur within personal, interpersonal, professional, and institutional domains, and therefore interventions can be implemented at one or more of these levels.
- Interventions aimed at both the individual (personal and professional life) and the healthcare system (institutional level) are likely to be necessary if we are going to effectively address this problem overall.

13.12 Useful Resources

13.12.1 Books

The Burnout Prevention Matrix—by Dike Drummond M.D.
Now Discover Your Strengths—by Marcus Buckingham and Donald O. Clifton
Free course on mindfulness
www.palousemindfulness.com

13.12.2 Help for Physicians to Prevent Burnout

www.thehappymd.com
http://theheartofmedicine.org/
http://www.commonweal.org/
http://www.rishiprograms.org/programs/all-healthcare-professionals/
http://cppr.com/
http://www.johnhenrypfifferling.com/
http://www.valuesbasedleader.com/6-questions-to-ignite-engagement-and-prevent-burnout/

13.12.3 Physician Assistance Programs

http://www.menningerclinic.com/patient-care/inpatient-treatment/professionals-in-crisis-program
http://healthandwellness.vanderbilt.edu/work-life/faculty-physician-wellness/assistance-programs.php

References

Allen R, Judkins-Cohn T, de Velasco R et al (2013) Moral distress among healthcare professionals at a health system. JONAS Healthc Law Ethics Regul 15(3):111–118. quiz 119–120

Alpern F, Correnti CE, Dolan TE, Llufrio MC, Sill A (1992) A survey of recovering Maryland physicians. *Md Med J.* 41(4):301–303
Austin W, Kelecevic J, Goble E, Mekechuk J (2009) An overview of moral distress and the paediatric intensive care team. Nurs Ethics 16(1):57–68
Aycock N, Boyle D (2009) Interventions to manage compassion fatigue in oncology nursing. Clin J Oncol Nurs 13(2):183–191
Balboni TA, Balboni M, Enzinger AC et al (2013) Provision of spiritual support to patients with advanced cancer by religious communities and associations with medical care at the end of life. JAMA Intern Med. 173(12):1109–1117
Bath PDH (1992) Spiritual dimensions of nursing and patient care: Challenges and dilemmas for nursing education and clinical practice. Unpublished dissertation, Lancaster Theological Seminary, Lancaster, PA
Bauer-Wu S (2005) Seeds of hope, blossoms of meaning. Oncol Nurs Forum 32(5):927–933
Ben-Zur H, Michael K (2007) Burnout, social support, and coping at work among social workers, psychologists, and nurses: the role of challenge/control appraisals. Soc Work Health Care. 45(4):63–82
Bowden MJ, Mukherjee S, Williams LK, DeGraves S, Jackson M, McCarthy MC (2015) Work-related stress and reward: an Australian study of multidisciplinary pediatric oncology healthcare providers. Psychooncology 24(11):1432–1438
Browning DM (2010) Microethical and relational insights from pediatric palliative care. Virtual Mentor 12(7):540–547
Bruce CR, Miller SM, Zimmerman JL (2015) A qualitative study exploring moral distress in the ICU team: the importance of unit functionality and intrateam dynamics. Crit Care Med 43(4):823–831
Brumnquell D, Michaelson CM (2016) Moral hazard in pediatrics. Am J Bioeth 16(7):29–38
Burke LA, Neimeyer RA (2014) Spiritual distress in bereavement: evolution of a research program. Religions. 5(4):1087–1115
Bush NJ (2009) Compassion fatigue: are you at risk? Oncol Nurs Forum 36(1):24–27
Buxton D (2010) Pediatric palliative care: born of necessity. Virtual Mentor 12(7):519–521
Caldeira S, de Carvalho EC, Vieira M (2014) Between spiritual wellbeing and spiritual distress: possible related factors in elderly patients with cancer. Rev. Lat-Am Enferm. 22(1):28–34
Carter BS, Wocial LD (2012) Ethics and palliative care: which consultant and when? Am J Hosp Palliat Care 29(2):146–150
Clark JD, Dudzinski DM (2013) The culture of dysthanasia: attempting CPR in terminally ill children. Pediatrics 131(3):572–580
Cohen M, Gagin R (2005) Can skill-development training alleviate burnout in hospital social workers? Soc Work Health Care. 40(4):83–97
Collins W (2005) Embracing spirituality as an element of professional self-care. Soc Work Christianity 32(3):263–274
Dane B, Chachkes E (2001) The cost of caring for patients with an illness: contagion to the social worker. Soc Work Health Care. 33(2):31–51
Desbiens JF, Fillion L (2007) Coping strategies, emotional outcomes and spiritual quality of life in palliative care nurses. Int J Palliat Nurs. 13(6):291–300
Drummond D (2015) Physician burnout: its origin, symptoms, and five main causes. Fam Pract Manag. 22(5):42–47
Dudzinski DM (2016) Navigating moral distress using the moral distress map. J Med Ethics 42(5):321–324
Edmonds C, Lockwood GM, Bezjak A, Nyhof-Young J (2012) Alleviating emotional exhaustion in oncology nurses: an evaluation of Wellspring's "Care for the Professional Caregiver Program". J Cancer educ 27(1):27–36
Elpern EH, Covert B, Kleinpell R (2005) Moral distress of staff nurses in a medical intensive care unit. Am J Crit Care 14(6):523–530
Emanuel L, Ferris F, von Gunten C, Von Roenn J et al (2011) Combating compassion fatigue and burnout in cancer care. Medscape
Epstein EG, Hamric AB (2009) Moral distress, moral residue, and the crescendo effect. J Clin Ethics 20(4):330–342
Fanos JH (2007) "Coming through the fog, coming over the moors": the impact on pediatric oncologists of caring for seriously ill children. J Cancer Educ 22(2):119–123
Figley C (1995) Compassion fatigue: secondary traumatic stress disorders from treating the traumatized. New York, NY, Brunner-Routledge
Figley CR (2002) Compassion fatigue: psychotherapists' chronic lack of self care. J Clin Psychol. 58(11):1433–1441
Fourie C (2015) Moral distress and moral conflict in clinical ethics. Bioethics. 29(2):91–97
Frankl V (2014) Man's search for meaning. Beacon Press, Boston, MA
Friebert S (2010) Nondisclosure and emerging autonomy in a terminally ill teenager. Virtual Mentor 12(7):522–529
Garros D, Austin W, Carnevale FA (2015) Moral distress in pediatric intensive care. JAMA Pediatr 169(10):885–886
Gerow L, Conejo P, Alonzo A, Davis N, Rodgers S, Domian EW (2010) Creating a curtain of protection: nurses' experiences of grief following patient death. J Nurs Scholarsh 42(2):122–129
Gundersen L (2001) Physician burnout. Annals of Intern Med. 135(2):145–148
Gwyther LP, Altilio T, Blacker S et al (2005) Social work competencies in palliative and end-of-life care. J Soc Work End Life Palliat Care. 1(1):87–120
Halpern SD (2011) Perceived inappropriateness of care in the ICU: what to make of the clinician's perspective? JAMA 306(24):2725–2726
Hamric AB, Blackhall LJ (2007) Nurse-physician perspectives on the care of dying patients in intensive care units: collaboration, moral distress, and ethical climate. Crit Care Med 35(2):422–429

Hamric AB, Borchers CT, Epstein EG (2012) Development and testing of an instrument to measure moral distress in health care professionals. AJOB Prim Res 3(2):1–9
Hayes C, Ponte PR, Coakley A et al (2005) Retaining oncology nurses: strategies for today's nurse leaders. Oncol Nurs Forum 32(6):1087–1090
Hecktman HM (2012) Stress in Pediatric Oncology Nurses. J Pediatr Oncol Nurs 29(6):356–361
Henry BJ (2014) Nursing burnout interventions: what is being done? Clin J Oncol Nurs 18(2):211–214
Hinds PS, Quargnenti AG, Hickey SS, Mangum GH (1994) A comparison of the stress—response sequence in new and experienced pediatric oncology nurses. Cancer Nurs 17(1):61–71
Houston S, Casanova MA, Leveille M et al (2013) The intensity and frequency of moral distress among different healthcare disciplines. J Clin Ethics 24(2):98–112
Jameton A (1984) Nursing practice: the ethical issues. Prentice Hall, Inc., Englewood Cliffs, NJ
Johnson LM, Church CL, Metzger M, Baker JN (2015) Ethics consultation in pediatrics: long-term experience from a pediatric oncology center. Am J Bioeth 15(5):3–17
Joubert L, Hocking A, Hampson R (2013) Social work in oncology-managing vicarious trauma-the positive impact of professional supervision. Soc Work Health Care. 52(2–3):296–310
Kalvemark S, Hoglund AT, Hansson MG, Westerholm P, Arnetz B (2004) Living with conflicts-ethical dilemmas and moral distress in the health care system. Soc Sci Med 58(6):1075–1084
Kang J, Shin DW, Choi JY et al (2012) Addressing the religious and spiritual needs of dying patients by healthcare staff in Korea: patient perspectives in a multi-religious Asian country. Psycho-oncology. 21(4):374–381
Karanikola MN, Albarran JW, Drigo E et al (2014) Moral distress, autonomy and nurse-physician collaboration among intensive care unit nurses in Italy. J Nurs Manag. 22(4):472–484
Kaur D, Sambasivan M, Kumar N (2013) Effect of spiritual intelligence, emotional intelligence, psychological ownership and burnout on caring behaviour of nurses: a cross-sectional study. J Clin Nurs. 22(21–22):3192–3202
Keeler A (2010) Artificial hydration in pediatric end-of-life care. Virtual Mentor 12(7):558–563
Keene EA, Hutton N, Hall B, Rushton C (2010) Bereavement debriefing sessions: an intervention to support health care professionals in managing their grief after the death of a patient. Pediatr Nurs 36(4):185–189. quiz 190
Khamisa N, Peltzer K, Oldenburg B (2013) Burnout in relation to specific contributing factors and health outcomes among nurses: a systematic review. Int J Environ Res Public Health. 10(6):2214–2240
Kjeldmand D, Holmstroem I (2008) Balint groups as a means to increase job satisfaction and prevent burnout among general practitioners. Ann Fam Med. 6(2):138–145
Knight JR, Sanchez LT, Sherritt L, Bresnahan LR, Silveria JM, Fromson JA (2002) Monitoring physician drug problems: attitudes of participants. J Addict Dis. 21(4):27–36
Knight JR, Sanchez LT, Sherritt L, Bresnahan LR, Fromson JA (2007) Outcomes of a monitoring program for physicians with mental and behavioral health problems. J Psychiatr Pract. 13(1):25–32
Kushnick HL (2010) Trusting them with the truth-disclosure and the good death for children with terminal illness. Virtual Mentor 12(7):573–577
Lamiani G, Borghi L, Argentero P (2017) When healthcare professionals cannot do the right thing: a systematic review of moral distress and its correlates. J Health Psychol 22(1):51–67
Le Blanc PM, Hox JJ, Schaufeli WB, Taris TW, Peeters MC (2007) Take care! The evaluation of a team-based burnout intervention program for oncology care providers. J Appl Psychol 92(1):213–227
Lee KJ, Forbes ML, Lukasiewicz GJ et al (2015) Promoting staff resilience in the pediatric intensive care unit. Am J Crit Care 24(5):422–430
MacDonald DA, Friedman HL (2002) Assessment of humanistic, transpersonal, and spiritual constructs: state of the science. J Humanist Psychol. 42(4):102–125
Maslach C, Jackson SE (1981) Maslach Burnout Inventory. Consulting Psychologists Press, Palo Alto, CA
Maslach C, Leiter MP (2005) Reversing burnout: how to rekindle your passion for your work. Stanford Social Innovation Reveiw. Winter 2005. Leland Stanford Jr. University. Stanford, CA
Maslach C, Schaufeli WB, Leiter MP (2001) Job burnout. Annu Rev. Psychol. 52:397–422
McAndrew NS, Leske JS, Garcia A (2011) Influence of moral distress on the professional practice environment during prognostic conflict in critical care. J Trauma Nurs 18(4):221–230
Medland J, Howard-Ruben J, Whitaker E (2004) Fostering psychosocial wellness in oncology nurses: addressing burnout and social support in the workplace. Oncol Nurs Forum. 31(1):47–54
Mekechuk J (2006) Moral distress in the pediatric intensive care unit: the impact on pediatric nurses. Int J Health Care Qual Assur Inc Leadersh Health Serv 19(4–5):i–vi
Mobley MJ, Rady MY, Verheijde JL, Patel B, Larson JS (2007) The relationship between moral distress and perception of futile care in the critical care unit. Intensive Crit Care Nurs 23(5):256–263
Moody K, Kramer D, Santizo RO et al (2013) Helping the helpers: mindfulness training for burnout in pediatric oncology: a pilot program. J Pediatr Oncolo Nurs. 30(5):275–284
Morgan D (2009) Caring for dying children: assessing the needs of the pediatric palliative care nurse. Pediatr Nurs 35(2):86–90

Morse RM, Martin MA, Swenson WM, Niven RG (1984) Prognosis of physicians treated for alcoholism and drug dependence. JAMA. 251(6):743–746
Mougalian SS, Lessen DS, Levine RL et al (2013) Palliative care training and associations with burnout in oncology fellows. J Support Oncol. 11(2):95–102
Mukherjee S, Beresford B, Glaser A, Sloper P (2009) Burnout, psychiatric morbidity, and work-related sources of stress in paediatric oncology staff: a review of the literature. Psycho-oncology. 18(10):1019–1028
Mukherjee S, Beresford B, Tennant A (2014) Staff burnout in paediatric oncology: new tools to facilitate the development and evaluation of effective interventions. Eur J Cancer Care (Engl). 23(4):450–461
Musgrave CF, McFarlane EA (2003) Oncology and non-oncology nurses' spiritual well-being and attitudes toward spiritual care: a literature review. Oncol Nurs Forum. 30(3):523–527
Musto LC, Rodney PA, Vanderheide R (2015) Toward interventions to address moral distress: navigating structure and agency. Nursing Ethics 22(1):91–102
Myss C (1996) Anatomy of the spirit: the seven stages of power and healing. Three Rivers Press, New York, NY
Najjar N, Davis LW, Beck-Coon K, Carney DC (2009) Compassion fatigue: a review of the research to date and relevance to cancer-care providers. *J Health Psychol* 14(2):267–277
National Consensus Project (2013) Clinical practice guidelines for quality palliative care, 3rd edn. Pittsburgh, PA, National Consensus Project for Quality Palliative Care
Nedrow A, Steckler NA, Hardman J (2013) Physician resilience and burnout: can you make the switch? Fam Pract Manag. 20(1):25–30
Newell J, MacNeil G (2010) Professional burnout, vicarious trauma, secondary traumatic stress, and compassion fatigue. Best Pract Mental Health. 6(2):57–68
Nurses AAoCC (2008) Position statement on moral distress. Aliso Viejo, CA, AACN
Orlovsky C (2006) Compassion fatigue. Prairie Rose. 75(3):13
Papathanassoglou ED, Karanikola MN, Kalafati M, Giannakopoulou M, Lemonidou C, Albarran JW (2012) Professional autonomy, collaboration with physicians, and moral distress among European intensive care nurses. Am J Crit Care 21(2):e41–e52
Parker M, Gadbois S (2000) The fragmentation of community: part 1, the loss of belonging and commitment at work. J Nurs Adm 30(7–8):386–390
Parlakian R (2001) Look, listen, and learn: reflective supervision and relationship-based work. ZERO TO THREE: National Center for Infants, Toddlers and Families, Washington, DC
Pauly BM, Varcoe C, Storch J (2012) Framing the issues: moral distress in health care. HEC Forum 24(1):1–11
Pavlish C, Brown-Saltzman K, Jakel P, Fine A (2014) The nature of ethical conflicts and the meaning of moral community in oncology practice. Oncol Nurs Forum. 41(2):130–140
Pellebon DA, Anderson SC (1999) Understanding the life issues of spiritually-based clients. J Contemp Soc Serv 80(3):229–238
Pfifferling JH, Gilley K (1999) Putting 'life' back into your professional life. Fam Pract Manag. 6(6):36–42
Piers RD, Azoulay E, Ricou B et al (2011) Perceptions of appropriateness of care among European and Israeli intensive care unit nurses and physicians. JAMA. 306(24):2694–2703
Piles CL (1990) Providing spiritual care. Nurse Educ. 15(1):36–41
Poghosyan L, Aiken LH, Sloane DM (2009) Factor structure of the Maslach burnout inventory: an analysis of data from large scale cross-sectional surveys of nurses from eight countries. Int J Nurs Stud 46(7):894–902
Potter P, Deshields T, Divanbeigi J et al (2010) Compassion fatigue and burnout: prevalence among oncology nurses. Clin J Oncol Nur 14(5):E56–E62
Puchalski C, Ferrell B, Virani R et al (2009) Improving the quality of spiritual care as a dimension of palliative care: the report of the consensus conference. J Palliat Med 12(10):885–904
Puntillo KA, McAdam JL (2006) Communication between physicians and nurses as a target for improving end-of-life care in the intensive care unit: challenges and opportunities for moving forward. Critical Care Med 34(11 Suppl):S332–S340
Quill TE, Williamson PR (1990) Healthy approaches to physician stress. Arch Intern Med. 150(9):1857–1861
Ramondetta LM, Sun C, Surbone A et al (2013) Surprising results regarding MASCC members' beliefs about spiritual care. Support Care Cancer. 21(11):2991–2998
Repenshek M (2009) Moral distress: inability to act or discomfort with moral subjectivity? Nurs Ethics. 16(6):734–742
Ross L (1995) The spiritual dimension: its importance to patients' health, well-being and quality of life and its implications for nursing practice. Int J Nurs Stud 32(5):457–468
Rossi A, Cetrano G, Pertile R et al (2012) Burnout, compassion fatigue, and compassion satisfaction among staff in community-based mental health services. Psychiatry Res. 200(2–3):933–938
Roth M, Morrone K, Moody K et al (2011) Career burnout among pediatric oncologists. *Pediatr Blood Cancer* 57(7):1168–1173
Rourke MT (2007) Compassion fatigue in pediatric palliative care providers. Pediatr Clin North Am. 54(5):631–644
Ruotsalainen JH, Verbeek JH, Marine A, Serra C (2015) Preventing occupational stress in healthcare workers. Cochrane Database Syst Rev 4:CD002892
Rushton CH, Kurtz MJ (2015) Moral distress and you. Silver Spring, MD, American Nurses Association
Sabo BM (2006) Compassion fatigue and nursing work: can we accurately capture the consequences of caring work? Int J Nurs Pract. 12(3):136–142
Saunders JM, Valente SM (1994) Nurses' grief. Cancer Nurs 17(4):318–325

Shanafelt T, Dyrbye L (2012) Oncologist burnout: causes, consequences, and responses. J Clin Oncol 30(11):1235–1241
Shanafelt T, Chung H, White H, Lyckholm LJ (2006) Shaping your career to maximize personal satisfaction in the practice of oncology. J Clin Oncol 24(24):4020–4026
Shanafelt TD, Boone S, Tan L et al (2012) Burnout and satisfaction with work-life balance among US physicians relative to the general US population. Arch Intern Med. 172(18):1377–1385
Shanafelt TD, Gradishar WJ, Kosty M et al (2014) Burnout and career satisfaction among US oncologists. J Clin Oncol 32(7):678–686
Shanafelt TD, Hasan O, Dyrbye LN et al (2015a) Changes in burnout and satisfaction with work-life balance in physicians and the general US working population between 2011 and 2014. *Mayo Clin Proc.* 90(12):1600–1613
Shanafelt TD, Gorringe G, Menaker R et al (2015b) Impact of organizational leadership on physician burnout and satisfaction. Mayo Clin Proc. 90(4):432–440
Shepard A (2010) Moral distress: a consequence of caring. Clin J Oncol Nurs 14(1):25–27
Shore JH (1987) The Oregon experience with impaired physicians on probation. An eight-year follow-up. JAMA. 257(21):2931–2934
Simon CE, Pryce JG, Roff LL, Klemmack D (2005) Secondary traumatic stress and oncology social work: protecting compassion from fatigue and compromising the worker's worldview. J Psychosoc Oncol. 23(4):1–14
Slocum-Gori S, Hemsworth D, Chan WW, Carson A, Kazanjian A (2013) Understanding compassion satisfaction, compassion fatigue and burnout: a survey of the hospice palliative care workforce. Palliat Med 27(2):172–178
Spinetta JJ, Jankovic M, Ben Arush MW et al (2000) Guidelines for the recognition, prevention, and remediation of burnout in health care professionals participating in the care of children with cancer: report of the SIOP Working Committee on Psychosocial Issues in Pediatric Oncology. *Med Pediatr Oncol* 35(2):122–125
Tanyi RA (2002) Towards clarification of the meaning of spirituality. J Adv Nurs 39(5):500–509
Tanyi RA, McKenzie M, Chapek C (2009) How family practice physicians, nurse practitioners, and physician assistants incorporate spiritual care in practice. J Am Acad Nurse Pract. 21(12):690–697
Thompson A (2013) How Schwartz rounds can be used to combat compassion fatigue. Nurs Manag (Harrow). 20(4):16–20
Tillich P (2000) The courage to be, 2nd edn. Yale University Press, New Haven and London
Trotochaud K, Coleman JR, Krawiecki N, McCracken C (2015) Moral distress in pediatric healthcare providers. J Pediatr Nurs 30(6):908–914
Trufelli DC, Bensi CG, Garcia JB et al (2008) Burnout in cancer professionals: a systematic review and meta-analysis. Eur J Cancer Care (Engl). 17(6):524–531
Turnell A, Rasmussen V, Butow P et al (2016) An exploration of the prevalence and predictors of work-related well-being among psychosocial oncology professionals: an application of the job demands-resources model. Palliat Support Care. 14(1):33–41
Ulrich CM, Hamric AB, Grady C (2010) Moral distress: a growing problem in the health professions? Hastings Cent Rep 40(1):20–22
Van Berckelaer A (2011) Using Reflective Supervision to Support Trauma-Informed Systems for Children. A White Paper developed for the Multiplying Connections Initiative. Multiplying Connections, A Project of the Health Federation of Philadelphia. Philadelphia, PA
Varcoe C, Pauly B, Webster G, Storch J (2012) Moral distress: tensions as springboards for action. HEC Forum 24(1):51–62
Whitehead PB, Herbertson RK, Hamric AB, Epstein EG, Fisher JM (2015) Moral distress among healthcare professionals: report of an institution-wide survey. J Nurs Scholarsh 47(2):117–125
Wilson MA, Goettemoeller DM, Bevan NA, McCord JM (2013) Moral distress: levels, coping and preferred interventions in critical care and transitional care nurses. J Clin Nurs 22(9–10):1455–1466
Wocial LD (2008) An urgent call for ethics education. Am J Bioeth 8(4):21–23. author reply W21–22
Wocial LD (2016) Moral hazard analysis: illuminating the moral contribution of important stakeholders. Am J Bioeth 16(7):48–50
Wocial LD, Weaver MT (2013) Development and psychometric testing of a new tool for detecting moral distress: the moral distress thermometer. J Adv Nurs 69(1):167–174
Wocial LD, Hancock M, Bledsoe PD, Chamness AR, Helft PR (2010) An evaluation of unit-based ethics conversations. JONAS Healthc Law, Ethics Regul 12(2):48–54. quiz 55–46

14 Advancing Pediatric Palliative Oncology Through Innovation

Katharine Brock, Melissa Mark, Rachel Thienprayoon, and Christina Ullrich

14.1 Advancing Palliative Care Research in Pediatric Oncology

14.1.1 Need for an Evidence Base

Pediatric palliative care (PPC) is a recognized subspecialty, though the evidence base supporting this field is still in its early stage. Sound research is essential for continued progress in palliative care within pediatric oncology. Rigorous research addressing important questions is necessary to guide clinical care, promote its integration by increasing the relevance and credibility of the field, shape systems of care delivery, and drive and inform policy supporting its implementation. Acknowledging the needed knowledge, skills, and expertise to advance the field of PPC, the American Academy of Pediatrics (AAP) stated that continued development through research and education is essential for growth and improvement of PPC services (American Academy of Pediatrics 2000). Within the cancer care arena, the Institute of Medicine (IOM) report acknowledged the importance of research in its report on the role of the National Cancer Institute in palliative care. One of the IOM's ten recommendations was that every comprehensive cancer center be required to research palliative care and symptom control (Institute of Medicine 2001).

An evidence base for PPC in oncology must be further developed in the near future for several reasons. Until this occurs, care will be marked by theoretical equipoise (we are uncertain about efficacy of a treatment based on the evidence accumulated to date) or, worse, clinical equipoise (we truly have no knowledge of whether one treatment is better than another) (Casarett 2002). By replacing anecdotes, clinical experience, and local practice with evidence to guide the care we give children, we are more likely to provide current, safe, and effective care. Utilization of evidence-based interventions also adds to the legitimacy of both the field of PPC and PPC practitioners themselves. Mounting evidence will also spur further investigation, accelerating PPC research in this field. Finally, we must test interventions before

K. Brock, M.D., M.S.
Aflac Cancer & Blood Disorders Center, Pediatric Palliative Care, Children's Healthcare of Atlanta, Emory University, Atlanta, GA, USA
e-mail: katharinebrock@gmail.com

M. Mark, M.D. • R. Thienprayoon, M.D., M.S.C.S.
Cincinnati Children's Hospital Medical Center, 3333 Burnet Ave, ML-2001, Cincinnati, OH, USA
e-mail: Melissa.Mark@cchmc.org; Rachel.Thienprayoon@cchmc.org

C. Ullrich, M.D., M.P.H. (✉)
Harvard Medical School, Pediatric Hematology/Oncology and Palliative Care, Boston Children's Hospital/Dana Farber Cancer Institute, 450 Brookline Avenue, Boston, MA 02215, USA
e-mail: christina_ullrich@dfci.harvard.edu

J. Wolfe et al. (eds.), *Palliative Care in Pediatric Oncology*, Pediatric Oncology,
https://doi.org/10.1007/978-3-319-61391-8_14

clinical practice drifts too far from an evidence base and they are incorporated into practice, rendering study of them in the clinical setting impossible (Casarett 2002). Research is also necessary to understand access to PPC, unmet needs, and PPC delivery in various settings.

14.1.2 Key Research Questions and Priorities

In this nascent field, research efforts could be directed in numerous directions. With limited resources, it is important to identify priority areas that will address the most urgent questions and serve as groundwork for future research. In 2003, Institute of Medicine recommendations for PPC included the development of priorities for research (Institute of Medicine 2003; Downing et al. 2015).

In a Delphi study of Canadian PPC health professionals, participants identified four priority areas: (1) What matters most to patients and parents receiving PPC services? (2) What are the bereavement needs of families in PPC? (3) What are the best practice standards in pain and symptom management? (4) What are effective strategies to alleviate suffering at the end of life (Steele et al. 2008)? Baker and colleagues also conducted a Delphi study to prioritize the PPC research agenda though in addition to PPC experts, parents were also involved. Consensus identified 20 priorities, and these were grouped into five categories (decision-making, care coordination, symptom management, quality improvement, and education) (Baker et al. 2015). While rates of palliative oncology need are less than other palliative care needs (Alliance WPC, Organization WH 2014), the particular needs and research priorities warrant special consideration. For example, PPC experts and stakeholders identified the following priorities via consensus: (1) children's understanding of death and dying, (2) managing pain in children where there is no morphine, (3) funding, (4) training, and (5) assessment of the World Health Organization (WHO) two-step analgesic ladder for pain management in children (Downing et al. 2015).

Despite these efforts, there have not as of yet been systematic efforts to identify priorities for PPC research within the pediatric oncology population. For children with cancer at end of life, Hinds and colleagues delineated five key areas where research is needed. Somewhat similar to the priorities above, they include (1) the characteristic of cancer-related death and the profiles of survivorship in bereaved family members and healthcare providers, (2) the trajectory of dying in children and adolescents and a comparison of care delivery preferred by the family and that actually delivered, (3) end-of-life decision-making, (4) the financial costs of a child or adolescent dying a cancer-related death and associated policy making, and (5) outcomes of symptom-directed or bereavement interventions (Hinds et al. 2004).

While PPC includes end-of-life care, it extends well beyond it. To guide research in the provision of PPC for children with cancer throughout the care continuum (not limited to end of life), one might consider topics that have already been studied in adults with cancer, with findings that could be reasonably extrapolated to children, the focusing on remaining areas of focus. Due to a host of factors such as physiologic and developmental considerations (e.g., needs of neonates and adolescents are both very different from those of adults), differences in family structure and emphasis on disease-directed treatment late in the illness trajectory, and particular need for concurrent care, some research focused on the unique needs of children and their families is necessary.

Research on the palliative care needs of children with cancer should therefore focus on the unique characteristics and needs of the pediatric population (Ullrich and Morrison 2013). Pediatric-specific areas in need of further inquiry include non-pain symptoms experienced by children, child-reported outcomes, decision-making processes (e.g., surrogate or shared) involving children, sibling concerns, and cost-effectiveness of pediatric palliative care in either the hospital, community, or home setting (Ullrich and Morrison 2013).

14.1.3 State of the Science

The state of the science for the field of oncology (e.g., screening, diagnosis, up-front cancer-directed treatment) has reached a highly developed state. Oncology trials increasingly have endpoints beyond survival, and symptom or health-related quality of life (HRQL) endpoints are now prevalent (Buchanan et al. 2007). This has been stimulated by a growing awareness of the import and relevance of these outcomes. This increase in recognition of these outcomes is exemplified by the US Food and Drug Administration's adoption of patient-reported outcomes (PRO) to support drug approvals and label claims and creation of the Study Endpoints and Labeling Development (SEALD) group, which identified recommended methodology for rigorous PRO measure use and interpretation (McLeod et al. 2011).

Despite this progress, the evidence base for palliative and end-of-life care in oncology is less developed. According to one review of the palliative oncology literature, the most common topics were physical symptoms, health services research, and psychosocial issues (Hui et al. 2011). Less than 5% of the literature was comprised of communication, decision-making, spirituality, education, and research methodologies. While the proportion of original research studies has increased, though there have been no significant changes in study design or research topic, the majority of papers are case series/reports, as opposed to analytical studies (cohort studies and randomized controlled trials) (Hui et al. 2011).

Similar to the palliative oncology literature, the palliative care literature as a whole is predominated by observational studies, with few randomized or prospective evaluations of interventions (Kaasa et al. 2006; Wee et al. 2008; Knapp 2009). Many studies are retrospective in nature, are susceptible to recall bias and limited by the data available for analysis, and demonstrate associations as opposed to causality. Others are limited by sample size and heterogeneity between study populations. Interpretation of studies is also challenged by variation in study design and outcome reporting. The findings of a review of Cochrane reviews in palliative care summed up the literature with its determination that the Cochrane reviews cannot "provide good evidence for clinical practice because the primary studies are few in number, small, clinically heterogeneous, and of poor quality and external validity. They are useful in highlighting the weakness of the evidence base and problems in performing trials in palliative care" (Wee et al. 2008).

With regard to pediatric studies, the evidence base is even more limited. For example, <3% of studies published in palliative care journals from 2006 to 2010 were pediatric studies; among them, none were randomized controlled trials or systematic reviews (Kumar 2011).

14.1.4 Research Challenges and Innovative Opportunities

The pace of PPC research is challenged by a wide range of factors. Fortunately, most are not insuperable, and investigators can surmount them with creativity and ingenuity. In the end, these challenges do not exempt PPC research from widely held standards for research methodology. Like research in other fields, it must be of high quality to inform practice, policy, and future research and to ultimately advance the field.

14.1.4.1 Outcomes and Measurement

PPC research is challenged by a lack of consensus around definitions (e.g., "Who does the palliative care population include?" "How is the end-of-life period defined?"), as well as the outcomes that matter most. The ideal outcomes of interest must be balanced by reality, that is, what is actually measurable. For example, while self-report is often considered the gold standard with regard to PROs, developmental considerations, cognitive impairment, and illness can impair a child's ability to comprehend questions or respond for himself/herself. In such instances, investigators must rely on behavioral observation or proxy reports. A better understanding of how self- and proxy reports differ and the reliability and validity of proxy report is therefore a critical question. Innovative, technological methods with interfaces based on universal design principles to give children who are challenged to provide written or verbal responses an opportunity to convey their experience would expand opportunities for them to report their own experience. That being said, there will be instances, such as at the very end of life, in which self-report in real time is not possible, and outcomes must be obtained from proxies (in real time, or more likely, retrospectively).

There is a great need for standard metrics, utilizing measurement tools demonstrated to be valid and sensitive to change. The evidence supporting extant HRQL measures is poor, with many lacking reported psychometric properties (Coombes et al. 2016). The most widespread instrument is the PedsQL, which has been validated in numerous groups of children with specific PPC conditions. However, analysis of the psychometric properties of a cohort of children eligible for PPC (not disease specific) found that it was not a valid instrument in that population (Huang et al. 2010). The diversity of the PPC population, even when limited to the subgroup of children with cancer, makes it difficult to develop one single, encompassing measure. Ongoing work to adapt measures that exist or create ones de novo followed by validation work is needed. Application of adult instruments to pediatric populations without analysis of their performance will yield questionable results. In addition, though some widely used instruments such as the PedsQL have validated non-English versions (http://www.pedsql.org/translations.html), standard metrics that are in languages other than English and applicable to non-Western cultures are also needed.

A more promising approach would be to identify outcomes that are most meaningful and can most practicably be measured using a multidisciplinary approach involving a range of experts and stakeholders, including children and parents. In the end, an overall approach utilizing a combination of generic measures (which may not be relevant to all children) and disease-specific measures (relevant to only a specific subpopulation) will likely be most fruitful.

14.1.4.2 Study Population and Study Design

Recruitment and Data Collection: Of all research populations within PPC, the oncology population is one of the more homogeneous. This is in fact why many PPC studies have relied on this population. However, the population of children with advanced cancer is still relatively small and to some degree heterogeneous. These features can challenge the development of an appropriate comparison group. Investigators must also be aware that these characteristics can introduce variability in outcomes, thereby decreasing the precision of estimates (e.g., wide standard deviations and confidence intervals). With less apparent differences between groups, the power of a study is reduced, and a difference between groups may not be detected, even when one exists (i.e., type II error). Initial investment in efforts to obtain sample size calculations and effect estimates are therefore well worth the effort before embarking on a full-scale study. Such efforts are especially important in small sample sizes in order to make the best possible use of potential research participants.

Children with advanced cancer may bear a high burden of illness, and their families may face a high degree of stressors. The child's course may also be uncertain. These factors can both individually and collectively have a significant impact on study participation. It is advisable to minimize the burden of data collection whenever possible, using the simplest instruments and fewest in number as possible and avoiding repetitive questions (i.e., justify every question posed). These characteristics of this population can also lead to difficulty in recruiting, enrolling, and retaining participants, threatening the power of the study, and potentially introducing bias from a nonrepresentative sample. As above, investigators are well served by considering sampling strategies to avoid bias and taking into account attrition in planning sample size, study duration, and analytic methods. In PPC research it is particularly important to take into account sources of bias, including response bias, loss to follow-up, or missing data, particularly data not missing at random.

Given the challenges presented by research in this population, investigators must consider innovative strategies to overcome them. Effective strategies are rooted in a strong focus on the perspectives and needs of participants themselves, much as the practice of palliative care lends a focus on the lived experience of children and their families. With regard to data collection, web-based data collection systems can increase flexibility in terms of when, where, and how assessments are (Wolfe et al. 2015). Item response theory and computerized adaptive tests (CAT) are innovative methods of capturing HRQL in children that circumvent issues such as relevance and burden. For example, either CAT or short form surveys can be constructed using items in a large pediatric item bank developed by the Patient-Reported Outcomes Measurement Information System project (Irwin et al. 2009). Strategies to enhance recruitment and enrollment are presented in Box 14.1.

Multi-method Approaches: A key point is that whether it is to evaluate study design, feasibility, and recruitment time or to estimate sample size and usability of data collection methods or interventions, it is hard to overemphasize the involvement of patients and families. The value of qualitative approaches in generating rich data to drive hypotheses and inform theory is well known. Qualitative data from focus groups or one-on-one interviews to engage participant representatives and optimize study procedures are well worth the up-front investment. Participatory research may also reap rewards in terms of promoting engagement and participation and enhancing adherence to study procedures (Institute of Medicine (US) and National Research Council (US) National Cancer Policy Board et al. 2001). Qualitative preparatory work is particularly important before embarking on intervention studies, informing study conceptualization, providing information regarding feasibility, evaluating acceptability, and assessing the face validity of new interventions (Akard et al. 2013; Farquhar et al. 2011, 2013).

Observational Studies: These studies draw inferences about the effect of an exposure, which play an important role in describing unmet needs and provision of and gaps in care, including access and disparities. Rigorous observational studies should utilize the correct comparison groups, be of adequate size to make meaningful inferences, adjust for potential confounders, and mitigate bias whenever possible. Larger and more diverse sample sizes and utilization of multiple sites enhance reproducibility and generalizability. Observational study samples should be thoroughly described so that generalizability to other populations can be evaluated.

A limitation of observational studies is that receipt of an exposure is often not random and observed differences in outcomes between groups may depend on factors that influence whether or not they receive the exposure, instead of the exposure itself. Randomized controlled trials (RCTs) account for such factors via randomization, creating balanced groups and allowing estimation of treatment effects. However, randomization is not always possible in the advanced cancer population, as discussed below. In such instances, observational studies using sound design and innovative methods can shed light on causal relationships and estimates of effect. Such methods include instrumental variable methods and propensity score matching. Matching creates group that received the treatment and is comparable to a group on all observed covariates that did not receive the treatment. A limitation of propensity score matching is that utilization of <5000 observations can yield inconsistent estimates.

Intervention Studies: Randomized placebo-controlled trials (RCTs) are often considered the gold standard for evaluating interventions. For example, the FDA frequently requires new drug applications to include RTCs in the pediatric age group if the drug is indicated for this age group (Berde et al. 2012). They do so by balancing known and unknown factors, so that the intervention is the only known difference between groups. In general, they utilize both highly selected populations and specific outcomes and avoid contamination from other variables potentially impacting results. Because of these measures, RCTs assess efficacy of an intervention under ideal conditions, as opposed to effectiveness of an intervention implemented in real-world circumstances. To evaluate whether RCT findings are likely to apply to real-world settings (i.e., their generalizability), the study sample should be well characterized and the intervention well defined. An alternative framework is that of pragmatic trials in which oftentimes more than one variable is evaluated in real-world conditions (Grande and Todd 2000). In such studies it is particularly important to focus on structure, process, and outcomes together by (1) clearly defining the intervention, (2) describing study processes and adherence in detail, and (3) evaluating a variety of outcomes from a range of perspectives.

RCTs were developed to investigate pharmacologic treatments and are not practicable or suitable for every intervention research question or clinical context. Non-pharmacologic interventions, such as palliative care interventions, which tend to be complex services or care models, are not always conducive to RCTs. In sum, RCTs are often limited in their ability to take into account the complex nature of clinical care and, moreover, serious illness (Aoun and Kristjanson 2005). Other RCT characteristics that warrant special consideration with regard to palliative care populations or interventions are presented in Table 14.1.

To surmount some of the challenges presented by RCT investigators have devised variations in RCT methodology that remain rooted in random allocation. Crossover studies make efficient use of participants by allowing participants to cross over between the intervention and control groups and are useful when a given condition is stable and intervention effects are rapidly "on" and "off." N-of-1 trials are crossover studies that evaluate an intervention for an individual, using each individual as a test participant as well as their own control. They similarly make use of participants in an efficient manner. In many ways, they are ideal for palliative care populations where heterogeneity is common and interventions are tailored to individuals. Furthermore, they can directly benefit participants by providing them with a clinically definite answer in real time (Guyatt et al. 1990).

Another variation on the RCT theme is the fast-track trial, an adaptation of the "wait list design." It is useful when there is incomplete equipoise about the intervention, though it does require participants to have longer prognoses. Because all participants are offered the intervention, this design may be more acceptable to patients, clinicians, and institutional review boards (IRBs) alike (Higginson and Booth 2011). Open-label extension trials also provide participants with an opportunity to receive the treatment; however, analyses should be limited to assessments of adverse effects, rather than efficacy, due to threats to internal validity such as inability to control for placebo effects (Berde et al. 2012). In adaptive randomization, the probability of assignment to an arm during the study changes and is similarly useful when equipoise is in question.

14.1.4.3 Beyond Investigation: Advancing Research as a Whole

Beyond innovation and rigor in the conduct of studies, there are other facets of scientific inquiry that warrant attention if we are to actually advance the field of palliative care in oncology. A foremost need is that of research capacity. There are few investigators with expertise in this population. In recent years, fellowships in palliative care research have been developed to train investigators who are well versed in common challenges and strategies to surmount them. Established investigators must also have adequate protected time and funding. A 2009 survey of US palliative care research demonstrated that only 20% of investigators who published extramurally funded studies were supported by federal funds (Gelfman and Morrison 2008). Those within palliative care and oncology must advocate not only for clinical services and clinical training but also support for resources to support research. Importantly, the research community must be an active participant in this cause, including advocating for research training opportunities, funding and palliative care study sections across federal funders, and serving on study sections to provide expert review of palliative care research.

Table 14.1 Pediatric Palliative Care Considerations for Randomized Controlled Trials

Study population	Considerations
Adequacy of sample size	• Inadequate sample sizes can prevent random allocation necessary for equal distribution of confounders (Grande and Todd (2000))
	• Small sample sizes create risk for inadequate statistical power, limiting detection of differences between groups (type II error)
Homogeneity of sample	• Difficult to achieve in populations of children with advanced illness, especially those with rapidly changing clinical situations
Well-defined population	• Terms such as "palliative chemotherapy" and "end of life" are frequently not clearly nor universally defined
Design	
Goal: test efficacy under prescribed conditions	• Real-world effectiveness not proven
Highly controlled (i.e., selected or "clean") populations	• Avoids those with characteristics that could interfere with detecting an intervention effect
Utilizes measurable, specified outcomes	• Important outcomes may be difficult to define and/or measure
	• What can be measured is not necessarily what matters most
Clinical equipoise	• New services at risk for being perceived as being more desirable
	• Equipoise not possible if intervention has already been accepted and adopted into practice
	• Can make the RCT the only way to gain access to the intervention
	• Alternatively, can randomize more individuals to the intervention arm (Grande and Todd 2000)
Randomization	• May not be ethical with withhold treatment from one group
Intervention	
Standardized, defined intervention	• Goal is usually uniform intervention across participants
	• By definition palliative care interventions are holistic and tailored to individuals (Aoun and Kristjanson 2005)
Use of placebo	• Provides comparison so efficacy of intervention can be derived
	• If use of a placebo could lead to uncontrolled symptoms such as pain or nausea, consider use of immediate rescue design, with drug sparing rather than symptom scores as the primary outcome (Berde et al. 2012)
Blinding to intervention	• Without blinding as to treatment group assignment, expectations can bias the results (Grande and Todd 2000)
	• Especially important when outcomes are subjective, as they often are in palliative care setting and with patient-reported outcomes
	• When two treatments being compared are very different (e.g., oral versus intravenous formulations), double dummy technique is useful
	• Not always feasible for service or care model interventions
	• Not necessary for pragmatic trials

Fortunately, innovative programs such as the National Palliative Care Research Center, founded by palliative care investigators and supported by private and federal funding, have responded to this need.

Well-trained and resourced investigators will be most productive with local and national structures to support collaborative and complementary research. Infrastructure including research networks, such as the Palliative Care Research Network and the Pediatric Palliative Care Research Network, promote investigator career development and foster multisite collaborations that have already shown great success. PPC research within oncology will also require well-coordinated efforts between PC and oncology worlds. These two disciplines must combine forces to heighten awareness of the need for funding and the benefit of sound research in providing quality care for children with cancer. In general, a collaborative approach, in which innovative approaches, methodologies, materials, and expertise are shared, will further accelerate research progress.

PPC researchers are especially challenged by the lack of large datasets. For example, adult palliative care investigators have large databases [e.g., Medicare, Surveillance, Epidemiology, and End Results (SEER)] for evaluating patterns and costs of care at end-of-life care. For children, there is little information on costs; those data that exist are largely limited to in-hospital care or location of death (Knapp and Madden 2010). In the absence of a national healthcare system and variation between states in Concurrent Care for Children provisions, cost analyses can only be performed on subpopulations. Because there is limited ability to conduct multistate or multi-plan analyses, the data that do exist in Medicare or Medicaid or single health plans are largely inaccessible (Knapp and Madden 2010). Research on costs of care can produce findings highly relevant to policy makers and healthcare administrators. PPC investigators must engage with these stakeholders to make needed data accessible.

14.1.4.4 Using Research to Advance the Field of PPC in Oncology

Dissemination: Acting on research is also challenged by how hard it is to keep up with the literature (Hui et al. 2011) because relevant papers are published in a wide range of journals, covering heterogeneous research topics (Tieman et al. 2009). Furthermore, the interdisciplinary and interprofessional nature of palliative care means that pertinent journal articles span a host of disciplines and are published by investigators representing many professions. In fact, palliative care nursing and social work journals have the highest percentage of pediatric publications, as compared to more general palliative care journals (Kumar 2011). Bibliographic and database searches are further complicated by the inclusion of papers on "palliative chemotherapy" or "palliative radiotherapy." Biomedical libraries can assist with more advanced searches to exclude these papers.

While many PC publications focus on cancer, the proportion of oncology studies that focus on PC is very small (<1%). Oncologists mainly read oncology journals and may therefore encounter little PC content. In addition to partnerships with librarians, services that scan the medical literature for relevant publications can address this gap. For example, PC-FACS (Fast Article Critical Summaries for Clinicians in Palliative Care) is an electronic publication that summarizes impactful publications in non-palliative care journals and provides a corresponding commentary.

14.1.5 Ethical Considerations

IRBs/Research Ethics Committees (RECs) are charged with protecting "vulnerable" populations. In general, children are regarded as vulnerable in that they may not be able to fully represent their own views and interests. Children with advanced cancer (intrinsic vulnerability), including those at end of life, and bereaved parents are historically regarded as particularly vulnerable due to personal factors or external circumstances (extrinsic vulnerability). Their vulnerability may also be relational, stemming from interactions or relationships with the care team or investigator. However, many children in fact can understand the purpose of research and what participation entails (Hinds et al. 2005).

Anecdotal evidence suggests that in their effort to protect perceived vulnerable subjects, IRBs/RECs either disapprove research in these populations, mandate modifications to study design (e.g., require opt-in as opposed to opt-out approaches, prohibiting recruitment of newly bereaved parents), or entail lengthy review procedures before approval. In addition, excluding certain participants or delaying their involvement may introduce bias.

Bereaved parents have also historically been viewed as a vulnerable group. However, the fact that recruitment rates are often well under 100% suggests that parents do have the ability to consider participation and decline if so desired. In many respects, offering parents the opportunity to participate respects their autonomy, affording them (with sensitivity) the ability to determine for themselves whether they will participate.

In such instances investigators are well served to approach IRBs/RECs as collaborators who, like them, have the well-being of the child/family as their primary goal. IRB/REC reviewers will appreciate the provision of data describing how similar research participants have largely found the experience to be both valuable and meaningful and that little harm has been documented (Table 14.2). It should, however, be noted that those who did not participate to begin with might have viewed participation less favorably. IT is

Table 14.2 Participation in research

Reference	Study design	Findings
Scott et al. (2002)	Eighty-one of 97 families who had previously completed an in-depth interview as part of a national case-control study of Ewing's sarcoma	98% believed their involvement would benefit others and were glad to have participated
		92% would recommend to others in their position that they participate in similar studies
		7% felt interview was more painful than expected
		64% felt a benefit was they could talk about their child's illness
		Parents who had completed the interview <1 year before recalled it as being more painful than those who had completed it >1 year before
Dyregrov (2004)	Study in Norway of parents whose child died due to an accident, suicide, or SIDS	100% of parents experienced participation as "positive"/"very positive"
	Subsample completed short questionnaire evaluating participation in a study involving in-depth interviews	None regretted participating
		They linked positive experiences to being allowed to tell their complete story, the interview format, and a hope that they might help others
		Three-quarters of the interviewees reported that it was to some degree painful to talk about the traumatic loss
Kreicbergs et al. (2004)	Pilot study to assess harm and benefit of a questionnaire to Swedish parents whose child died of cancer	95% of parents found the pilot study valuable
	Pilot followed by a main study consisting of a nationwide survey about the child's care and death and the parents' perceptions of the study	423 (99%) parents found the investigation valuable
		285 (68%) were positively affected
		123 (28%) were negatively affected [10 (2%) of whom, very much]
Hynson et al. (2006)	In-depth interviews with bereaved parents of children who had died from a range of conditions	Participating in research was viewed positively
		Parents reported their experience was enhanced by the sensitivity of the initial approach to them
		Although the majority of parents primarily chose to participate for altruistic reasons, many described the research process as personally beneficial
		Careful attention to timing, approach, and the interviewer's skills were underpinnings of a positive experience
Mongeau et al. (2007)	Report of two participatory research studies of a respite program; both studies involved parents throughout all phases of the study, including data collection and analysis	Investigators report that participation of healthcare professionals, volunteers, and parents benefitted all through their active engagement. Participatory approach allowed them to voice concerns and supported a sense of empowerment
		Of note, the participatory process enhanced the impact of the research, its social relevancy, and rigor of the research

(continued)

Table 14.2 (continued)

Reference	Study design	Findings
Eilegard et al. (2013)	Swedish nationwide study on avoidable and modifiable healthcare-related factors in pediatric oncology among bereaved siblings who lost a brother or sister to cancer	174 of 240 (73%) responded
		None thought their participation would affect them negatively long term
		13% (21/168) stated it was a negative experience to fill out the questionnaire
		84% (142/169) found it to be a positive experience
Baker et al. (2013)	Prospective multicenter study to collect tumor tissue by autopsy of children with diffuse intrinsic pontine glioma. Parents completed questionnaire after child's death to describe the purpose for, hopes for, and regrets about their participation in autopsy-related research	Parents reported no regrets and cited benefits
		All parents felt that study participation was the right decision
		None regretted it
		91% agreed that they would make the choice again
Steele et al. (2014)	Survey of caregivers of children with a life-threatening illness regarding their experience in one of two observational studies	None regretting having participated
		75% found participation not at all painful
		50% reported it had at least some positive effect
Starks et al. (2016)	PPC intervention to reduce family stress symptoms while in the ICU through early palliative care Questionnaire burden assessed on a 1–10 scale Open-ended comments were analyzed to describe the participants' experience in the study	Questionnaire burden was low: mean (SD) scores were 1.1 (1.6), 0.7 (1.5), and 0.9 (1.6) for the baseline, discharge, and follow-up questionnaires
		Participation beneficial by (1) promoting reflection and self-awareness about stress, coping, and resilience and (2) feeling cared for because the intervention and questionnaires focused on their own well-being

worth noting pointing out that intervention studies can also *directly* benefit participants (Hays et al. 2006; Wolfe et al. 2014; Breen 2006).

14.2 Quality Improvement in Palliative Care

In 2001, a meeting of the National Consensus Project (NCP) founded the initial efforts toward defining quality in the field of palliative care (http://www.nationalconsensusproject.org). This collaborative of six major hospice and palliative care organizations included the AAHPM (American Academy of Hospice and Palliative Medicine), CAPC (Center to Advance Palliative Care), HPNA (Hospice and Palliative Nurses Association), NHPCO (National Hospice and Palliative Care Organization), NASW (National Association of Social Workers), and NPCRC. The meeting resulted in the Clinical Guidelines for Quality Palliative Care, which described the core concepts and structures for quality palliative care and defined eight domains of practice. The third edition of these guidelines was released in 2013 and explicitly includes neonates, children, and adolescents (Table 14.3) (http://www.nationalconsensusproject.org).

The eight domains of care identified by the NCP were utilized by the Measuring What Matters (MWM) campaign (Dy et al. 2015), a consensus project of the AAHPM and HPNA, which aimed to recommend a concise portfolio of valid, clinically relevant, crosscutting indicators for internal measurement of hospice and palliative care. The MWM campaign identified ten indicators or specific tools that quantitatively assess specific healthcare structures, processes, or outcomes that mapped to five of the domains of care identified in the NCP guidelines. These indicators were published in 2015 (Dy et al. 2015). NCP domains and MWM indicators mapping to each domain, with suggested

Table 14.3 National Consensus Project domains of care for palliative care

1. Structure and processes of care	Guidelines within this domain detail the meaning of interdisciplinary teams and family-centered care. All families should have access to palliative care expertise and staff 24 h a day, 7 days a week, and respite services should be available
2. Physical aspects of care	The interdisciplinary team should assess and manage pain and other symptoms based on best available evidence within the context of disease status. This includes the use of validated measurement tools appropriate for the age of the child. Treatment of distressing symptoms and side effects should include a broad spectrum of pharmacologic, behavioral, and complementary or integrative therapies including referral to appropriate specialists as needed
3. Psychological and psychiatric aspects of care	Care should include regular, ongoing assessment of psychological reactions related to illness including stress, coping strategies, and anticipatory grieving as well as evaluation for psychiatric conditions, especially anxiety and depression. Grief and bereavement support should be provided to all families
4. Social aspects of care	The interdisciplinary team should perform a comprehensive social assessment to identify the social strengths, needs, and goals of each patient and family
5. Spiritual, religious, and existential aspects of care	Communication with the patient and family should be respectful of religious and spiritual beliefs, rituals, and practices. All members of the care team should recognize spiritual distress when present and attend to this distress within their scope of practice. All patients should have access to spiritual care professionals
6. Cultural aspects of care	Each patient receives care in a culturally and linguistically appropriate manner. Professional interpreter services should be utilized, and written materials should be available in the patient/family's preferred language
7. Care of the patient at the end of life	Care of any patient at the end of life is time and detail intensive. This is especially true for pediatric patients. The interdisciplinary team should assess the patient for symptoms and proactively prepare the family on the recognition and management of potential symptoms and concerns. Care planning at this stage may include a hospice referral if this option is congruent with the patient and family's goals of care
8. Ethical and legal aspects of care	The interdisciplinary team should educate the patient and family about advanced care planning documents to promote clear communication of care preferences across the continuum of care. These documents may include designation of a healthcare proxy, inpatient and/or outpatient orders for limited resuscitation, and advanced directives. Knowledge of state-specific documentation as well as guidelines for the use of such documents by minors is imperative. Ethical clinical issues should be documented and appropriate ethics consultation utilized to assist in conflict resolution as well as policy development. All care should be provided in accordance with professional, state, and federal laws, regulations, and current accepted standards of care

measurement sources, are summarized in Table 14.4.

The Palliative Care Quality Network (PCQN), founded in 2009, is one example of a quality improvement network in palliative care. The PCQN is a continuous learning collaborative committed to improving the quality of palliative care services provided to patients and their families (https://www.pcqn.org/about/). PCQN and its members use shared data collection and analytic strategies to drive quality improvement initiatives, identify and disseminate best practices, and foster a professional community that contributes to the growth and future direction of palliative care (https://www.pcqn.org/about/). Generally speaking, PCQN and similar initiatives are focused on palliative care in the adult world, as thus far, the domains and indicators identified by NCP and MWM have not been evaluated specifically in pediatric palliative and hospice care. But there is a high level of interest in quality improvement in the pediatric palliative care community, and research aiming to validate these domains of care for children pediatrics is ongoing. In 2016, the Pediatric Palliative Improvement Network (PPIN) was created with six initial member institutions, with the global aim of decreasing suffering in children with serious illness and in their families. Efforts are underway, through PPIN, to utilize infrastructure offered by the AAP to allow shared data collec-

Table 14.4 Measuring What Matters quality indicators mapping to NCP domains, with validated sources for measurement

National consensus project domain	Measuring What Matters indicator	Source
1. Structure and processes of care	Comprehensive assessment Hospice: % of patients enrolled for more than 7 days for whom a comprehensive assessment was completed within 5 days of admission (documentation of prognosis, functional assessment, screening for physical and psychological symptoms, and assessment of social and spiritual concerns) Seriously ill patients receiving specialty palliative care in an acute hospital setting: % of patients admitted for more than 1 day who had a comprehensive assessment (screening for physical symptoms and discussion of patient/family's emotional or psychological needs) completed within 24 h of admission	PEACE Set Schenck et al. (2010, 2014), Hanson et al. (2010)
2. Physical aspects of care	Screening for physical symptoms % of seriously ill patients receiving specialty PC in an acute hospital setting for more than 1 day or patients enrolled in hospice for more than 7 days who had a screening for physical symptoms (pain, dyspnea, nausea, constipation) during admission visit	PEACE Set Schenck et al. (2010, 2014), Hanson et al. (2010)
	Pain treatment % of seriously ill patients receiving specialty PC in an acute hospital setting for more than 1 day or patients enrolled in hospice for more than 7 days who screened positive for moderate to severe pain on admission, % with medication or non-medication treatment within 24 h of screening	PEACE Set Schenck et al. (2010, 2014), Hanson et al. (2010)
	Dyspnea screening and management % of patients with advanced chronic or serious life-threatening illnesses who are screened for dyspnea. For those who are diagnosed with moderate or severe dyspnea, % with a documented plan of care to manage dyspnea	AMA-PCPI/NCQA American Medical Association (2008)
3. Psychological and psychiatric aspects of care	Discussion of emotional or psychological needs % of seriously ill patients receiving specialty PC in an acute hospital setting for more than 1 day or patients enrolled in hospice for more than 7 days with chart documentation of a discussion of emotional or psychological needs	PEACE Set Schenck et al. (2010, 2014), Hanson et al. (2010)
4. Social aspects of care	No indicators	
5. Spiritual, religious, and existential aspects of care	Discussion of spiritual/religious concerns % of hospice patients with documentation of a discussion of spiritual/religious concerns or documentation that patient/caregiver/family did not want to discuss	Deyta, LLC/NQF#1647
6. Cultural aspects of care	No indicators	
7. Care of the patient at the end of life	No indicators	

Table 14.4 (continued)

National consensus project domain	Measuring What Matters indicator	Source
8. Ethical and legal aspects of care	Documentation of surrogate % of seriously ill patients receiving specialty PC in an acute hospital setting for more than 1 day or patients enrolled in hospice for more than 7 days with name and contact information for surrogate decision-maker in the chart or documentation that there is no surrogate	PEACE Set Schenck et al. (2010, 2014), Hanson et al. (2010)
	Treatment preferences % of seriously ill patients receiving specialty PC in an acute hospital setting for more than 1 day or patients enrolled in hospice for more than 7 days with chart documentation of preferences for life-sustaining treatments	PEACE Set Schenck et al. (2010, 2014), Hanson et al. (2010)/NQF#1641
	Care consistency with documented care preferences If a vulnerable elder has specific treatment preferences documented in a medical record, then these treatment preferences should be followed	ACOVE PC and EOL Care Lorenz et al. (2007), Walling et al. (2010)
Global measure	No specific measure endorsed, but committee, panels, membership, and stakeholders agreed that patient and/or family assessments of quality are a key part of measuring quality for any setting caring for palliative or hospice care patients	

tion and quality improvement initiatives from organizations across our field. As the field matures, we anticipate that both systems-level processes and patient- and family-level outcomes will be defined, benchmarked, and measured across pediatric palliative care programs.

14.2.1 Collaboration, Communication, and Connection Through Technology

14.2.1.1 Telehealth and Pediatric Palliative Care

Many children who are eligible for palliative care and live in rural locations have to travel a great distance to reach their subspecialty providers in larger pediatric hospitals. For families of children with complex and chronic conditions, especially those who rely on technology to support their lives, travel of any kind can be uniquely challenging. These challenges become even more amplified, and the importance of being at home more dear, as a child's end of life approaches. Thus, geographical dislocation between the palliative care teams and patients they care for can present a major challenge (Bensink et al. 2009).

Telemedicine has been defined as "the use of medical information exchanged from one site to another via electronic communications to improve a patient's health status" (http://www.americantelemed.org/about-telemedicine/what-is-telemedicine#.V8B6FWV7WA8). Telehealth has historically had a broader definition, encompassing telemedicine's clinical care for patients and tele-education, tele-research, and disaster response (Burke and Hall 2015). For the purposes of this chapter, "telehealth" can be defined as the internet-based use of real-time audiovisual communication between patients and healthcare providers. Telehealth offers the opportunity for patients to remain in the comfort of their homes and still communicate effectively with their doctors and other providers at a distance. Telepractice does not replace the face-to-face visit, but rather adds to it (Burke and Hall 2015). Studies have found that the important components of a pediatric palliative medicine consultation can be completed using telehealth (Bradford et al. 2014a), that telehealth is an economical means of accomplishing PPC (Bradford et al. 2014b), and that using telehealth in this manner increases the equity of access to care (Bradford et al. 2010).

A successful telehealth encounter requires some infrastructure. The technical needs of a telehealth program depend on the type of telemedicine an organization intends to practice; synchronous or live telemedicine involves a real-time interaction between the participants at two or more sites (Burke and Hall 2015). For PPC these sites typically include the child in his or her home and the provider in his or her office or hospital. Families must have internet access and a web camera in their homes; in some cases, home care or hospice nurses may utilize laptop computers or tablets which are brought into the home for this purpose. Figure 14.1 shows a pediatric palliative care physician communicating with a patient in his home in Cincinnati, OH. Providers need access to a secure, encrypted, videoconferencing system to connect to the patient and family, and as the quality of the encounter depends on the quality of the connection, the organization or hospital should provide adequate bandwidth to support the provider's needs (Burke and Hall 2015). See Fig. 14.2 for an example of a telehealth cart, which includes a web camera, monitors, and keyboard for documentation, for use in an ambulatory clinic at Cincinnati Children's Hospital Medical Center.

Documentation of a telehealth encounter should follow the standards of documentation for a typical outpatient encounter. Physical examination findings may be supplemented by a home care nurse examining the child in real time or through technologies which allow physicians to monitor vital signs, examine a child's ears, etc. While billing and reimbursement for telehealth encounters has been cited as a historical barrier to use and sustainability, it is possible to receive

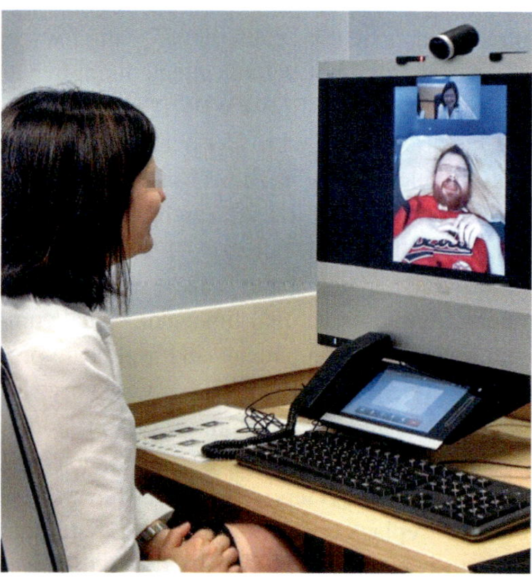

Fig. 14.1 A telehealth encounter between a pediatric palliative care physician and patient in his home in Cincinnati, OH. Photo courtesy of the Telehealth Center at Cincinnati Children's Hospital Medical Center

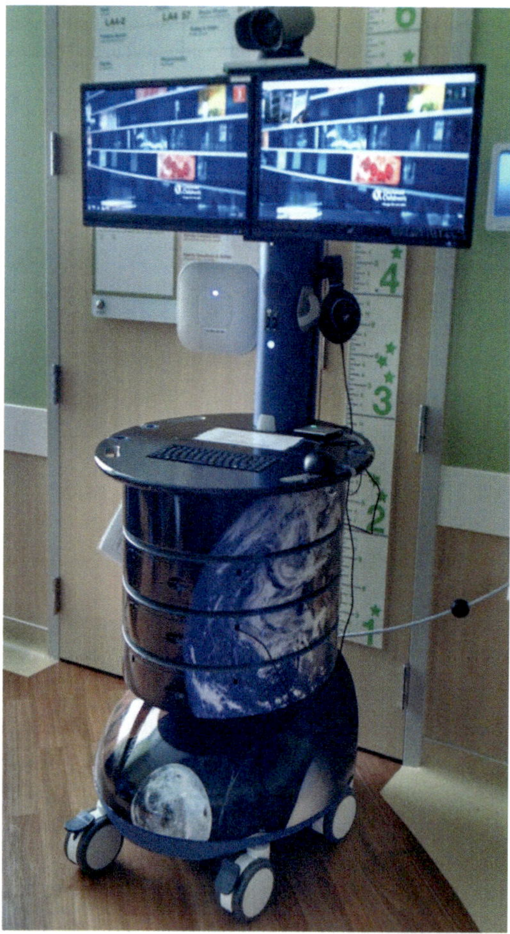

Fig. 14.2 A telehealth cart, which includes a web camera, monitors, and keyboard for documentation, for use in an ambulatory clinic. Photo courtesy of the Telehealth Center at Cincinnati Children's Hospital Medical Center

reimbursement for telehealth encounters, and coding for telemedical care is remarkably straightforward (Burke and Hall 2015). For more information regarding coding and billing for telemedicine encounters, references include:

The American Telemedicine Association website (www.americantelemed.org)

The July 2014 report "State Telehealth Laws and Reimbursement Policies: A Comprehensive Scan of the 50 States and the District of Columbia" (http://cchpca.org/sites/default/files/resources/State%20Laws%20and%20Reimbursement%20Policies%20Report%20Feb%20%202015.pdf)

14.2.1.2 Health Information Technology

Good communication is at the heart of high-quality palliative care, and communication between patients, providers, and other families can be augmented using health information technologies. Many health information technology platforms are available for use by children and families eligible for palliative care (Madhavan et al. 2011). The electronic health record (EHR) and the patient portal of the EHR are specific technologies intended to support the exchange of clinical information. The EHR is generally used by and between providers, while patient portals offer the patient and family the ability to remotely access subsets of data, such as lab results or radiology scan results, to request appointments, and to directly contact a physician or other providers (Madhavan et al. 2011). The EHR can be used in myriad ways to make clear a patient or family's goals, through specific code status orders on the inpatient and ambulatory side, documentation of advance directive conversations, and uploading of advance directive or Medical (physician) Orders for Life-Sustaining Treatment (MOLST/POLST) documents. Ideally in the future, the patient portal will also allow families and patients' access to resources to communicate their goals of care to the teams caring for them and will be able to interact with smartphone technology to accomplish the same goal.

Technologies designed to offer social support include information sharing portals, online peer-to-peer support groups, social media, and email list serves. Information sharing portals such as CaringBridge (www.caringbridge.org) are available for patients and families to share their stories and allow them to share news with many by only entering information once (Madhavan et al. 2011). Online peer-to-peer support groups or networks, available through websites such as Facebook, provide a medium for families to engage with others experiencing similar illnesses, to seek support from one another, and to share their stories (Madhavan et al. 2011). These networks allow families experiencing rare illnesses to contact one another directly and effectively, which would have been virtually impossible only a few years ago. One peer-to-peer support site specific to PPC is the Courageous Parents Network (https://courageousparentsnetwork.org) which was created by parents to support other parents through all stages of a child's illness. The palliative care community—providers and patients alike—has been at the forefront in using social media in the form of Twitter, Instagram, and other applications to connect with one another, to lobby for legislation which will impact palliative care, and to generally grow the field. "Hashtags" such as #hpm, #palliativecare, #hospice, or #EOL are used to continue an ongoing conversation about palliative care; #pedpc is specific to pediatric palliative care. Finally, for palliative care providers seeking more direct support from one another, one commonly used technology is email list serves, which allow a provider to contact a large group through a single email. The AAP Section of Hospice and Palliative Medicine list serve is available to anyone who joins the section. Providers may use the list serve to seek clinical support in treating symptoms, psychosocial support in thinking through difficult cases, or support for patients who are transferring to other areas of the country.

14.2.2 Thinking Outside the Box

Location of Care at the Time of Death: When families have the ability to plan a child's location of death, children are more likely to die at home, and parents report feeling more prepared for the circumstances surrounding the child's death

(Dussel et al. 2009). Death at home has been signaled as an indicator of good quality end-of-life care (Dussel et al. 2009), but historically for children in the intensive care unit, death at home has not been an option. Recently the advent of pediatric palliative transport (PPT), the medical transport to home or an inpatient hospice with the support of a critical care transport team, has allowed for a critically ill child's death outside of the hospital (Nelson et al. 2015). With PPT, the child is transported home on all life-sustaining treatments offered in the critical care unit, with the expectation of discontinuing those treatments at home and the likelihood that death will occur soon after. Interviews of parents whose children died following PPT found that for these families, the hospital was an undesirable location of death; parents were commonly motivated by the idea that a return home held potential to be a more proper way for their child to die (Nelson et al. 2015). For parents of newborns, being home created a "sense of normalcy," and parents had the opportunity to hold their babies without tubes and to use things that were waiting at home for the baby (Nelson et al. 2015). PPT does require a critical care transport team, which may not be available in smaller centers or may be required elsewhere when a family desires to return home. Yet parents' recollections of their experiences with PPT indicate that transport and death at home enhanced the quality of life for the family and the child; parents were given some control at a moment when they felt most vulnerable (Nelson et al. 2015).

Integrative Innovations in Pediatric Palliative Care: Integrative therapies such as music therapy, art therapy, pet therapy, and child life therapy are critical components to caring for "the whole child" and are ripe for innovation. One novel approach in music therapy in pediatric palliative and hospice medicine is the use of "heartbeat therapy," pioneered by Brian Schreck, MA, MT-BC, a music therapist at Cincinnati Children's Hospital Medical Center (Fig. 14.3). In heartbeat therapy, a microphone is woven into a stethoscope, or a digital stethoscope capable of recording the heartbeat is used. The child's heartbeat is recorded, sometimes at the end of life, and it provides a rhythm to a piece of music chosen by the family. The music is played over the sound of the heartbeat and the recording is given to the family. Music can be added to the initial track as the family grieves, and the composition becomes illustrative of their journey over time, each as unique as the child and family for whom it was created. Some families opt to add the sound of the heartbeat to a stuffed animal or toy for siblings, or for children of a decedent parent. Other families may have all of their heartbeats recorded and woven together behind the music. For women who are enrolled in perinatal hospice programs, whose infants are unlikely to survive through delivery, a

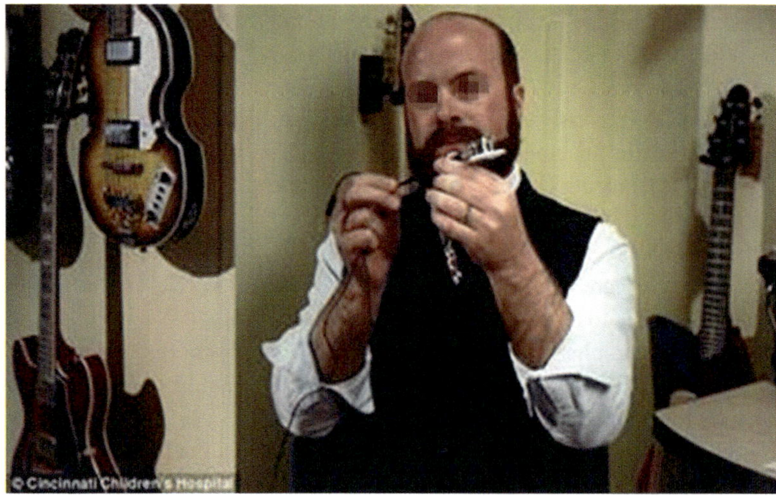

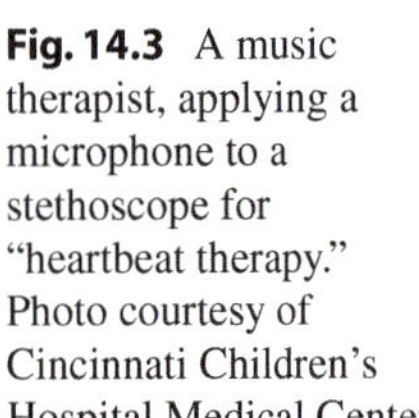

Fig. 14.3 A music therapist, applying a microphone to a stethoscope for "heartbeat therapy." Photo courtesy of Cincinnati Children's Hospital Medical Center

Doppler can be used to record the infant's heartbeat and the same techniques applied to build legacy of the baby's life. Many families request to have the "heartbeat music" played or shared at the child's funeral.

Animal-assisted therapy (AAT) can be a significant part of treatment for people with a physical, social, emotional, or cognitive diagnoses, and patients who are eligible for palliative care, and is a part of the overarching treatment plan of the patient (Goddard and Gilmer 2015). AAT requires stated goals for each session, and the treatment is often individualized to the patient and documented in the medical record (Goddard and Gilmer 2015). In 2014, the American Humane Association and Zoetis, Inc launched the first clinical trial evaluating the impact of animal-assisted therapy in the care of children with cancer. Entitled the "Canines and Childhood Cancer" study, the study will examine how animal-assisted therapy affects stress and anxiety among children with cancer and their parents/guardians, as well as health-related quality of life for patients (http://www.americanhumane.org/clinical-trial-launches-documenting-efficacy-of-animal-assisted-therapy.html). Animal-assisted therapy is a growing field in the care of seriously ill children, and several children's hospitals now have on-site therapy dogs to meet with patients in multiple settings. Some children's hospitals also offer "pet visitation areas" where children can reunite with their own pets while they are admitted to the hospital. Finally, hospice groups frequently offer pet therapy visits to the homes of patients who are enrolled in their programs.

Spiritual care is an integral part of palliative care. In pediatrics, recognizing and celebrating the spirituality of children and giving them a language to speak of their experiences of the transcendent allow meaning making and hope. Godly Play© is a method that seeks to give children a language that can help them explore and make meaning around their existential limits or those things that threaten to "box us in" simply because we are human: the limits of aloneness, freedom, questions of meaning or purpose, and death (Minor and Campbell 2016). Through Godly Play© methodology, children gain an increased awareness of their existential limits in a safe and supportive environment and are able to express their consciousness of these limits within the relationships they have with themselves, their community, the world around them, and their spiritual and religious beliefs (Minor and Campbell 2016). It is thought that facilitating these spiritual expressions through these relational dynamics, and within the context of their existential limits, leads to spiritual and emotional well-being (Minor and Campbell 2016). For children experiencing serious illness or who are approaching the end of life, Godly Play© may offer an additional opportunity to nurture their spirituality and to foster emotional well-being.

14.3 Advancing Education and Training

Developing innovative changes in palliative oncology research and clinical care will first require an innovative transformation in how we train and educate the interdisciplinary pediatric oncology and pediatric palliative care teams. This ranges from development and measurement of new educational models to the integration and crossover of palliative care and oncology education, as well as preparing oncologists to conduct high-quality palliative care, medical education, and psychosocial research.

The AAP, IOM, WHO, and American Society of Clinical Oncology have all recommended that physicians and health professionals who care for seriously ill patients have basic palliative care skills, including competency in pain and symptom management, end-of-life care, communication, decision-making support, ethics, and psychological and spiritual dimensions of care (Institute of Medicine 2003, 2014; American Academy of Pediatrics Section on Hospice and Palliative Medicine and Committee on Hospital Care 2013; National Cancer Control Programmes 2002; Smith et al. 2012; Roth et al. 2009). The Association of Pediatric Hematology/Oncology Nurses has similarly issued a position paper on the role of pediatric hematology/oncology nurses in pain management for children with cancer at the end of life (http://aphon.org/education/clinical-practice). Palliative care skills should be learned and performed by all members of a patient's care team; when performed by pediatric oncologists, this is referred to as primary palliative care, and when performed by a board-certified pediatric palliative care team, this is referred to as secondary or specialty palliative care (Institute of Medicine 2014).

Current trainees and program directors have recognized the need for superior palliative care education (Roth et al. 2009; Baker et al. 2007). Despite recommendations from our professional societies and research citing a desire for improved training, most pediatric hematology/oncology fellowships lack formalized palliative care and end-of-life education (Roth et al. 2009; Baker et al. 2007; File et al. 2014; Feraco et al. 2016). When education is provided, it has traditionally been lecture based (Roth et al. 2009; File et al. 2014; McCabe et al. 2008; Kersun et al. 2009; Litrivis et al. 2012; Boss et al. 2009; Schiffman et al. 2008) despite the knowledge that most clinicians prefer experiential training and that lecture-based education is unlikely to affect skills performance.

As the cure rates for many pediatric cancers have risen over the previous decades, the current generation of pediatric hematology/oncology fellows and advanced practice providers encounters less patients that relapse and die than those that trained in previous decades. Currently, pediatric trainees have fewer opportunities to practice palliative care skills on the job—conducting few palliative care conversations, caring for a small number of patients who die, and receiving performance feedback of inconsistent quality (Baker et al. 2007; McCabe et al. 2008). Few clinicians are able to rotate with an experienced interdisciplinary pediatric palliative care team, perform home visits, or perform concurrent visits with a hospice team. The 'see one, do one, teach one' method of learning may be harmful to patients and families, and has led to the lack of palliative care experience, knowledge, competence, and respectful communication skills in many pediatric specialists (Baker et al. 2007; McCabe et al. 2008; Meert et al. 2008; Contro et al. 2002, 2004; Kolarik et al. 2006; Liben et al. 2008; Serwint et al. 2006; Michelson et al. 2009; Sheetz and Bowman 2008; Rider et al. 2008; Orgel et al. 2010; Levetown 2008).

14.3.1 Simulation-Based Models of Teaching Palliative Care

What is our most common procedure performed in pediatric hematology/oncology? Lumbar puncture? Bone marrow aspiration? These procedures are routinely taught, monitored, and performed in a systematic fashion. They are highly reproducible across providers. However, high-stakes communication is performed many times per day by clinicians interacting with patients, families, staff, and other clinicians. We bring a wealth of styles, personalities, and cultures, all of which influence our patient-physician encounters.

Simulation-based learning has the potential to change the understanding and implementation of PC in pediatric hematology/oncology (Cheng et al. 2007; Boulet et al. 1998). Simulations are scenarios or environments designed to closely approximate real-world situations, usually for the purposes of training or evaluation. Simulation plays a large role in the education of personnel in industries in which there are inherent risks of catastrophic error (i.e., NASA, airline industry, military, anesthesia, and emergency medicine) and where training in the real world is too costly or dangerous (Cheng et al. 2007). Simulation-based education relies on "suspending disbelief," allowing students to immerse themselves in a learning experience that closely matches what they encounter in the clinical setting (Cheng et al. 2007).

In medicine, simulation-based education has been used commonly in areas of high-stakes communication (resuscitation) and procedural skills. Several innovative models at the institutional, national, and international levels have used role-play and video-recorded simulation (Brown et al. 2012; Tobler et al. 2014; Carter and Swan 2012; Haut et al. 2012; Lindsay 2010; Youngblood et al.

2012; Brock et al. 2015a). These models encompass tasks such as breaking bad news, disclosing medical errors, as well as having discussions about relapse and end-of-life care. We will highlight a few of these national models here.

EPEC: Pediatrics: EPEC (Education in Palliative and End-of-life Care) began in the late 1990s as a novel "train the trainer educational intervention" developed by the American Medical Association and the Robert Wood Johnson Foundation (VanGeest 2001). Since that time, it has had multiple iterations and has expanded into other subspecialty areas, including pediatrics. The inaugural pediatric session was held in 2012, with sessions to follow in conjunction with ASPHO to target pediatric oncologists. The curriculum is comprised of 6 in person conference sessions along with 20 distance learning online modules. One unique aspect of the EPEC curriculum is the focus on teaching methodology. Details of the program, which was developed and implemented with NIH funding, can be found at http://epec.net/epec_pediatrics.php.

VitalTalk: VitalTalk (the parent organization of Oncotalk) is a series of intensive 2-day courses with the purpose of learning communication skills and expressions of empathy in the same way other skills in medicine are learned: watching skilled practitioners and then practicing with supervision (Back et al. 2007; Fryer-Edwards et al. 2006). VitalTalk courses are divided into multiple sessions; each session starts with didactic teaching of new communication skills (such as identifying when emotion is driving patient responses, dealing with emotion, picking up on empathic cues, and responding empathically). Participants practice and develop these newly learned skills. Trained facilitators present a clinical scenario, and one person at a time interacts with the actor, while the remaining members and facilitators watch, listen, and give feedback. When a participant is struggling, "time-outs" and "do-overs" are encouraged so that continuous and rapid improvement is achieved. In addition, VitalTalk offers faculty development courses designed for attending level instruction on being a better bedside teacher and gaining the skills to be a VitalTalk instructor.

VitalTalk had previously had individual curricula in oncology (Oncotalk), nephrology (NephroTalk), geriatrics (Geritalk), fellow learning (Fellowtalk), and an online toolbox (Tough Talk), all of which highlight core teaching and communication skills. While extraordinarily successful and widely disseminated (including an app for mobile use), all versions of VitalTalk are focused on adult clinicians who can communicate directly with their patients. No pediatric version of this curriculum has been developed, and this represents an opportunity for future program development and investigation (http://vitaltalk.org/).

Comfort Codes: Medical practitioners react immediately for a Code Blue—physicians running down the hall, nurses maneuvering to give patients medications, and pharmacists expertly manning the code cart. One rarely sees this level of resource mobilization for patients suffering in a different way—from pain, dyspnea, delirium, anxiety, or other symptoms that are causing intense suffering. Code comforts were designed to provide a sense of urgency to suffering patients and providers that providing relief is now a top priority. The goal is to provide immediate, intensive relief of suffering using a clearly defined process that requires rapid-response teamwork. This team can involve the primary team, palliative care physicians, nurses, respiratory therapists, chaplains, and child life specialists (https://hbr.org/2014/12/code-comfort-a-code-blue-alternative-for-patients-with-dnrs).

Successful implementation of a comfort code would require deliberate and repeated practice, similar to training required for responding to a Code Blue. Future research should incorporate multidisciplinary simulations involving physicians, nurses, pharmacists, chaplains, and child life specialists. A palliative care "code cart" could be developed and utilized. A combined high- and low-fidelity simulation model could enhance learning in this capacity; high-fidelity simulation mannequins could have pain, dyspnea, or other symptoms and would "respond" to the interventions provided, while other team members could be speaking to the family (patient actors) in the low-fidelity component.

14.3.2 Primary Pediatric Palliative Care Skills for Pediatric Oncology Fellows

Palliative Care Curriculum in Hematology/Oncology Training: The simplest, most easily implemented, and cost-effective method of teaching palliative care skills to pediatric oncology fellows is to incorporate palliative care training into the didactic curriculum that fellows complete through their 3 years of training. This training should address the American Academy of Pediatrics core competencies of providing basic pain and symptom management for children and to request timely palliative care consultation (American Academy of Pediatrics Section on Hospice and Palliative Medicine and Committee on Hospital Care 2013; Mack and Wolfe 2006). More specifically, fellows should be instructed on using pharmacologic and non-pharmacologic methods to manage pain and symptoms, providing end-of-life care, enhancing communication skills, supporting decision-making, recognizing ethical issues, and addressing psychological and spiritual dimensions of life and illness (American Academy of Pediatrics Section on Hospice and Palliative Medicine and Committee on Hospital Care 2013). As fellows become emotionally attached to families they care for and as children die, fellows' feelings of grief and anxiety should be openly addressed and supported (Granek et al. 2015).

Training for fellows should occur in a variety of ways. Medication management for pain, fatigue, constipation, nausea, vomiting, insomnia, anxiety, and depression can be taught in a didactic forum, whereas communication skills should be addressed through experiential education, including role-playing, simulation, workshops, and direct feedback over the course of the fellowship (Baughcum et al. 2007; Harris et al. 2015; Gerhardt et al. 2009). Although not universally offered, a 2–4 week palliative care rotation with a specialist palliative care team can also be of benefit (Singh et al. 2016). Addressing the spiritual, psychological, and ethical dimensions of illness may be better taught by board-certified chaplains, psychiatrists, psychologists, and ethicists (Robinson et al. 2016; Baker et al. 2016). Training programs should also consider incorporating bereaved family members into the educational curriculum as their perspectives are being more widely reported (Contro et al. 2002; Snaman et al. 2016a).

Fellowship Training: Beyond "primary pediatric palliative care," some pediatric oncology fellows may choose to concentrate their focus in oncology to the area of palliative care. Historically this was done purely by interest, and many of the first pediatric palliative care physicians were oncologists; 2012 was the last year that physicians could sit for the hospice and palliative medicine boards based on practice experience. From that point forward, a 1-year formal fellowship in palliative care has been required in order to become board eligible. Board certification examinations are offered through various related boards, including American Board of Pediatrics (ABP). Certification by the ABP requires that all hospice and palliative medicine candidates hold certification in general pediatrics or a subspecialty of pediatrics (i.e., pediatric oncology) in order to be eligible (https://www.abp.org/content/hospice-and-palliative-medicine-certification). Some pediatricians may choose to complete palliative care fellowship directly after residency training, after some years of practice, or after completing a traditional 3-year subspecialty fellowship.

Pediatric palliative care fellowship training programs currently vary widely across programs, with most programs supporting 1–2 physician fellows per year. The Harvard Interprofessional Palliative Care Fellowship Program is one example of a training program that incorporates and integrates training for physician, nurse practitioner, and social work fellows. The pediatric portion of the fellowship, now over 10 years old, includes two to three pediatric fellows, a nurse practitioner fellow, and a social work fellow who train together. More programs like this will be needed to ensure we are training an interdisciplinary workforce in pediatric palliative care.

Integrated Fellowship: Alternatively, an integrated model exists, developed by Justin Baker, MD (Snaman et al. 2016b). In this model, a pediatric oncology fellow with an interest in palliative care would complete their first clinical year of hematology/oncology and during their second year of fellowship go on to do their palliative care training. During this year of palliative care, the fellow continues to see their primary oncology patients in clinic ½ day per week in order to maintain continuity. They would then go on to complete the final 2 "research" years of fellowship with a focus on palliative care within oncology. While this was first done by Baker and colleagues at St. Jude Children's Research Hospital, it has since been adapted by other pediatric oncology training programs. Advantages of this training model include expanded research in the field and an unparalleled opportunity to integrate palliative care and oncology on a much deeper and intimate level (Snaman et al. 2016b).

Training Oncologists in Palliative Care Research: Some pediatric oncologist may choose to have a focus area in palliative care without doing an additional year of fellowship. These fellows would have the opportunity to explore these topics as part of their traditional research experience within oncology training, usually in the second and third year of fellowship. Potential research mentors might include a trained palliative care physician if an oncologist without specific expertise or interests is available at their institution. Opportunities for research collaboration outside a specific institution are also viable options.

Doctoral and Other Palliative Care Training Models: The current model of palliative care fellowship is a 1-year clinical fellowship, without any specific research requirement. This is in contrast to the more traditional model of pediatric oncology training that is usually 3 years in length. The first year is usually heavily clinical, followed by 2 years of a research focus with lighter clinical responsibilities. For those who do palliative care fellowship outside of other subspecialty training, this leaves little opportunity or path to hone research skills or have dedicated research time. Alternatives may include grant funding through career development awards and/or institutional support. Future training options in the USA may include pediatric palliative care fellowships that offer a research track for those who wish to pursue a career in academia. Graduate programs focusing on palliative care are available for those who want a more intensive palliative care training experience. For example, for social work trainees, palliative care training programs such as the 2-year Zelda Foster Studies Program exist (Gardner et al. 2015). For all disciplines, the need for more community-based palliative care research and research training must be balanced with the need for pediatric palliative care physicians outside of large tertiary referral centers.

14.3.3 Palliative Care Outcomes and Measurement in Pediatric Oncology

As palliative oncology and palliative care medical education research continues to grow, investigators, program directors, and division chairs will need measurement tools for assessing resident, fellow, faculty, and staff palliative care comfort, confidence, competence, knowledge, skill acquisition, and retention over time.

Better Ways to Measure Effectiveness of Novel Models: Current measurement tools will likely be insufficient for measuring patient, family, provider, and educational outcomes. At present, there are few well-established, reliable, and valid measurement tools for assessing and tracking different aspects of palliative education (Quinn et al. 2008; Ferrell and McCaffery 2014; Lazenby et al. 2012; Williams et al. 2009; Brown et al. 2011; Makoul 2001; Nakazawa et al. 2009, 2010; Baile et al. 2000; Brock et al. 2015b; Calhoun et al. 2009, 2010; Peterson et al. 2014; Street 1991). Many are geared toward undergraduate medical education (SEGUE and SPIKES models) or resident populations with fewer survey tools for attending physician skill assessment. Medical education studies of novel palliative care interventions have historically been limited in their data collection and analysis by tools that have been adapted for pediatric care or compiled from multiple surveys and therefore lack data on their reliability and validity. Few pediatric studies have tracked participants over a prolonged time, and the test-retest reliability of a questionnaire will need to be assessed (Baughcum et al. 2007; Gerhardt et al. 2009).

More Validated and Reliable Tools for Measurement of Fellow, Attending, Clinician Skills: Current measurement tools are also limited in their ability to measure multiple team members simultaneously, assessing individual member's abilities to work and communicate within an interdisciplinary team. Future survey and assessment tools should incorporate not only the ability of the clinician to interact with the patient and family but also the quality of the interaction with other health professionals, such as advanced practice providers, social workers, care coordinators, chaplains, and medical interpreters.

In taking education one step further, educators could "keep the camera rolling" and obtain video of attending physicians providing feedback to junior residents and fellows. In this way, you can continue to "teach the teacher" or "train the trainer."

Lastly, there is a growing role for the direct observation and feedback by patients and their family members (Street 1991). A growing body of literature supports that many families have endured poor end-of-life experiences, much of which has been centered on communication within the hospital (Contro et al. 2002; Mack et al. 2005; Kassam et al. 2013). While many fellowships have parents or caregivers' complete informal questionnaires, feedback is highly skewed toward positive scores with few comments geared toward improvement. This arises if patients are uncertain how to give high-quality advice, or there is fear of retribution or mistreatment if poor marks were to be assigned.

Conclusion

A range of methodologies and strategies are needed to develop and deliver innovative palliative care within pediatric oncology. A robust scientific foundation is needed to address the many gaps in the current knowledge base supporting practice and policy. High-quality, forward-facing care necessitates rigorous quality improvement efforts, technological ingenuity, and a commitment to novel educational techniques to promote both primary palliative care skills in pediatric oncology clinicians and pediatric palliative care (PPC) subspecialists across all disciplines (e.g., physicians, nurses, psychosocial clinicians). To meet these needs and drive the practice of palliative care forward, innovation, originality, openness to novel approaches and new technologies, and striving for continual improvement are necessities.

Box 14.1 Strategies to Increase Sample Size by Facilitating Recruitment and Reducing Attrition

Recruitment Strategies

1. Seek enrollment early (before or at the time of eligibility).
2. Use electronic databases to track potential participants and reasons for refusal, if possible.
3. Use multiple strategies to identify all eligible participants:
   (a) Regular information sessions with providers
   (b) Presence of "project recruiters" in referring disease programs
   (c) Permit referrals from participants already included
   (d) Advertisements directly to potential participants (e.g., Facebook advertising)
4. Consider use of social media (e.g., Twitter, Facebook) (Akard et al. 2015).
5. Pre-consent (or pre-education)—useful in complex or highly stressful recruitment scenarios. Consent is sought in advance of eligibility criteria all being met. Allows education of family about a study in a controlled environment (Nimmer et al. 2016). While acceptability to IRBs is variable, pre-education is an alternative when pre-consent is not permitted.
6. Secure clinician buy-in (especially gatekeeping clinicians). Ensure they regard study as justified and useful and are committed to it.

7. Offer to provide a copy of aggregated results at the end of the study (e.g., copy of manuscript).

Strategies to Reduce Attrition

(a) Keep evaluation periods as short as possible.
(b) Optional re-enrollment: enroll participants for an initial (short) period of time, and then later revisit their willingness to continue for subsequent enrollment periods.
(c) Tokens of appreciation for participation.
(d) Regular communications from study team regarding study progress (e.g., milestones achieved) and updates on relevant literature in the field.

Box 14.2 Case Vignette

Dr. Noah Pruvel is planning a study in which he will conduct one-on-one interviews with parents of children who underwent bone marrow transplantation in order to better understand their end-of-life experience. He will mail letters of invitation to parents after first obtaining permission from the child's physician to contact them. He involved bereaved parents in the design of the study and preparation of recruitment materials and interview guide.

How can he address concerns that his institution's IRB might have when reviewing his protocol?

- Participation of patients and families in research design from the start demonstrates a sensitivity to needs and vulnerabilities of research participants. It should be noted that this approach can address concerns of clinician gatekeepers as well.
- Outlining (1) a sensitive and respectful approach to the recruitment and consent process and (2) a plan to mitigate distress and attend to it once it occurs also reassures IRBs about the potential burdens and risks of participation. It is also useful to clearly delineate the difference between causing distress (due to study participation) and incidental distress (due to parent circumstances).
- Preparation of a letter to the IRB summarizing the experience of bereaved parents in research, which includes finding value and meaning in participation, can educate IRB members about the positive aspects of participation in research.
- If IRB concerns persist, speaking with the IRB chair or IRB reviewer (if permitted) or offering to attend an IRB meeting in person to address concerns can be very effective. Oftentimes direct communication clarifies issues and resolves concerns.

References

Akard TF, Gilmer MJ, Friedman DL, Given B, Hendricks-Ferguson VL, Hinds PS (2013) From qualitative work to intervention development in pediatric oncology palliative care research. J Pediatr Oncol Nurs 30:153–160

Akard TF, Wray S, Gilmer MJ (2015) Facebook advertisements recruit parents of children with cancer for an online survey of web-based research preferences. Cancer Nurs 38:155–161

Alliance WPC, Organization WH (2014) Global atlas of palliative care at the end of life. In: Alliance WPC, ed. i; 19–25

American Academy of Pediatrics (2000) Committee on bioethics and committee on hospital care. Palliative care for children. Pediatrics 106:351–357

American Academy of Pediatrics Section on Hospice and Palliative Medicine and Committee on Hospital Care (2013) Pediatric palliative care and hospice care commitments, guidelines, and recommendations. Pediatrics 132:966–972

American Medical Association (2008) Physician consortium on performance improvement palliative and end of life care physician performance measurement set 2008. (Accessed August 9, 2016, at http://www.amaassn.org/ama/pub/physician-resources/physician-consortium-performance-improvement/pcpi-measures.page)
Aoun SM, Kristjanson LJ (2005) Challenging the framework for evidence in palliative care research. Palliat Med 19:461–465
Back AL, Arnold RM, Baile WF et al (2007) Efficacy of communication skills training for giving bad news and discussing transitions to palliative care. Arch Inter Med 167:453–460
Baile WF, Buckman R, Lenzi R, Glober G, Beale EA, Kudelka AP (2000) SPIKES-A six-step protocol for delivering bad news: application to the patient with cancer. Oncologist 5:302–311
Baker JN, Torkildson C, Baillargeon JG, Olney CA, Kane JR (2007) National survey of pediatric residency program directors and residents regarding education in palliative medicine and end-of-life care. J Palliat Med 10:420–429
Baker JN, Windham JA, Hinds PS et al (2013) Bereaved parents' intentions and suggestions about research autopsies in children with lethal brain tumors. J Pediatr 163:581–586
Baker JN, Levine DR, Hinds PS et al (2015) Research priorities in pediatric palliative care. J Pediatr 167:467–70.e3
Baker HB, McQuilling JP, King NM (2016) Ethical considerations in tissue engineering research: case studies in translation. Methods 99:135–144
Baughcum AE, Gerhardt CA, Young-Saleme T, Stefanik R, Klopfenstein KJ (2007) Evaluation of a pediatric palliative care educational workshop for oncology fellows. Pediatr Blood Cancer 49:154–159
Bensink ME, Armfield NR, Pinkerton R et al (2009) Using videotelephony to support paediatric oncology-related palliative care in the home: from abandoned RCT to acceptability study. Palliat Med 23:228–237
Berde CB, Walco GA, Krane EJ et al (2012) Pediatric analgesic clinical trial designs, measures, and extrapolation: report of an FDA scientific workshop. Pediatrics 129:354–364
Boss RD, Hutton N, Donohue PK, Arnold RM (2009) Neonatologist training to guide family decision making for critically ill infants. Arch Pediatr Adolesc Med 163:783–788
Boulet JR, Ben-David MF, Ziv A et al (1998) Using standardized patients to assess the interpersonal skills of physicians. Acad Med: J Assoc Am Med Coll 73:S94–S96
Bradford N, Herbert A, Walker R et al (2010) Home telemedicine for paediatric palliative care. Stud Health Technol Inform 161:10–19
Bradford NK, Armfield NR, Young J, Herbert A, Mott C, Smith AC (2014a) Principles of a paediatric palliative care consultation can be achieved with home telemedicine. J Telemed Telecare 20:360–364
Bradford NK, Armfield NR, Young J, Smith AC (2014b) Paediatric palliative care by video consultation at home: a cost minimisation analysis. BMC Health Serv Res 14:328
Breen M (2006) An evaluation of two subcutaneous infusion devices in children receiving palliative care. Paediat Nurs 18:38–40
Brock K, Cohen H, Sourkes B et al (2015a) Teaching pediatric fellows palliative care through simulation and video intervention: a practical guide to implementation. MedEdPORTAL, Washington, DC
Brock KE, Cohen HJ, Popat RA, Halamek LP (2015b) Reliability and validity of the pediatric palliative care questionnaire for measuring self-efficacy, knowledge, and adequacy of prior medical education among pediatric fellows. J Palliat Med 18:842–848
Brown C, Gephardt G, Lloyd C, Swearingen C, Boateng B (2011) Teaching palliative care skills using simulated family encounters. MedEdPORTAL, Washington, DC
Brown CM, Lloyd EC, Swearingen CJ, Boateng BA (2012) Improving resident self-efficacy in pediatric palliative care through clinical simulation. J Palliat Care 28:157–163
Buchanan DR, O'Mara AM, Kelaghan JW, Sgambati M, McCaskill-Stevens W, Minasian L (2007) Challenges and recommendations for advancing the state-of-the-science of quality of life assessment in symptom management trials. Cancer 110:1621–1628
Burke BL Jr, Hall RW (2015) Section on telehealth care. Telemedicine: pediatric applications. Pediatrics 136:e293–e308
Calhoun AW, Rider EA, Meyer EC, Lamiani G, Truog RD (2009) Assessment of communication skills and self-appraisal in the simulated environment: feasibility of multirater feedback with gap analysis. Simul Healthc 4:22–29
Calhoun AW, Rider EA, Peterson E, Meyer EC (2010) Multi-rater feedback with gap analysis: an innovative means to assess communication skill and self-insight. Patient Educ Couns 80:321–326
Carter BS, Swan R (2012) Pediatric palliative care instruction for residents: an introduction to IPPC. Am J Hosp Palliat Care 29:375–378
Casarett D (2002) 'Randomize the first patient': old advice for a new field. AAHPM Bull 2:4–5
Cheng A, Duff J, Grant E, Kissoon N, Grant VJ (2007) Simulation in paediatrics: an educational revolution. Paediatr Child Health 12:465–468
Clinical Practice (2017) at http://aphon.org/education/clinical-practice
Clinical Trial Launches to Document Efficacy of Animal-Assisted Therapy for Child Cancer Patients and Their Families (2014) (Accessed August 30, 2016, at http://www.americanhumane.org/clinical-trial-launches-documenting-efficacy-of-animal-assisted-therapy.html)
Contro N, Larson J, Scofield S, Sourkes B, Cohen H (2002) Family perspectives on the quality of pediatric palliative care. Arch Pediatr Adolesc Med 156:14–19

Contro NA, Larson J, Scofield S, Sourkes B, Cohen HJ (2004) Hospital staff and family perspectives regarding quality of pediatric palliative care. Pediatrics 114:1248–1252

Coombes LH, Wiseman T, Lucas G, Sangha A, Murtagh FE (2016) Health-related quality-of-life outcome measures in paediatric palliative care: a systematic review of psychometric properties and feasibility of use. Palliat Med 30(10):935–949

Downing J, Knapp C, Muckaden MA, Fowler-Kerry S, Marston J (2015) Priorities for global research into children's palliative care: results of an International Delphi study. BMC Palliat Care 14:36

Dussel V, Kreicbergs U, Hilden JM et al (2009) Looking beyond where children die: determinants and effects of planning a child's location of death. J Pain Symptom Manag 37:33–43

Dy SM, Kiley KB, Ast K et al (2015) Measuring what matters: top-ranked quality indicators for hospice and palliative care from the american academy of hospice and palliative medicine and hospice and palliative nurses association. J Pain Symptom Manag 49:773–781

Dyregrov K (2004) Bereaved parents' experience of research participation. Soc Sci Med 58:391–400

Eilegard A, Steineck G, Nyberg T, Kreicbergs U (2013) Bereaved siblings' perception of participating in research—a nationwide study. Psycho-Oncology 22:411–416

Farquhar MC, Ewing G, Booth S (2011) Using mixed methods to develop and evaluate complex interventions in palliative care research. Palliat Med 25:748–757

Farquhar M, Preston N, Evans CJ et al (2013) Mixed methods research in the development and evaluation of complex interventions in palliative and end-of-life care: report on the MORECare consensus exercise. J Palliat Med 16:1550–1560

Feraco AM, Brand SR, Mack JW, Kesselheim JC, Block SD, Wolfe J (2016) Communication skills training in pediatric oncology: moving beyond role modeling. Pediatr Blood Cancer 63(6):966–972

Ferrell B, McCaffery M (2014) Knowledge and attitudes survey regarding pain

File W, Bylund CL, Kesselheim J, Leonard D, Leavey P (2014) Do pediatric hematology/oncology (PHO) fellows receive communication training? Pediatr Blood Cancer 61:502–506

Fryer-Edwards K, Arnold RM, Baile W, Tulsky JA, Petracca F, Back A (2006) Reflective teaching practices: an approach to teaching communication skills in a small-group setting. Acad Med 81:638–644

Gardner DS, Gerbino S, Walls JW, Chachkes E, Doherty MJ (2015) Mentoring the next generation of social workers in palliative and end-of-life care: the zelda foster studies program. J Soc Work End Life Palliat Care 11:107–131

Gelfman LP, Morrison RS (2008) Research funding for palliative medicine. J Palliat Med 11:36–43

Gerhardt CA, Grollman JA, Baughcum AE, Young-Saleme T, Stefanik R, Klopfenstein KJ (2009) Longitudinal evaluation of a pediatric palliative care educational workshop for oncology fellows. J Palliat Med 12:323–328

Goddard A, Gilmer MJ (2015) The role and impact of animals with pediatric patients. Pediat Nurs 41(2):65–71

Grande GE, Todd CJ (2000) Why are trials in palliative care so difficult? Palliat Med 14:69–74

Granek L, Bartels U, Barrera M, Scheinemann K (2015) Challenges faced by pediatric oncology fellows when patients die during their training. J Oncol Pract 11:e182–e189

Guyatt GH, Keller JL, Jaeschke R, Rosenbloom D, Adachi JD, Newhouse MT (1990) The n-of-1 randomized controlled trial: clinical usefulness. Our three-year experience. Ann Inter Med 112:293–299

Hanson LC, Scheunemann LP, Zimmerman S, Rokoske FS, Schenck AP (2010) The PEACE project review of clinical instruments for hospice and palliative care. J Palliat Med 13:1253–1260

Harris LL, Placencia FX, Arnold JL, Minard CG, Harris TB, Haidet PM (2015) A structured end-of-life curriculum for neonatal-perinatal postdoctoral fellows. Am J Hosp Palliat Care 32:253–261

Haut C, Michael M, Moloney-Harmon P (2012) Implementing a program to improve pediatric and pediatric ICU nurses' knowledge of and attitudes toward palliative care. J Hosp Palliat Nurs 14:71–79

Hays RM, Valentine J, Haynes G et al (2006) The seattle pediatric palliative care project: effects on family satisfaction and health-related quality of life. J Palliat Med 9:716–728

Higginson IJ, Booth S (2011) The randomized fast-track trial in palliative care: role, utility and ethics in the evaluation of interventions in palliative care? Palliat Med 25:741–747

Hinds PS, Pritchard M, Harper J (2004) End-of-life research as a priority for pediatric oncology. J Pediatr Oncol Nurs 21:175–179

Hinds PS, Drew D, Oakes LL et al (2005) End-of-life care preferences of pediatric patients with cancer. J Clin Oncol 23:9146–9154

Huang IC, Shenkman EA, Madden VL, Vadaparampil S, Quinn G, Knapp CA (2010) Measuring quality of life in pediatric palliative care: challenges and potential solutions. Palliat Med 24:175–182

Hui D, Parsons HA, Damani S et al (2011) Quantity, design, and scope of the palliative oncology literature. Oncologist 16:694–703

Hynson JL, Aroni R, Bauld C, Sawyer SM (2006) Research with bereaved parents: a question of how not why. Palliat Med 20:805–811

Improving the Quality of Caring (Accessed August 30, 2016 at https://www.pcqn.org/about/)

Institute of Medicine (2001) National research council national cancer policy B. In: Foley KM, Gelband H (eds) Improving palliative care for cancer: summary and recommendations. National Academies, Washington, DC, Copyright 2001 by the National Academy of Sciences. All rights reserved

Institute of Medicine (2003) When children die: improving palliative and end-of-life care for children and their families—summary. The National Academies, Washington, DC

Institute of Medicine (2014) Dying in America: improving quality and honoring individual preferences near the end of life. The National Academies, Washington, DC

Institute of Medicine (US) and National Research Council (US) National Cancer Policy Board (2001) In: Foley KM, Gelband H (eds) Improving palliative care for cancer: summary and recommendations. National Academies, Washington, DC

Irwin DE, Varni JW, Yeatts K, DeWalt DA (2009) Cognitive interviewing methodology in the development of a pediatric item bank: a patient reported outcomes measurement information system (PROMIS) study. Health Qual Life Outcomes 7:3

Kaasa S, Hjermstad MJ, Loge JH (2006) Methodological and structural challenges in palliative care research: how have we fared in the last decades? Palliat Med 20:727–734

Kassam A, Skiadaresis J, Habib S, Alexander S, Wolfe J (2013) Moving toward quality palliative cancer care: parent and clinician perspectives on gaps between what matters and what is accessible. J Clin Oncol 31:910–915

Kersun L, Gyi L, Morrison WE (2009) Training in difficult conversations: a national survey of pediatric hematology-oncology and pediatric critical care physicians. J Palliative Med 12:525–530

Knapp CA (2009) Research in pediatric palliative care: closing the gap between what is and is not known. Am J Hosp Palliat Care 26:392–398

Knapp C, Madden V (2010) Conducting outcomes research in pediatric palliative care. Am J Hosp Palliat Care 27:277–281

Kolarik RC, Walker G, Arnold RM (2006) Pediatric resident education in palliative care: a needs assessment. Pediatrics 117:1949–1954

Kreicbergs U, Valdimarsdottir U, Steineck G, Henter JI (2004) A population-based nationwide study of parents' perceptions of a questionnaire on their child's death due to cancer. Lancet 364:787–789

Kumar SP (2011) Reporting of pediatric palliative care: a systematic review and quantitative analysis of research publications in palliative care journals. Indian J Palliat Care 17:202–209

Lazenby M, Ercolano E, Schulman-Green D, McCorkle R (2012) Validity of the end-of-life professional caregiver survey to assess for multidisciplinary educational needs. J Palliat Med 15:427–431

Levetown M, American Academy of Pediatrics Committee on B (2008) Communicating with children and families: from everyday interactions to skill in conveying distressing information. Pediatrics 121:e1441–e1460

Liben S, Papadatou D, Wolfe J (2008) Paediatric palliative care: challenges and emerging ideas. Lancet 371:852–864

Lindsay J (2010) Introducing nursing students to pediatric end-of-life issues using simulation. Dimens Crit Care Nurs 29:175–178

Litrivis E, Singh AL, Moonian A, Mahadeo KM (2012) An assessment of end-of-life-care training: should we consider a cross-fellowship, competency-based simulated program? J Pediatr Hematol Oncol 34:488–489

Lorenz KA, Rosenfeld K, Wenger N (2007) Quality indicators for palliative and end-of-life care in vulnerable elders. J Am Geriatr Soc 55(Suppl 2):S318–S326

Mack JW, Wolfe J (2006) Early integration of pediatric palliative care: for some children, palliative care starts at diagnosis. Curr Opin Pediatr 18:10–14

Mack JW, Hilden JM, Watterson J et al (2005) Parent and physician perspectives on quality of care at the end of life in children with cancer. J Clin Oncol 23:9155–9161

Madhavan S, Sanders AE, Chou WY et al (2011) Pediatric palliative care and eHealth opportunities for patient-centered care. Am J Prev Med 40:S208–S216

Makoul G (2001) The SEGUE framework for teaching and assessing communication skills. Patient Educ Couns 45:23–34

McCabe ME, Hunt EA, Serwint JR (2008) Pediatric residents' clinical and educational experiences with end-of-life care. Pediatrics 121:e731–e737

McLeod LD, Coon CD, Martin SA, Fehnel SE, Hays RD (2011) Interpreting patient-reported outcome results: US FDA guidance and emerging methods. Expert Rev Pharmacoecon Outcomes Res 11:163–169

Meert KL, Eggly S, Pollack M et al (2008) Parents' perspectives on physician-parent communication near the time of a child's death in the pediatric intensive care unit. Pediatr Crit Care Med 9:2–7

Michelson KN, Ryan AD, Jovanovic B, Frader J (2009) Pediatric residents' and fellows' perspectives on palliative care education. J Palliat Med 12:451–457

Minor CV, Campbell R (2016) The parable of the sower: a case study examining the use of the Godly Play© (R) method as a spiritual intervention on a psychiatric unit of a major children's hospital. Int J Child Spiritual 21:38–51

Mongeau S, Champagne M, Liben S (2007) Participatory research in pediatric palliative care: benefits and challenges. J Palliat Care 23:5–13

Nakazawa Y, Miyashita M, Morita T, Umeda M, Oyagi Y, Ogasawara T (2009) The palliative care knowledge test: reliability and validity of an instrument to measure palliative care knowledge among health professionals. Palliat Med 23:754–766

Nakazawa Y, Miyashita M, Morita T, Umeda M, Oyagi Y, Ogasawara T (2010) The palliative care self-reported practices scale and the palliative care difficulties scale: reliability and validity of two scales evaluating self-reported practices and difficulties experienced in palliative care by health professionals. J Palliat Med 13:427–437

National Cancer Control Programmes (2002) Policies and Managerial Guidelines. World Health Organization, Geneva

National Consensus Project Guidelines for Quality Palliative Care (2013) Clinical practice guidelines for quality palliative care, 3rd edn. (Accessed August 19, 2015, at http://www.nationalconsensusproject.org)

Nelson H, Mott S, Kleinman ME, Goldstein RD (2015) Parents' experiences of pediatric palliative transports: a qualitative case series. J Pain Symptom Manag 50:375–380

Nimmer M, Czachor J, Turner L et al (2016) The benefits and challenges of preconsent in a multisite, pediatric sickle cell intervention trial. Pediatr Blood Cancer 63:1649–1652

Orgel E, McCarter R, Jacobs S (2010) A failing medical educational model: a self-assessment by physicians at all levels of training of ability and comfort to deliver bad news. J Palliat Med 13:677–683

Peterson EB, Calhoun AW, Rider EA (2014) The reliability of a modified Kalamazoo Consensus statement checklist for assessing the communication skills of multidisciplinary clinicians in the simulated environment. Patient Educ Couns 96:411–418

Quinn K, Hudson P, Ashby M, Thomas K (2008) "Palliative care: the essentials": evaluation of a multidisciplinary education program. J Palliat Med 11:1122–1129

Rider EA, Volkan K, Hafler JP (2008) Pediatric residents' perceptions of communication competencies: implications for teaching. Med Teach 30:e208–ee17

Robinson MR, Thiel MM, Shirkey K, Zurakowski D, Meyer EC (2016) Efficacy of training interprofessional spiritual care generalists. J Palliat Med 19(8):814–821

Roth M, Wang D, Kim M, Moody K (2009) An assessment of the current state of palliative care education in pediatric hematology/oncology fellowship training. Pediatr Blood Cancer 53:647–651

Schenck AP, Rokoske FS, Durham DD, Cagle JG, Hanson LC (2010) The PEACE project: identification of quality measures for hospice and palliative care. J Palliat Med 13:1451–1459

Schenck AP, Rokoske FS, Durham D, Cagle JG, Hanson LC (2014) Quality measures for hospice and palliative care: piloting the PEACE measures. J Palliat Med 17:769–775

Schiffman JD, Chamberlain LJ, Palmer L, Contro N, Sourkes B, Sectish TC (2008) Introduction of a pediatric palliative care curriculum for pediatric residents. J Palliat Med 11:164–170

Scott DA, Valery PC, Boyle FM, Bain CJ (2002) Does research into sensitive areas do harm? Experiences of research participation after a child's diagnosis with Ewing's sarcoma. Med J Aust 177:507–510

Serwint JR, Rutherford LE, Hutton N (2006) Personal and professional experiences of pediatric residents concerning death. J Palliat Med 9:70–81

Sheetz MJ, Bowman MA (2008) Pediatric palliative care: an assessment of physicians' confidence in skills, desire for training, and willingness to refer for end-of-life care. Am J Hosp Palliat Care 25:100–105

Singh AL, Klick JC, McCracken CE, Hebbar KB (2016) Evaluating hospice and palliative medicine education in pediatric training programs. Am J Hosp Palliat Care 34(7):603–610

Smith TJ, Temin S, Alesi ER et al (2012) American society of clinical oncology provisional clinical opinion: the integration of palliative care into standard oncology care. J Clin Oncol 30:880–887

Snaman JM, Torres C, Duffy B, Levine DR, Gibson DV, Baker JN (2016a) Parental perspectives of communication at the end of life at a pediatric oncology institution. J Palliat Med 19:326–332

Snaman JM, Kaye EC, Levine DR et al (2016b) Pediatric palliative oncology: a new training model for an emerging field. J Clin Oncol 34:288–289

Starks H, Doorenbos A, Lindhorst T et al (2016) The family communication study: a randomized trial of prospective pediatric palliative care consultation, study methodology and perceptions of participation burden. Contemp Clin Trials 49:15–20

State telehealth laws and reimbursement policies report 2014 (Accessed August 26, 2016, at http://cchpca.org/sites/default/files/resources/State%20Laws%20and%20Reimbursement%20Policies%20Report%20Feb%20%202015.pdf)

Steele R, Bosma H, Johnston MF et al (2008) Research priorities in pediatric palliative care: a Delphi study. J Palliat Care 24:229–239

Steele R, Cadell S, Siden H, Andrews G, Smit Quosai T, Feichtinger L (2014) Impact of research participation on parents of seriously ill children. J Palliat Med 17:788–796

Street RL Jr (1991) Physicians' communication and parents' evaluations of pediatric consultations. Med Care 29:1146–1152

The PedsQL (2017) Measurement model for the pediatric quality of life inventory, at http://www.pedsql.org/translations.html

Tieman JJ, Sladek RM, Currow DC (2009) Multiple sources: mapping the literature of palliative care. Palliat Med 23:425–431

Tobler K, Grant E, Marczinski C (2014) Evaluation of the impact of a simulation-enhanced breaking bad news workshop in pediatrics. Simul Healthc 9:213–219

Ullrich C, Morrison RS (2013) Pediatric palliative care research comes of age: what we stand to learn from children with life-threatening illness. J Palliat Med 16:334–336

VanGeest JB (2001) Process evaluation of an educational intervention to improve end-of-life care: the education for physicians on End-of-Life Care (EPEC) program. Am J Hosp Palliat Med 18:233–238

Walling AM, Asch SM, Lorenz KA et al (2010) The quality of care provided to hospitalized patients at the end of life. Arch Inter Med 170:1057–1063

Wee B, Hadley G, Derry S (2008) How useful are systematic reviews for informing palliative care practice? Survey of 25 cochrane systematic reviews. BMC Palliat Care 7:13

What is telemedicine? (Accessed August 26, 2016 at http://www.americantelemed.org/about-telemedicine/what-is-telemedicine#.V8B6FWV7WA8)

Williams D, Fisicaro T, Hargraves R, Berg D (2009) End-of-Life communication education program for internal medicine residents. MedEdPORTAL, Washington, DC

Wolfe J, Orellana L, Cook EF et al (2014) Improving the care of children with advanced cancer by using an electronic patient-reported feedback intervention: results from the PediQUEST randomized controlled trial. J Clin Oncol 32:1119–1126

Wolfe J, Orellana L, Ullrich C et al (2015) Symptoms and distress in children with advanced cancer: prospective patient-reported outcomes from the PediQUEST study. J Clin Oncol 33:1928–1935

Youngblood AQ, Zinkan JL, Tofil NM, White ML (2012) Multidisciplinary simulation in pediatric critical care: the death of a child. Crit Care Nurse 32:55–61

GPSR Compliance

The European Union's (EU) General Product Safety Regulation (GPSR) is a set of rules that requires consumer products to be safe and our obligations to ensure this.

If you have any concerns about our products, you can contact us on ProductSafety@springernature.com

In case Publisher is established outside the EU, the EU authorized representative is:

Springer Nature Customer Service Center GmbH
Europaplatz 3
69115 Heidelberg, Germany

Batch number: 10371063

Printed by Printforce, the Netherlands